ACUTE ISCHEMIC STROKE

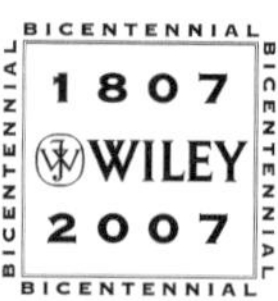

THE WILEY BICENTENNIAL–KNOWLEDGE FOR GENERATIONS

Each generation has its unique needs and aspirations. When Charles Wiley first opened his small printing shop in lower Manhattan in 1807, it was a generation of boundless potential searching for an identity. And we were there, helping to define a new American literary tradition. Over half a century later, in the midst of the Second Industrial Revolution, it was a generation focused on building the future. Once again, we were there, supplying the critical scientific, technical, and engineering knowledge that helped frame the world. Throughout the 20th Century, and into the new millennium, nations began to reach out beyond their own borders and a new international community was born. Wiley was there, expanding its operations around the world to enable a global exchange of ideas, opinions, and know-how.

For 200 years, Wiley has been an integral part of each generation's journey, enabling the flow of information and understanding necessary to meet their needs and fulfill their aspirations. Today, bold new technologies are changing the way we live and learn. Wiley will be there, providing you the must-have knowledge you need to imagine new worlds, new possibilities, and new opportunities.

Generations come and go, but you can always count on Wiley to provide you the knowledge you need, when and where you need it!

WILLIAM J. PESCE
PRESIDENT AND CHIEF EXECUTIVE OFFICER

PETER BOOTH WILEY
CHAIRMAN OF THE BOARD

ACUTE ISCHEMIC STROKE

An Evidence-based Approach

EDITED BY

DAVID M. GREER

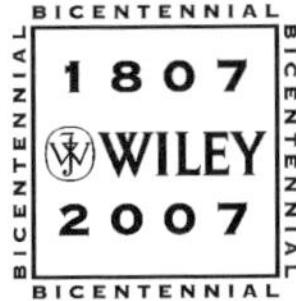

WILEY-LISS
A JOHN WILEY & SONS, INC., PUBLICATION

Published by John Wiley & Sons, Inc., Hoboken, New Jersey
Published simultaneously in Canada

For general information on our other products and services or for technical support, please contact our Customer Care Department within the United States at 877-762-2974, outside the United States at 317-572-3993 or fax 317-572-4002.

Wiley also publishes its books in a variety of electronic formats. Some content that appears in print may not be available in electronic formats. For more information about Wiley products, visit our web site at www.wiley.com.

Wiley Bicentennial Logo: Richard J. Pacifico

Library of Congress Cataloging-in-Publication Data:

Acute ischemic stroke : an evidence-based approach / [edited by] David M. Greer.
p. ; cm.
Includes bibliographical references.
ISBN 978-0-470-06807-6 (cloth)
1. Cerebrovascular disease–Treatment. 2. Cerebral ischemia–Treatment.
3. Evidence-based medicine. I. Greer, David M., 1966-
[DNLM: 1. Cerebrovascular Accident–therapy. 2. Evidence-Based Medicine.
WL 355 A1891 2008]
RC388.5.A283 2008
616.8'1–dc22

2007013702

Printed in the United States of America
10 9 8 7 6 5 4 3 2 1

CONTENTS

PREFACE

For many years, physicians have been plagued by a paucity of available treatments for patients with acute ischemic stroke. The therapies we had to offer were either potentially quite hazardous, sometimes leading to poor outcomes, or so benign as to seem to offer little benefit. However, with advances in our understanding of stroke mechanisms, different patient populations, timing of therapy, and modern medicines and techniques, we have gained the ability to successfully treat acute ischemic stroke in a manner that has proven beneficial over broad categories of patients.

We now have the opportunity to make our treatment of acute stroke "evidence based"—we can be guided by many large randomized trials looking at thrombolytic agents, antithrombotic agents, and neuroprotective agents. The evidence has taken us a great distance, but has sometimes raised more questions than it has answered. This book provides the reader with an excellent review of the evidence to support the current treatment of acute ischemic stroke and provides an avenue for discovery by highlighting the future directions of research.

I am greatly indebted to the authors of this book, who have painstakingly waded through the data to provide a comprehensive and thorough evaluation of the literature. We hope that you will find herein a guide to support your practice and research interests, and perhaps a clue to how we might together further the field of acute stroke treatment.

David M. Greer, MD, MA

CONTRIBUTORS

Alim P. Mitha, MD Massachusetts General Hospital

Aneesh B. Singhal, MD Massachusetts General Hospital

Carlos E. Sanchez, MD Massachusetts General Hospital

Christopher S. Ogilvy, MD Massachusetts General Hospital

David M. Greer, MD, MA Massachusetts General Hospital

Eric E. Smith, MD, MPH, FRCPC Massachusetts General Hospital

Eric S. Rosenthal, MD Massachusetts General Hospital

Guilherme C. Dabus, MD Massachusetts General Hospital

Joshua A. Hirsch, MD Massachusetts General Hospital

Joshua M. Levine, MD Hospital of the University of Pennsylvania

Karen L. Furie, MD, MPH Massachusetts General Hospital

Kevin N. Sheth, MD Massachusetts General Hospital

Larami MacKenzie, MD Hospital of the University of Pennsylvania

Lee H. Schwamm, MD Massachusetts General Hospital

Magdy Selim, MD, PhD Beth Israel Hospital, Boston

Michael H. Lev, MD Massachusetts General Hospital

Orla Sheehan, MD, BAO, BCh, MRCPI Mater University Hospital and University College, Dublin, Ireland

Peter Kelly, MD, MS, FRCPI Mater University Hospital and University College, Dublin, Ireland

Raul G. Nogueira, MD Massachusetts General Hospital

Sherry H.-Y. Chou, MD Massachusetts General Hospital

Walter J. Koroshetz, MD National Institute of Health, National Institute of Neurologic Disorders and Stroke

William A. Copen, MD Massachusetts General Hospital

1

STROKE: HISTORICAL PERSPECTIVES AND FUTURE DIRECTIONS

MAGDY SELIM

Recent years have witnessed increasing recognition and interest in stroke as a major public health problem. However, stroke is an ancient disease. Imhotep, the founder of Egyptian medicine, described stroke in one of the world's earliest medical documents, the Edwin Smith papyrus, around 3000 BC. More detailed description of this condition followed in AD 1600s when Thomas Willis identified the arterial supply of the brain, "the circle of Willis," and used the term "apoplexy" to describe stroke. In the 1800s, anatomists Matthew and Cruveilher illustrated the lesions in stroke; Dechambre described the small cavity that remains after a small stroke and termed it "lacune"; and Virchow introduced the elements of "Virchow's triad" and reported on thromboembolism as a cause of vascular occlusion, marking the true beginning of the understanding of this condition. In the 1900s, Charles Foix analyzed the distribution of infarcts in various arterial territories and correlated brain lesions with clinical findings, sparking interest in stroke as a clinical entity. Clinical observations by astute physicians, like Foix and Broca, during the nineteenth century provided the basis for clinical anatomical correlates of stroke. The introduction of computerized axial tomography and angiography during the twentieth century made it possible to define the potentially causative vascular lesions.

The modern period in the history of stroke began in the 1960s when C. Miller Fisher described detailed clinical and pathological observations on the features of lacunar strokes, carotid artery disease, transient ischemic attacks, and intracerebral hemorrhage. His student Louis Caplan established one of the first stroke registry

Acute Ischemic Stroke: An Evidence-based Approach, Edited by David M. Greer.

databases to collect and analyze important epidemiological, clinical, radiological, and pathological data. Stroke treatment was rudimentary and often nihilistic. Stroke victims might have been treated with maggots or leeches in order to improve blood supply to the brain in hopes of restoring its functions. In 1961, Thomas Dawbe introduced the term "risk factors" to describe the contribution of specific conditions to cardiovascular disease. Shortly thereafter, the Framingham heart study highlighted the link between cardiovascular risk factors and stroke. The risk factors were refined and they provided insights into the biology of stroke. The concept of stroke prevention was introduced, and antithrombotics and antihypertensives were used to reduce stroke risk.

Remarkable advances in the field of stroke occurred during the past 50 years. Advances in basic sciences uncovered the intricate pathophysiology of stroke and cerebral ischemia. Various steps in the ischemic cascade were identified, and the concept of neuroprotection evolved, generating several therapeutic agents for clinical investigation. The adoption of organized clinical trials methodology led to the approval of intravenous recombinant tissue-plasminogen activator (rt-PA) as the first proven effective treatment for acute ischemic stroke in 1996. The introduction of new brain-imaging techniques, such as diffusion- and perfusion-weighted magnetic resonance imaging (MRI), enabled the study of the evolution of brain ischemia *in vivo*. The concept of the ischemic penumbra and its brief duration led to fundamental changes in the way we treat acute stroke patients. The term "time is brain" evolved to highlight that there is a small window of opportunity following stroke to intervene. Stroke became a medical emergency, and consensus emerged that thrombolytic and neuroprotective therapies would only be effective if delivered early after stroke onset. Endovascular interventionalists with neurological expertise are increasingly taking a hand in the acute management of stroke patients, marking a new chapter in the history of this challenging condition.

Unfortunately, the management of stroke remains suboptimal despite years of dedicated research and increasing attention. Clinical trials for the evaluation of novel therapies, however, have undergone considerable improvements and have become increasingly sophisticated over the years. Potentially promising investigations of novel neuroprotective compounds, hypothermia, oxygen therapy, brain stimulation, and regenerative therapy are currently underway. The stage is now set to identify new therapies that can significantly improve recovery in stroke patients. This book elucidates the evidence to support our care of acute stroke patients to date, and sets the stage for future areas of study. We have come a long way in our understanding of stroke, and the coming decades are likely to reveal amazing improvements in the care of this devastating condition.

2

NEUROIMAGING OF THE ACUTE STROKE PATIENT

William A. Copen and Michael H. Lev

INTRODUCTION

Acute stroke imaging is one of the most dynamically evolving areas of neuroradiology. Two decades ago, state-of-the-art computed tomography (CT) and magnetic resonance imaging (MRI) techniques were notoriously insensitive in detecting acute stroke, and the diagnosis was often a presumptive one. In the 1990s, widespread implementation of diffusion-weighted MRI provided neurologists and neuroradiologists with the first highly sensitive tool that could visualize acutely ischemic brain tissue. Currently, CT and MRI still form the backbone of clinical acute stroke imaging, but widely available techniques now provide ever-increasing diagnostic power.

In this chapter, we begin by considering the ways in which routinely used and investigational neuroimaging techniques provide three types of information that are important to the care of the acute stroke patient. First, they establish the diagnosis of ischemic stroke and exclude hemorrhage and other potential causes of an acute neurologic deficit. Second, they identify the vascular lesion responsible for the ischemic event. Third, they provide additional characterization of brain tissue that may guide stroke therapy by determining the viability of different regions of the brain and distinguishing between irreversibly infarcted tissue and potentially salvageable tissue.

Acute Ischemic Stroke: An Evidence-based Approach, Edited by David M. Greer.

ESTABLISHING THE DIAGNOSIS OF ISCHEMIC STROKE

Recent years have seen the emergence of successful treatment strategies for ischemic stroke, but these are most effective only when initiated within several hours after stroke onset. Therefore, extremely rapid diagnosis and initiation of treatment are critical in avoiding death or severe disability.

Unfortunately, there are a variety of other clinical conditions that may mimic the presentation of acute ischemic stroke. These include intracranial hemorrhage, seizure, sepsis, cardiogenic syncope, complicated migraine, dementia, nonischemic spinal cord lesion, peripheral neuropathy, transient global amnesia, and brain tumor, among others. One recent study found that, of patients presenting to a hospital with stroke-like symptoms, the diagnosis of stroke or transient ischemic attack was never established confidently in 31%, and alternative diagnoses were ultimately made in 19%.[1] Modern imaging techniques are capable of establishing the diagnosis with a high degree of certainty, and of doing so in the very rapid time frame required for emergent treatment.

Noncontrast CT

CT scanners are now nearly ubiquitous in or near the emergency departments of most North American hospitals. With multislice scanners, a noncontrast CT (NCCT) examination of the brain can be performed in well under 1 minute, with the newest scanners able to scan the head in 10 seconds or less. In most centers, the first (and sometimes only) imaging study undertaken for patients with suspected acute stroke is NCCT.

The primary purpose of NCCT in the acute stroke setting is not necessarily to diagnose ischemic stroke, but rather to exclude acute intracranial hemorrhage, whose presentation may mimic that of ischemic stroke. One large study found that, among patients with symptoms of acute stroke, NCCT achieved sensitivity and specificity of 90% and 99%, respectively, in detecting intracranial hemorrhage.[2] Detection of hemorrhage marks a critical decision point in the care of the acute stroke patient. Ischemic stroke therapies such as anticoagulation, thrombolysis, and induced hypertension could have disastrous effects if mistakenly administered to a patient with acute hemorrhage.

In the absence of hemorrhage, ischemic brain tissue may become slightly hypodense in NCCT images within the first 3–6 hours after stroke onset, for perhaps a variety of pathophysiologic reasons.[3] This early hypodensity is variably present. In one 1991 study, parenchymal hypodensity was detected in 44% of patients scanned within 5 hours after stroke onset.[4] It is likely that early parenchymal hypodensity is appreciated somewhat more frequently in current NCCT scans, partly because modern CT scanners produce higher quality images and partly because CT images are now often viewed not on film but on computer monitors, which allow for manipulation of window and level settings to produce higher contrast images. In one study, sensitivity for detection of acute stroke (less than 6 hours after onset) increased from 57% to 71% when high-contrast settings were used.[5]

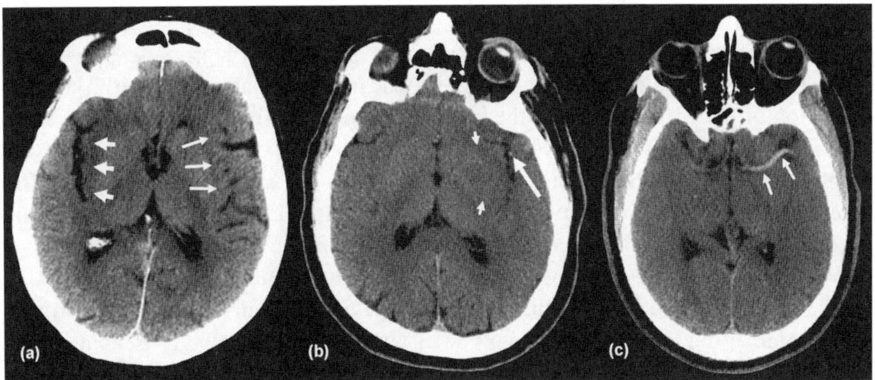

FIGURE 2.1 Early ischemic signs in NCCT images. The insular ribbon sign is shown in image (**a**). On the left, the relatively hyperdense ribbon of insular cortical gray matter can be distinguished from the adjacent subinsular white matter (long thin arrows). However, on the right, the insular ribbon cannot be distinguished from the underlying gray matter (short thick arrows), signifying the presence of a very early infarct. In image (**b**), the lateral margin of the left putamen cannot be seen (short arrows). This image also demonstrates hyperdense embolic material in a Sylvian branch of the middle cerebral artery (the "MCA dot sign," long arrow). Image (**c**) shows hyperdense embolic material in the middle cerebral artery stem (the "hyperdense MCA sign," arrows).

Early decreases in the CT density of ischemic tissue are often appreciated only indirectly. The process seems initially to affect gray matter more noticeably than white matter, decreasing the radiodensity of affected gray matter slightly, so that it approaches that of adjacent white matter. Therefore, loss of gray matter–white matter differentiation is a commonly described sign of acute infarction on NCCT. When infarction is in the territory of the middle cerebral artery (MCA), this is often manifested as obscuration of the basal ganglia (Fig. 2.1b) or as the "insular ribbon sign," in which the ribbon of gray matter in the insular cortex becomes indistinguishable from the subcortical white matter (Fig. 2.1a). Early edema is also sometimes visible because the increase in volume of slightly edematous brain tissue causes effacement of nearby cerebral sulci, cisterns, or ventricles.

Occasionally, the diagnosis of acute ischemia can be established by NCCT because embolic material can be visualized directly, usually in the MCA or its branches. Emboli are often more radiodense than normal brain tissue, and therefore an affected proximal MCA may appear as a linear hyperdensity ("hyperdense middle cerebral artery sign" or HMCA sign, Fig. 2.1c). One study found that the HMCA sign was 100% specific for MCA occlusion, but only 27% sensitive, probably because the density of embolic material is often indistinguishable from that of the normal MCA.[6]

Hyperdense embolic material in a more distal MCA branch, within the Sylvian fissure and oriented perpendicular rather than parallel to the axial plane of imaging, may appear as a small, rounded hyperdensity ("MCA dot sign," Fig. 2.1b). One study found that the MCA dot sign was present in 16% of patients scanned within 3 hours of onset of stroke symptoms, whereas the HMCA sign was seen in only 5%.[7] The HMCA sign portends a poor prognosis,[8,9] probably because it signifies occlusion of the MCA stem and therefore ischemia affecting a large volume of tissue. The MCA dot sign has been associated with better post-thrombolytic outcome than the HMCA sign,[7] perhaps because emboli in smaller arteries are more amenable to thrombolytic approaches, or because embolic occlusion of a more distal vessel results in ischemic damage affecting a smaller volume of tissue.

Despite the variety of ways in which acute infarction may be manifested in NCCT images, the overall sensitivity of NCCT is lower than that of other currently available imaging techniques that will be discussed below. The signs of acute stroke on NCCT are usually subtle and equivocal, such that inter- and even intraobserver agreements are low.[10–12] In one study, radiologists' sensitivity for detecting these signs increased from 38% to 52% when the clinical history provided raised their suspicions by suggesting stroke.[12]

The Alberta Stroke Programme Early CT Score (ASPECTS) represents one effort to improve intra- and inter-rater reliability, even among "nonexpert" readers, by providing a framework for quantifying the extent of ischemic hypodensity in early NCCT scans.[13] In ASPECTS, each of the 10 distinct regions in the territory of the MCA is assigned a score of 0 or 1 depending on the presence (1) or absence (0) of ischemic hypodensity, and the total number of ischemic regions is subtracted from 10. Thus, a score of 10 indicates no apparent hypodensity, whereas a score of 0 reflects hypodensity in the entire MCA territory. Measures like ASPECTS may be helpful not only in diagnosing acute stroke, but also in helping decide whether or not thrombolytic therapy should be initiated. Although one large study found that early ischemic signs in NCCT images were not independently associated with adverse outcomes after thrombolysis,[14]ASPECTS scores of 7 or less, indicating the presence of hypodensity in more than one third of the MCA territory, have been associated with a substantially increased risk of thrombolysis-related parenchymal hemorrhage.[15]

Because of the difficulty in detecting acute stroke using NCCT alone, in many centers the presence of a sufficiently suspicious clinical history, along with definite onset of symptoms within 3 hours and a negative NCCT exam, is considered strong enough evidence of acute stroke to warrant treatment with potentially dangerous intravenous thrombolysis. Indeed, such a treatment algorithm has been shown to result in an overall improvement in patient outcomes.[16] However, more advanced CT- and MR-based techniques, which will be discussed ahead, can establish the diagnosis of acute stroke with greater sensitivity and specificity.

MRI

The first clinical MRI images of the brain used to detect acute stroke were generally either T2-weighted or proton density-weighted images. These "conventional" MR images, like NCCT, are capable of detecting parenchymal changes in acute ischemic stroke because of vasogenic edema, which introduces new, relatively mobile water protons into ischemic tissue, resulting in increased signal intensity. However, because vasogenic edema is minimal in acute stroke, parenchymal hyperintensity may be difficult to detect and is often apparent only in cortical or deep gray matter.[17] A subsequently developed technique, T2-weighted fluid-attenuated inversion recovery (FLAIR) imaging, may provide increased sensitivity, but still achieved an overall sensitivity of only 29% within the first 6 hours of stroke onset in one study.[18] Besides parenchymal hyperintensity, other signs of acute stroke on MRI include loss of vascular flow voids, arterial hyperintensity in FLAIR images, vascular contrast enhancement signifying stasis of blood, and effacement of sulci, cisterns, and ventricles due to mild swelling.

A major breakthrough in stroke imaging occurred with the development of diffusion-weighted MRI (DWI). DWI produces images that are T2-weighted, but are also diffusion-weighted, in that different parts of the brain appear brighter or darker depending on the rate of water diffusion within them. In this context, diffusion refers to "self-diffusion," also known as Brownian motion, which is the random motion that all molecules exhibit when at temperatures above absolute zero. In brain tissue, this motion is constrained by physical obstacles such as cell membranes and cytoskeletal macromolecules. Therefore, DWI is able to depict microscopic pathologic changes by demonstrating changes in water diffusion.

In ischemic brain tissue, diffusion of water molecules becomes markedly restricted, within minutes of the onset of ischemia, because of cytotoxic edema. Cytotoxic edema, which is distinct from vasogenic edema, occurs because of failure of cell membrane ion pumps, leading to an accumulation of ions in the intracellular space. Water follows the ions by osmosis, leading to cellular swelling, but not overall tissue swelling, as there is no net addition of water. Although this process results in no detectable change in T2-weighted images, it is associated with a decrease in the apparent rate of water diffusion, which is depicted as a hyperintense lesion in diffusion-weighted images.

The sensitivity and specificity of DWI depend to some extent on the technique being used and the amount of imaging time that can be dedicated to the DWI sequence. DWI pulse sequences typically require between approximately 30 seconds and 4 minutes of imaging time to image the entire brain and achieve sensitivity and specificity approaching 100% (Fig. 2.2).[18–26] The rare infarcts that are not apparent on DWI are usually very small and are often located in the brainstem.

Some have questioned the specificity of DWI in delineating particular areas of the brain that are destined for infarction, noting that some DWI lesions resolve at least partially in follow-up studies. However, it appears that reversibility of DWI lesions is quite unusual[27] and typically involves only a small portion of initially abnormal tissue.[28] One study found that reversal of a DWI abnormality occurred in 33% of patients following intra-arterial thrombolysis. However, in this study, the areas of reversal nevertheless went on to infarction in the majority of patients.[29]

Besides establishing the diagnosis of ischemic stroke, DWI also offers the capability of measuring the approximate age of infarcts. The apparent diffusion coefficient (ADC) of water, a measure of diffusion that can be derived easily from DWI images, follows a typical sequence of changes in evolving infarcts.[30–41] ADC

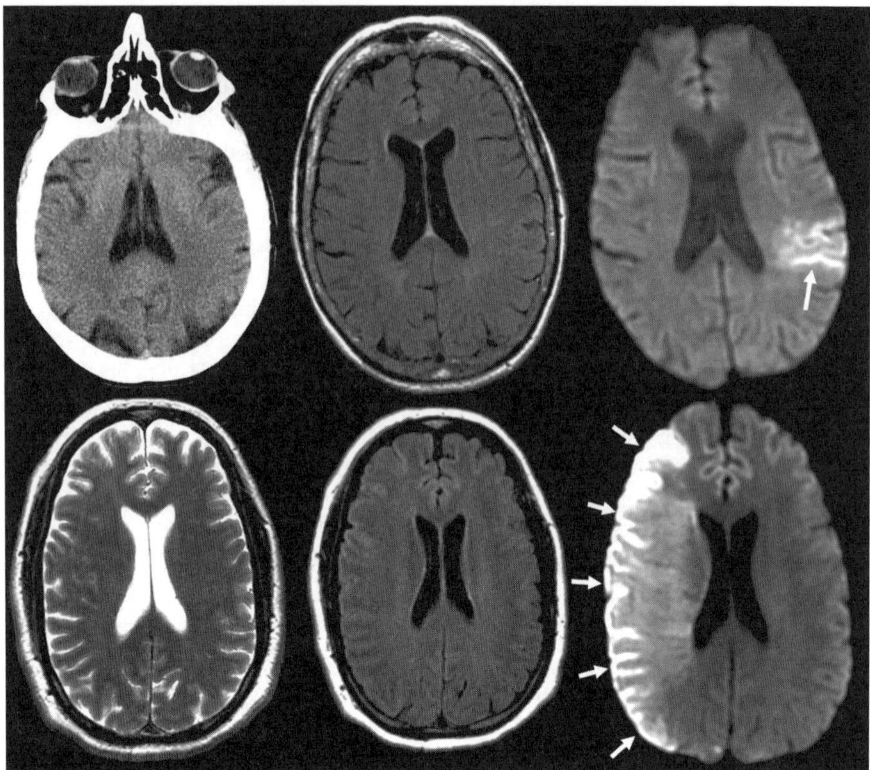

FIGURE 2.2 Sensitivity of DWI for detection of acute stroke. In one acute stroke patient (top row), an early NCCT image (top left) is normal. A T2-weighted FLAIR MRI image (top middle) shows very subtle parenchymal hyperintensity. The patient's acute infarct is far more conspicuous in a DWI image (top right, arrow). In a second patient (bottom row), both conventional T2-weighted images (bottom left) and T2-weighted FLAIR images (bottom middle) are nearly normal, but a DWI image (bottom right) shows a very large infarct affecting the entire right middle cerebral artery territory (arrows).

rapidly falls to below-normal levels, reaching a minimum value approximately 1 day after the onset of infarction. ADC then begins to rise again because vasogenic edema begins to introduce new water molecules that expand the interstitial space. ADC passes through normal values approximately 9 days after stroke onset.[40]

Although there is great variation in the pace of these ADC changes, it is generally true that infarcts with lower-than-normal ADC are less than approximately 2 weeks in age and those with low ADC and little or no associated abnormality in T2-weighted images are less than approximately 6 hours in age. These observations can be helpful in distinguishing acute infarcts from T2-hyperintense lesions of other etiologies and in determining which of multiple infarcts, if any, is the acute infarct that may be responsible for a patient's new symptoms.

IDENTIFYING THE VASCULAR LESION

Ischemic stroke occurs because of impairments in microvascular perfusion of affected brain tissue. However, the vascular event that results in impaired perfusion often occurs in a macroscopically visible vessel. Imaging studies that can study these vessels provide several kinds of important information to the stroke neurologist. First, by definitively demonstrating a vascular lesion that could be responsible for ischemic symptoms, vascular imaging can help to cement the diagnosis of an acute ischemic stroke, especially when DWI is not available and other studies are equivocal or negative. Second, the location of the vascular lesion conveys important prognostic information. In general, vascular lesions that involve larger, more proximal arteries that serve larger volumes of tissues cause infarcts that result in more severe neurologic deficits and a greater likelihood of hemorrhagic transformation. Finally, vascular imaging can be essential in guiding therapy. Intra-arterial thrombolysis or mechanical clot disruption can be undertaken only if a sufficiently proximal arterial lesion can be identified. Even when only intravenous thrombolysis is considered, vascular imaging helps to predict the likelihood of successful thrombolysis, as well as the likelihood of severe injury if thrombolysis is not attempted.

Catheter Angiography

Catheter angiography is the oldest vascular imaging technique, and although it remains the gold standard for vascular imaging, it is seldom used diagnostically in the acute stroke setting. In this technique, the patient is brought to an operating room-like fluoroscopy suite and sedated. A catheter is inserted into a femoral artery and is then fluoroscopically guided into the aortic arch. The catheter is then advanced into one of the carotid or vertebral arteries, and a radio-opaque, iodine-based contrast material is injected, while high-resolution images of the neck or brain are acquired at a rate of several frames per second.

Catheter angiography provides exquisite image detail and can visualize vessels as small as 0.1 mm in diameter, considerably smaller than those seen by CT- and MR-based vascular imaging techniques. Catheter angiography also provides high temporal resolution, which can help to distinguish arteries from veins and to detect prolonged intravascular stasis of blood.

Despite its advantages, diagnostic catheter angiography is now almost never performed for evaluation of acute stroke in institutions that have access to modern CT and MR scanners. There are several reasons for this. Catheter angiography requires the presence of highly trained angiographers, technologists, and sometimes anesthesiologists, some of whom may not be immediately available at all times of the day. It is a relatively time-consuming technique, and it may unacceptably delay the initiation of therapy in the acute stroke patient. The iodinated contrast used for catheter angiography can result in nephrotoxicity and allergic reactions, which are discussed in the next section. Also, catheter angiography is a highly invasive and somewhat risky procedure. Complications may occur if atherosclerotic plaques are dislodged from the aorta during catheter passage or if small thrombi form on the tip of the catheter and travel into the brain. The rate of neurologic complications related to cerebral angiography is approximately 0.5–4%. Most of these are transient, with permanent neurologic deficits occurring in only 0.1–0.5% of patients who undergo an angiogram.[42]

CT Angiography

CT angiography (CTA) is a technique that provides high-resolution vascular images using the same CT scanners that are used for conventional CT imaging and the same iodine-based contrast agents that are used for catheter angiography and conventional contrast-enhanced CT. CTA is much less invasive than catheter angiography, as it involves injection of a bolus of contrast agent through a standard intravenous catheter in a peripheral vein, rather than into a centrally placed arterial catheter. CT images of the head and neck are obtained and are carefully timed to acquire images as the contrast material passes through the arteries (Fig. 2.3). Many CTA protocols also allow for excellent visualization of cervico-cranial venous structures.

The amount of contrast material required for CTA is comparable to that used for conventional contrast-enhanced CT imaging. The amount of scanning time required for a CTA examination of the head and neck, such as is usually performed for acute

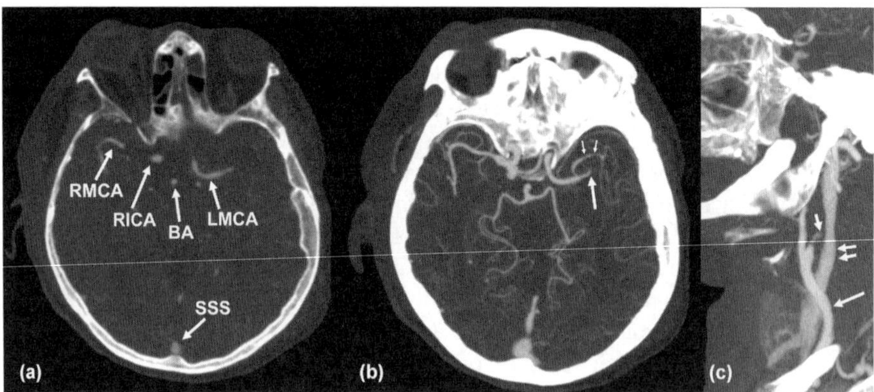

FIGURE 2.3 CT angiography. CTA is performed by acquiring axial CT images while an intravenously injected bolus of contrast material passes through the arteries. In one such image (**a**), portions of the contrast-filled right and left middle cerebral arteries (RMCA, LMCA) are clearly seen, as well as the right internal carotid artery (RICA) and basilar artery (BA). Note that major venous structures, including the superior sagittal sinus (SSS), are also seen. CTA images are often combined to form projections, such as image (**b**), which shows abrupt cutoff of one of the two middle cerebral artery divisions (large arrow) due to embolic occlusion. There is also irregular narrowing of the other division (small arrows). Another projection of CTA images of the neck from the same examination (**c**) shows the bifurcation of the left common carotid artery (single long arrow) into the external and internal (single short arrow) carotid arteries. The latter is acutely occluded due to dissection. Note the internal jugular vein (double arrows) passing close to the carotid arteries.

stroke patients, varies depending on the scanner being used. With a 16-slice CT scanner, less than 30 seconds of imaging time is typically needed, allowing the examination to occur during a single breath-hold, which reduces motion artifacts related to breathing. Thirty-two- and 64-slice scanners allow for even faster imaging, while using even less contrast material.

CTA offers many attractive features that have made it a very widely used technique in acute stroke imaging. As discussed above, CT scanners are widely available, and emergency patients can usually be brought to and from a scanner with minimal delay. CT scanners, unlike MRI scanners, allow for metallic equipment to be brought safely into the scanner room, allowing for easier monitoring of potentially unstable acute stroke patients, most notably those receiving intravenous recombinant tissue-plasminogen activator (rt-PA). The speed of the CTA technique also makes CTA images relatively resistant to degradation by artifact related to patient motion, which is a significant problem when scanning acute stroke patients who may be neurologically impaired, critically ill, or uncooperative. Although CTA does not usually offer catheter angiography's ability to show the movement of blood from arteries to veins over time and cannot show tiny blood vessels with the same spatial resolution provided by catheter angiography, CTA does produce vascular images with detail greater than that of other vascular imaging techniques such as magnetic resonance angiography (MRA). Furthermore, emerging CTA techniques may potentially allow for serial imaging of limited parts of the neurovascular anatomy, with tracking of the passage of contrast material from large arteries into veins.

CTA suffers from only a few disadvantages that weigh against these desirable attributes. Chief among them is the fact that CTA requires injection of iodine-based contrast material. Iodinated contrast is nephrotoxic and may result in transient or permanent renal failure, particularly in patients whose renal function is already impaired. The incidence and severity of contrast-induced nephropathy is low when adequate renal function is confirmed by means of prescan serum creatinine measurement[43] or preferably computation of the glomerular filtration rate. However, waiting for laboratory values to become available may unacceptably delay diagnosis and treatment in the acute stroke setting. Although drugs such as sodium bicarbonate and *N*-acetylcysteine have advanced the prevention of contrast-induced nephropathy in patients with impaired renal function, the mainstay of prevention remains adequate pre- and postcontrast hydration.

Besides impairment of renal function, injection of iodinated contrast triggers allergic adverse reactions in some patients. Some studies have reported that the incidence of such reactions is between 4.9% and 8.02% when high-osmolar ionic contrast agents are used.[44] However, the reported incidence of adverse reactions is much lower when nonionic monomeric contrast agents are used, falling to 0.59% in one study, with only 0.01% of patients suffering severe reactions.[45] In another study, the incidence of adverse reactions to nonionic contrast agents was 3.13%, with 0.04% of reactions classified as severe.[46]

With modern multislice scanners and optimized protocols,[47] CTA images can provide excellent visualization of the primary intracranial arteries (i.e., the proximal anterior, middle, and posterior cerebral arteries), their smaller secondary branches (e.g., the superior and inferior divisions of the MCA, and the pericallosal and callosomarginal arteries), and often even smaller tertiary branches. In one study of 44 acute stroke patients who were intra-arterial thrombolysis candidates and who underwent both CTA and catheter angiography studies, CTA was 98.4% sensitive and 98.1% specific in detecting occlusion of large intracranial arteries.[48]

Besides establishing the diagnosis of stroke, CTA can help to determine an acute stroke patient's prognosis by determining whether vascular lesions are in large primary intracranial arteries, where they tend to cause more widespread ischemic damage, or in smaller secondary and tertiary arteries. In one study of 74 acute stroke patients who were subsequently treated by intravenous or intra-arterial thrombolysis, the presence of a "carotid T lesion," in which an embolus occludes the top of the internal carotid artery and extends into the middle and anterior cerebral arteries, was a better predictor of early death than hypodensity more than one third of the (MCA) territory, which is often taken to be an indicator of advanced early injury and poor prognosis.[49] In that study, catheter angiography rather than CTA was used to identify the vascular lesion. Another study, which used CTA, found that occlusion of a large intracranial artery was one of the two factors that independently predicted poor outcome in acute stroke patients (the other was poor initial neurologic status).[50]

At the other extreme are those acute stroke patients who have no visible arterial occlusion whatsoever, presumably because their infarcts were due to lesions in small arteries that cannot be imaged, or because an embolus in a large proximal artery has broken up spontaneously. Several studies (again using catheter angiography rather than CTA) have shown that such patients generally enjoy relatively favorable outcomes.[51,52]

Besides merely predicting outcome, CTA plays a critical role in directing acute therapy by detecting occlusion of proximal intracranial arteries that are accessible by endovascular microcatheterization and therefore may be treated by intra-arterial thrombolysis or mechanical clot disruption. Indeed, studies using both catheter angiography and CTA suggest that proximal occlusions *should* be treated with intra-arterial rather than or in addition to intravenous thrombolysis, if possible, because intravenous thrombolysis is less effective in treating proximal lesions than in treating distal ones.[6,53,54]

Finally, besides visualizing blood vessels, CTA images may be more useful than NCCT in evaluating the brain parenchyma. In CTA, not only large vessels but also the microvasculature becomes opacified by contrast-containing blood. Therefore, in CT images used for CTA (sometimes called CTA source images or CTA-SI), hypoperfused brain tissue may become visibly hypodense, and CTA-SI allows for more sensitive detection of acute stroke than CT.[55–57] In one study, CTA-SI increased the utility of the ASPECTS metric in predicting the clinical outcomes of acute stroke patients.[58] Under idealized clinical scanning conditions,[59] CTA-SI can theoretically measure regional cerebral blood volume, thereby helping to identify tissue that may be irreversibly destined for infarction (see discussion of cerebral perfusion below).

Magnetic Resonance Angiography

MRA describes any of the several MRI techniques that are used to depict arteries. These can be divided into contrast-based techniques and noncontrast-based techniques.

There are two widely used noncontrast-based MRA techniques: time-of-flight (TOF) MRA and phase contrast (PC) MRA. The physical principles underlying both techniques are far more complicated than those underlying catheter angiography and CTA and are beyond the scope of this chapter. Both are unlike other vascular imaging techniques used in acute stroke, in that they are completely noninvasive, requiring no exogenous contrast material whatsoever, thereby obviating concerns regarding contrast allergies and contrast-induced nephropathy (Fig. 2.4). Unlike catheter angiography and CTA, MRI uses no ionizing radiation. Like catheter angiography (but not CTA), both TOF and PC MRA can be used to demonstrate the direction of blood flow, which can be helpful in assessing the direction of flow in a vessel providing collateral perfusion or in situations such as suspected subclavian steal. Additionally, PC MRA can quantitatively measure the velocity of flow, an ability shared only by ultrasound, a modality that is usually not used in acute stroke. All of these features represent potential advantages of noncontrast-based MRA over CTA.

However, noncontrast-based MRA suffers from several disadvantages. First among these are the logistical difficulties involved in moving an acute stroke patient to and from an MRI scanner, which have been discussed above. TOF and PC MRA are relatively time consuming, requiring approximately 3–8 minutes to produce images of either the cervical or intracranial arteries. Also, MRA images are more

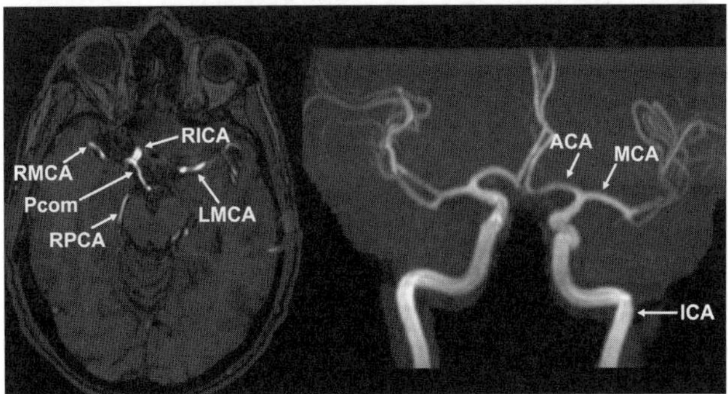

FIGURE 2.4 Noncontrast MR angiography. A noncontrast MRA examination of the head was performed in a patient with suspected acute stroke, resulting in axial images like that seen on the left, which shows portions of the patient right and left middle cerebral arteries (RMCA, LMCA), the right internal carotid artery (RICA), the right posterior cerebral artery (RPCA), and the right posterior communicating artery (Pcom). Like CTA images, MRA images are often combined to yield projections such as the one on the right, in which the internal carotid (ICA), middle cerebral (MCA), and anterior cerebral (ACA) arteries are more clearly visualized by computationally removing the arteries of the posterior circulation.

sensitive to degradation by patient motion than are CTA images, and this represents a significant disadvantage in imaging the acute stroke patient. Finally, both TOF and PC rely on rapid, coherent motion of water molecules in blood to make arteries visible in MRA images. Therefore, these techniques often show artifactually diminished or absent blood flow when there is turbulent flow in a stenotic segment of an artery or slow flow distal to a stenosis. This problem, in combination with relatively inferior spatial resolution, makes TOF and PC prone to overestimating the degree of stenosis in a narrowed vessel.

MRA can also be performed with a contrast agent, using a technique that is conceptually similar to that used for CTA (Fig. 2.5). Essentially, T1-weighted images of the head or neck are obtained during the intravascular transit of an intravenously injected bolus of a gadolinium-based contrast material. The technique is more technically demanding than noncontrast MRA, because image acquisition must be timed to coincide with arterial enhancement. In depicting arteries, contrast-enhanced MRA relies not on the motion of water molecules, but instead on the distribution of the contrast agent. Therefore, contrast-enhanced MRA is less likely than noncontrast MRA to overestimate stenosis in regions of slow or turbulent

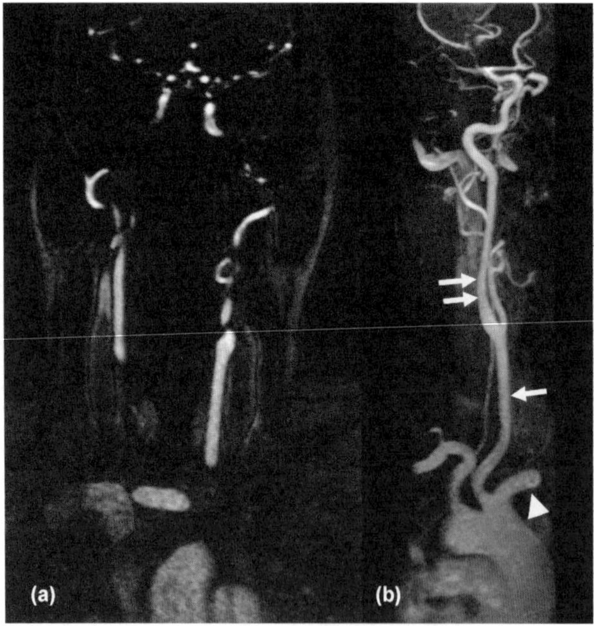

FIGURE 2.5 Contrast MR angiography. An MRA examination of the neck may be performed by acquiring coronal images (**a**) during bolus injection of a contrast agent. These images can be combined to yield projections (**b**), in this case showing the entire course of the left common (single arrow) and internal carotid arteries (double arrows), both of which are widely patient without evidence of stenosis. Note this patient's so-called "bovine arch," a normal anatomic variant in which the left common carotid artery and left subclavian artery (arrowhead) share a common origin from the aortic arch.

blood flow. Furthermore, contrast-enhanced MRA allows for imaging of a much larger field of view in a shorter amount of time. For these reasons, contrast-enhanced MRA is often used to image the arteries of the neck, and this can be accomplished in approximately 1–2 minutes. However, contrast-enhanced MRA suffers from even worse spatial resolution than that of noncontrast MRA, making the technique less suitable for imaging of the smaller vessels of the head.

The accuracy of MRA has been empirically compared most often to that of other neurovascular imaging techniques not in the setting of acute stroke, but in subacute diseases such as cervical carotid stenosis and aneurysm screening, where MRA is most often used. MRA has been found to be highly accurate in determining whether carotid stenosis is severe enough to warrant endarterectomy.[60] Other studies have suggested that MRA is also highly accurate in detecting intracranial arterial stenosis or occlusion.[61,62] However, from a practical standpoint, MRA images of the head and neck are generally inferior to CTA images, especially when acute stroke patients are scanned on an emergency basis, and motion artifact is particularly likely to be a problem.

TISSUE VIABILITY

This section discusses some of the most exciting and technologically complex techniques used in acute stroke imaging: those that study brain tissue not just to determine that an ischemic event has occurred in a particular part of the brain, but also to study the viability of ischemic tissue. This has become especially important with the widespread implementation of thrombolytic therapy, which can be very successful in saving brain tissue and dramatically improving outcomes for acute stroke patients, but can also result in catastrophic intracranial hemorrhage. By studying tissue viability, neuroradiologists hope to identify brain tissue that is threatened by ischemia and may be saved by timely reperfusion and to distinguish this tissue from tissue that already has undergone irreversible damage, cannot be saved, and may be at increased risk of hemorrhagic conversion. This helps the patient and the stroke neurologist to understand better the risks and potential benefits of thrombolysis or other therapies.

By far, the most widely used and most empirically studied tissue viability imaging techniques are those that study tissue perfusion, and discussion of perfusion imaging techniques will dominate this section. We will also mention a few emerging techniques that currently are not as widely used in the acute stroke setting, but show promise for the future.

Perfusion Imaging: Introduction and Review of Pathophysiology

Perfusion imaging techniques study pathophysiologic events that occur in capillaries and other microscopic blood vessels that cannot be seen by angiographic techniques like CTA or MRA. The perfusion imaging techniques in most widespread clinical use are performed using CT or MRI, and generally obtain or estimate three particular perfusion measurements in each part of the brain: cerebral blood flow (CBF), cerebral blood volume (CBV), and mean transit time (MTT).

Perfusion imaging performed in the acute stroke setting generally relies upon bolus-tracking techniques, in which a bolus of a standard contrast agent is injected rapidly via a peripheral intravenous catheter, and images of the brain are obtained repeatedly as the contrast agent passes through the brain. In the case of CT, brain tissue increases and then decreases again in density as an iodine-based contrast agent passes through the brain. With MRI, the signal intensity of the tissue decreases and then increases again, due to a transient susceptibility effect caused by a gadolinium-based contrast agent (hence the term dynamic susceptibility contrast imaging or DSC). In either case, the perfusion examination takes only approximately 1 minute to perform. The images obtained in the examination are converted by a computer to contrast agent concentration versus time curves, which are in turn analyzed to yield measurements of CBV, CBF, and MTT in each part of the brain (or approximations of those quantities) in each voxel. This process is illustrated in Figure 2.6.

A brief review of vascular pathophysiology may help to clarify why these measurements are helpful in distinguishing between salvageable and irreversibly injured tissue. When a global or local loss of cerebral perfusion pressure (CPP) exceeds the autoregulatory capacity of the cerebral vasculature, global or local CBF begins to fall. Further vasodilation and capillary recruitment have the effect of increasing the effective vascular cross-sectional surface area, resulting in a lower blood velocity at any given level of CBF. This is detected by perfusion imaging techniques as an increase in the average amount of time that each volume of blood spends in each imaging voxel, that is, an increase in MTT. A decrease in the velocity of blood as it passes through capillaries is adaptive,

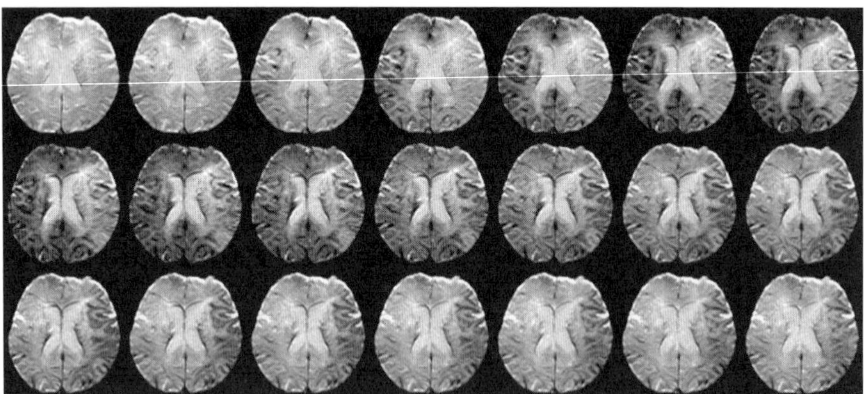

FIGURE 2.6 Dynamic susceptibility contrast imaging. Axial images of the brain are acquired repeatedly, in this case every 1.5 seconds. As a bolus of intravenously injected contrast material enters the brain, first arteries, then brain parenchyma, and finally veins demonstrate a transient loss of signal intensity. In this acute stroke patient, hypoperfusion of the left middle cerebral artery territory results in delayed arrival of the contrast bolus and prolonged stasis of contrast within the tissue.

as it allows time for a greater oxygen extraction fraction (OEF), that is, an increase in the fraction of oxygen molecules that have time to diffuse from erythrocytes into brain tissue.

With modest impairment of blood flow, this mechanism allows for preservation of oxidative metabolism without alteration in electrical function. However, when CPP and therefore CBF are sufficiently low, OEF reaches a maximum and cannot increase further. Brain tissue ceases to function electrically, resulting in a neurologic deficit. Microvascular collapse occurs, and CBV falls. If the oxygen supply falls low enough, the tissue dies. Of critical clinical importance is the observation that the amount of time it takes for tissue to suffer irreversible damage is inversely related to the severity of the ischemic insult. Tissue that is completely deprived of blood will die within a few minutes, but less severely hypoperfused tissue may survive for many hours, and may be saved by timely thrombolysis that restores perfusion, or perhaps by another therapeutic intervention.

To summarize this account of cerebrovascular pathophysiology, a mild decrease in CBF is accompanied by a concomitant increase in MTT and preserved or increased CBV. Tissue with severely decreased CBF also demonstrates increased MTT, but decreased CBV.

Perfusion Imaging: Interpretation of MRI Perfusion Images

At first glance, it might seem that perfusion imaging could distinguish salvageable tissue from irreversibly infarcted tissue simply by measuring levels of CBF and assuming that tissue with CBF below a certain level cannot be saved. Indeed, absolute quantification of perfusion parameters can be achieved with both CT-[63–67] and MRI-based[68–74] perfusion imaging techniques, and some have used absolute quantification to assess tissue viability.

However, in practice it may be difficult to draw conclusions from absolute measurements of perfusion parameters for at least three reasons. First, in patients with chronic atherosclerotic disease, tissue that has adapted to conditions of mild ischemia may have thresholds of viability that differ from those of normal tissue. Second, CBV and CBF are approximately two to three times greater in gray matter than in white matter, and these two types of brain tissue have very different thresholds of viability. Therefore, interpreting absolute measurements of perfusion parameters correctly requires distinguishing between gray matter and white matter. Because ischemic gray matter resembles normal white matter in CT images, it is probably impossible to do this with CT, and methods for doing it with MRI are not routinely used. Finally, absolute measurements of perfusion may not be as accurate as desired. Absolute measurements are made by first generating relative perfusion maps, in which perfusion in different parts of the brain is represented in arbitrary units without absolute meaning. These relative measurements are then converted to absolute ones by a scaling process that may introduce increased uncertainty and reduce the reliability of the measurements in assessing tissue viability.

For all of these reasons, neuroradiologists and stroke neurologists often interpret perfusion maps not by absolute measurement of perfusion levels, but by visually inspecting them for "lesions" representing abnormal CBV, CBF, or MTT. In this interpretation, the terms "infarct core" and "ischemic penumbra" are often used. The core, which often (but not always) lies near the center of the ischemic region, is defined as the tissue that has been irreversibly damaged and is unlikely to survive, regardless of therapeutic intervention. The term "ischemic penumbra," which originally had a slightly different meaning among neurologists and neuroscientists, is now often used to describe a region of tissue that is threatened by ischemia, but may be saved by rapid reperfusion. This only moderately ischemic tissue most often lies around the periphery of an ischemic lesion, where collateral vessels may serve to provide some degree of residual perfusion (Fig. 2.7).

Qualitative analysis of perfusion images is usually based on two assumptions that are derived from the pathophysiologic principles discussed above. First, tissue with visibly decreased CBV is so severely ischemic that it is unlikely to survive and lies within the "core" of the infarct. Second, tissue with decreased CBF or prolonged MTT may be mildly or severely ischemic and may or may not be salvageable. If this tissue does not appear abnormal in another, more specific type of image (such as CBV or DWI), it represents the "ischemic penumbra" and may potentially be rescued by immediate therapy.

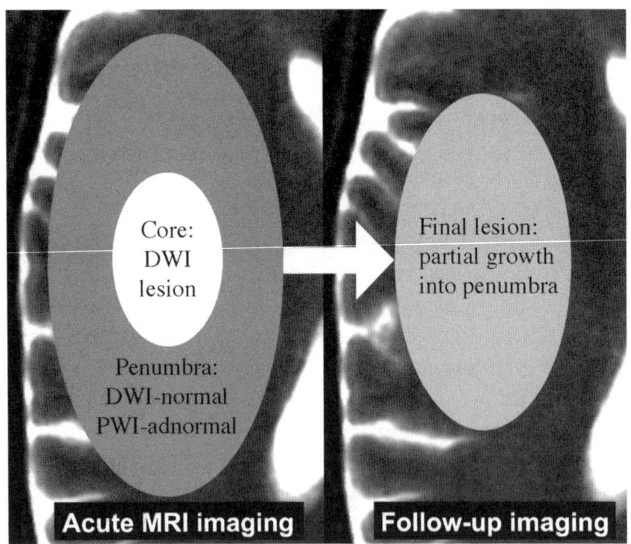

FIGURE 2.7 Core and penumbra in acute stroke imaging. The infarct core, presumptively identified by an abnormality in a DWI image or CBV map, represents tissue that cannot be salvaged. The ischemic penumbra represents tissue that is threatened by ischemia, but may still be saved by timely therapy. The penumbra is presumptively identified as that tissue that is normal in early DWI images or CBV maps, but abnormal in maps of CBF or MTT. According to the model that is often used in guiding stroke therapy, acute infarcts may grow, during the several days after stroke onset, to encompass some or all of the ischemic penumbra.

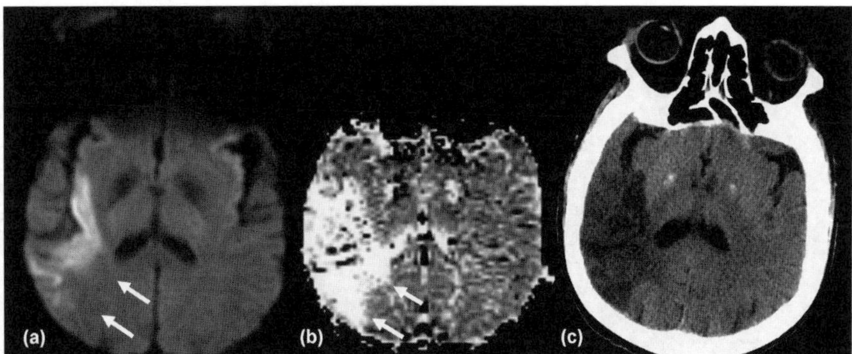

FIGURE 2.8 Growth of an acute infarct into a region of diffusion–perfusion mismatch. An early DWI image (**a**) shows an acute infarct in the right insula and temporal lobe. An MTT map (**b**) shows a somewhat larger perfusion abnormality, which extends posteriorly into a mismatch region (arrows) that appears normal in the DWI image. In a follow-up CT examination (**c**), the infarct has extended into the region of diffusion–perfusion mismatch.

These assumptions have been tested most often using MRI-based perfusion imaging (MRP), also called perfusion-weighted imaging or PWI, which has been in existence for a longer time than CT perfusion imaging (CTP). MRP images are usually interpreted in conjunction with DWI images that are concurrently obtained as part of a rapid MRI protocol that may require as little as 2 minutes of imaging time. In doing this, the lesion seen on early DWI images, rather than CBV maps, is usually taken to represent tissue at the core of the infarct, which is unlikely to recover. Examples of the interpretation of acute DWI and MRP images are shown in Figures 2.8–2.11.

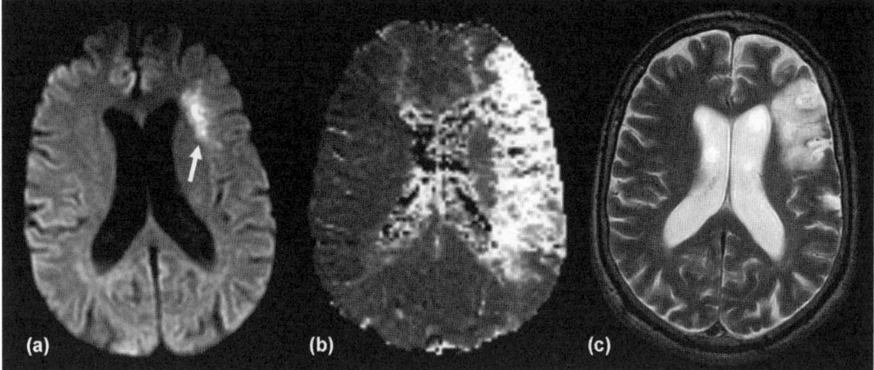

FIGURE 2.9 Partial growth of an acute infarct into a region of diffusion–perfusion mismatch. An early DWI image (**a**) shows a small acute infarct in the left frontal lobe (arrow). The MTT map (**b**) shows a much larger perfusion abnormality, theoretically reflecting a large volume of penumbral tissue at risk of infarction. A follow-up T2-weighted MRI image (**c**) shows that the infarct has grown to include some but not all of the threatened tissue.

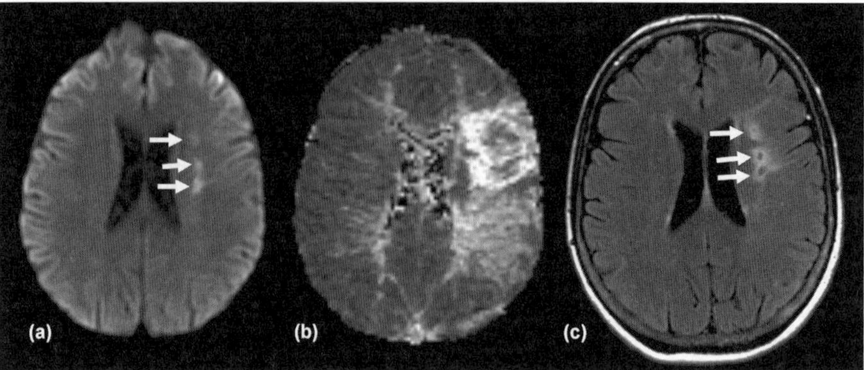

FIGURE 2.10 Failure of an acute infarct to grow into a region of diffusion–perfusion mismatch. An early DWI image (**a**) shows several small closely clustered acute infarcts in the left corona radiata. An MTT map (**b**) shows a much larger region of impaired perfusion, theoretically representing tissue at risk. However, a follow-up T2-weighted FLAIR image (**c**) shows that the infarct has not grown substantially. Preservation of penumbral tissue, as demonstrated by this case, is the goal of acute stroke therapy.

In most cases, the ultimate volume of an infarct is larger than that seen in initial DWI images,[37,75–80] encompassing both initially DWI-abnormal tissue and other tissue into which the infarct extends. The ultimate volume of an infarct also is usually larger than that seen in early CBV maps.[77,79,80] However, DWI images rather than CBV maps are usually used to identify the infarct core, both because infarcts are usually far more conspicuous in DWI images than in CBV maps, and because the DWI detects lesions that have been irreversibly damaged despite

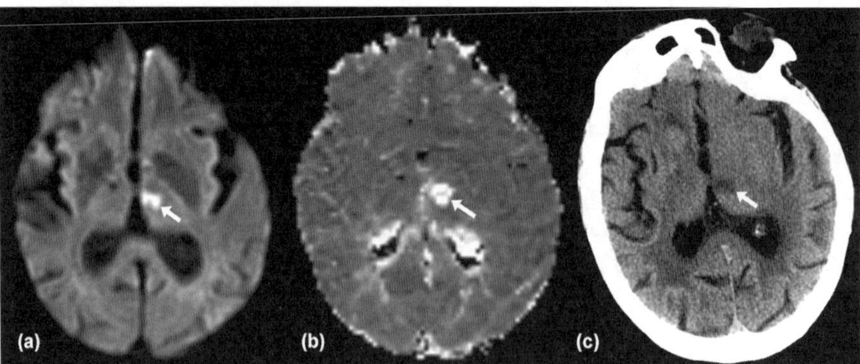

FIGURE 2.11 Matched diffusion and perfusion abnormalities. An early DWI image (**a**) shows an acute infarct in the left thalamus. An MTT map (**b**) shows a small perfusion abnormality that is no larger than the diffusion abnormality. When diffusion and perfusion lesions are matched, there is usually minimal if any infarct extension. Indeed, in this case, a follow-up CT scan (**c**) shows no enlargement of the infarct.

having undergone subsequent spontaneous reperfusion that makes them invisible in CBV maps.[80]

With MRP, the ischemic penumbra is usually defined for clinical purposes as the region of brain tissue that is abnormal in CBF or MTT maps, but normal in DWI images, that is, the region of so-called "diffusion–perfusion mismatch." This definition is congruent with the physiological observation that CBF reduction and MTT prolongation are more sensitive indicators of ischemia than CBV reduction. This definition is also consistent with empirical observations that the volume of a lesion seen in early CBF or MTT maps tends to overestimate the ultimate infarct volume and is less well correlated with final infarct volume than is the initial DWI or CBV lesion volume.[77,79,80] Usually, the MTT map is used for visual interpretation. This is because gray matter and white matter have markedly different CBF values, but quite similar MTT values. This makes MTT maps more homogeneous than CBF maps and increases the conspicuity of lesions in MTT maps.

The assumption that the ischemic penumbra is defined by the region of diffusion–perfusion mismatch has two important implications. First, it implies that patients with a large mismatch are most likely to demonstrate significant infarct growth in follow-up scans. Second, and perhaps of most direct relevance for the stroke neurologist, it implies that patients with a large diffusion–perfusion mismatch are most likely to benefit from thrombolytic therapy, because they have the largest volume of threatened tissue that may be saved by thrombolysis. Conversely, patients with little or no diffusion–perfusion mismatch should not receive thrombolytic therapy, because they have nothing to gain from such therapy, and should be spared the associated risk of hemorrhage.

The first of these hypotheses has been supported by several studies showing that infarcts tend to grow into the area of diffusion–perfusion mismatch, and that patients with larger mismatches tend to demonstrate more lesion growth.[37,81–85] It should be noted that, in two of these studies,[37,84] the perfusion parameter used to define the mismatch was not CBF or MTT, but instead the time it took for contrast concentration to reach peak concentration in each image voxel after contrast injection ("time to peak" or TTP). TTP measurements are often used as rough approximations of MTT measurements because calculation of CBF and MTT are somewhat complex, requiring a mathematical process called "deconvolution." The details of deconvolution are beyond the scope of this chapter, and the reader is referred to other sources for further explanation.[86,87] In many clinical settings, maps of parameters like TTP that do not require deconvolution may be available much more quickly than those that do require deconvolution. TTP is less specific than MTT in detecting underperfused tissue[88] because it does not distinguish between delayed contrast arrival time (such as that related to perfusion via collateral vessels) and truly prolonged intravascular transit time.

The second hypothesis, that patients should be selected for thrombolysis depending on whether or not they exhibit a diffusion–perfusion mismatch, may have enormous implications for stroke therapy in the near future, and is one of the most actively investigated and debated subjects in neuroimaging.

A group of studies investigating intravenous thrombolysis in acute stroke, considered together, provide indirect support for this hypothesis. In the National Institute of Neurological Disorders and Stroke (NINDS) rt-PA study,[16] patients who presented within 3 hours of stroke onset were treated with either intravenous rt-PA or placebo, based on clinical and NCCT criteria only, irrespective of whether or not they had diffusion–perfusion mismatch. In this study, patients who received the drug had significantly better outcomes after 3 months. However, the European Cooperative Acute Stroke study (ECASS), ECASS-II, and Alteplase Thrombolysis for Acute Noninterventional Therapy in Ischemic Stroke (ATLANTIS) studies, which used treatment windows of 0–6, 0–6, and 3–5 hours, respectively, found that thrombolysis resulted in worse outcomes than placebo.[89–91] These four studies, none of which used the presence of a diffusion–perfusion mismatch as an eligibility criterion, provided support for the Food and Drug Administration's (FDA) approval for intravenous thrombolysis for acute stroke patients, but only when those patients were known to be without symptoms no more than 3 hours before the time of initiation of treatment.

However, several important studies have shown that intravenous thrombolysis may be beneficial *more* than 3 hours after stroke onset, provided that only patients with a significant diffusion–perfusion mismatch are treated. In one such study, Ribo et al.[92] found that patients with a significant diffusion–perfusion mismatch could be treated safely and effectively in the 3–6-hour time period. In phase II of the desmoteplase in acute stroke (DIAS) trial, patients with diffusion–perfusion mismatch were treated with desmoteplase up to 9 hours after stroke onset, and showed better outcomes than patients given placebo, with only a minimal incidence of symptomatic hemorrhage.[22] Similar success was achieved in the same time window by the dose escalation study of desmoteplase in acute ischemic stroke (DEDAS).[93]

Another recent study[94] compared the outcomes of two groups of acute stroke patients who received intravenous or intra-arterial thrombolysis. In one group of patients, thrombolysis was initiated less than 6 hours after a known time of stroke onset. In the other group, the actual time of onset was not known, but thrombolysis was initiated within 6 hours of the time at which the patient became aware of his or her stroke. This was generally far more than 6 hours after the time at which the patient was last seen without symptoms. Patients in this second group were allowed to receive thrombolytic therapy only if an initial MRI examination showed a significant diffusion–perfusion mismatch. Their outcomes were actually slightly better than those in the group who were treated within 6 hours of onset, although the difference did not reach statistical significance.

These studies raise the possibility that, one day, imaging-based treatment protocols may allow for intravenous thrombolysis in patients well outside of the now-accepted 3-hour window, provided they demonstrate substantial diffusion–perfusion mismatch. Such protocols could allow for treatment of a vastly larger number of patients than are currently treated. It has been estimated that only 1–7% of acute stroke patients currently receive thrombolytic medication,[95–98] and that, in up to 95% of cases, they are ineligible because they present outside of the 3-hour time window.[99] As many as 80% of patients who present 6 hours after stroke onset may demonstrate a significant diffusion–perfusion mismatch.[100]

The echoplanar imaging thrombolysis evaluation trial (EPITHET) is the first large study designed specifically to assess whether the existence of a diffusion–perfusion mismatch should be an eligibility criterion for thrombolysis. Preliminary results published by the EPITHET investigators[88] failed to show a significant correlation between the volume of diffusion–perfusion mismatch and the extent of infarct expansion. The study is ongoing at the time of this writing.

Perfusion Imaging: Comparison of CTP and MRP

CTP is a relatively recent development in acute stroke imaging that is already in routine clinical use in many centers. CTP and MRP are similar in that both techniques are based on rapid serial image acquisition during intravenous injection of a bolus of contrast material. In both techniques, measurements of density over time (for CTP) or signal intensity over time (for MRP) are converted to contrast agent-versus-time curves, and these are processed in similar ways to yield the same perfusion measurements (most often CBV, CBF, and MTT). Example CTP images are shown in Figure 2.12.

Despite these similarities, CTP and MRP have some significant differences. Chief among CTP's advantages is its widespread availability and accessibility. As discussed above, CT scanners are far more widely available than MRI scanners in or near North American emergency departments, particularly after hours, when many MRI scanners are not operational. Furthermore, although some investigators have proposed that acute stroke patients may be safely directed to an MRI scanner without an initial CT scan,[2, 101] the clinical reality in most centers is that patients with suspected acute stroke undergo CT examination as a first study. Therefore, CTP offers the possibility of performing an examination that includes perfusion

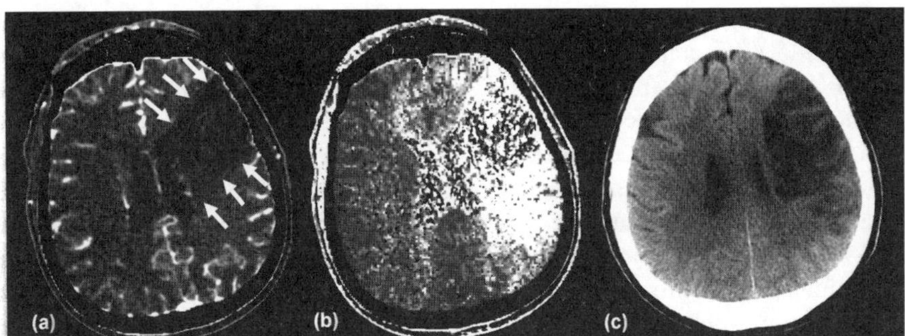

FIGURE 2.12 CT perfusion images. CTP images were acquired in this acute stroke patient who was unable to undergo MRI. A map of CBV (**a**) shows a well-defined region of decreased blood volume in the left frontal lobe. Because DWI images are not available, this region is presumed to represent the core of the infarct. MTT maps (**b**) show a much larger region of prolonged MTT, reflecting tissue at risk of infarction. In a follow-up CT scan (**c**), most but not all of the threatened tissue has progressed to infarction. Note that in some of the tissue that demonstrates low CBV, perfusion is so severely impaired that the amount of contrast agent that arrives is so small that MTT cannot be measured accurately, resulting in a noisy "speckled" appearance in the MTT map.

imaging without having to move to a second modality. As discussed above, CT allows for scanning of patients with pacemakers and other ferromagnetic implants, as well as monitoring of patients with ferromagnetic equipment that cannot be brought into an MRI scanner room.

Aside from CTP's use of potentially nephrotoxic contrast material and relatively large doses of ionizing radiation,[102] one of the main disadvantages of the technique is its limited coverage of the brain. The degree of coverage is highly dependent on the scanner being used, with multislice scanners affording much greater coverage. For example, our institution's current protocol for 16-slice CT scanners allows for imaging of two separate 2-cm axial slabs, resulting in coverage of 4 cm of the brain. However, our protocol for 64-slice scanners allows for imaging of two separate 4-cm slabs, which together cover most of the brain. By comparison, our current MRP protocol allows for acquisition of 16 slices of any desired thickness and orientation. As we usually choose to acquire axial MRP slices that are 5 mm thick and separated by 1 mm, this results in coverage of a 9.5-cm axial slab. Thus, with a 64-slice scanner, brain coverage with CTP approximates that of MRP, although evaluation of the posterior fossa may be somewhat compromised with CTP due to beam hardening artifacts at the skull base.

For both CTP and MRP, perfusion measurements are based on detection of a nondiffusible contrast agent that is confined to the 2–5% of each image voxel that is occupied by blood vessels.[103–106] Because CTP directly measures the quantity of contrast material in each image voxel, confinement of the contrast agent within vessels places an intrinsic limit on the degree of density change that can be measured by CTP, which is usually on the order of 10% or less. This fact, in conjunction with the intrinsically lower contrast-to-noise ratio of CT imaging, means that CTP maps are much noisier than MRP maps. Typically, CTP postprocessing algorithms perform extensive spatial averaging, in order to reduce noise by sacrificing some of CT's considerably superior spatial resolution.

MRP maps are less noisy than CTP maps because MRP detects the passage of gadolinium using susceptibility effects, which "bloom" out of each vessel, extending through a space whose radius is roughly proportional to the radius of the vessel. Thus, the susceptibility effect related to gadolinium in microscopic vessels blooms out of those vessels, reducing signal arising from all parts of each voxel, and resulting in a much larger measurable signal change as the gadolinium passes through brain, in the range of 20–40% in the gradient-echo images that are most often used for MRP. This blooming effect accounts for the superior contrast-to-noise ratio of MRP maps, and also for the fact that, unlike CTP maps, most MRP maps disproportionately weigh the presence of contrast in larger vessels.[107]

MRP can also be performed with spin-echo pulse sequences, which results in sensitivity to contrast in vessels of all sizes that more closely (but not perfectly) approximates the truly uniform sensitivity achieved by CTP.[107,108] However, this more uniform sensitivity comes at the expense of lower contrast, generally requiring twice the usual dose of gadolinium. Some researchers have used MRP pulse sequences that simultaneously acquire both spin-echo and gradient-echo images not only to correct for differences in sensitivity to vessels, but also to quantitatively distinguish between hemodynamic conditions of vessels of different sizes.[109] The clinical implications of differing sensitivities to vessels of different sizes have yet to be fully elucidated.

Perfusion Imaging: Interpretation of CT Perfusion Images

CTP is clearly superior to NCCT in detecting acute stroke. In one study, the overall accuracy of CTP maps ranged from 75.7% to 86.0%, compared to 66.2% for NCCT. This accuracy was achieved due to the superior sensitivity of MTT maps to NCCT (77.6% for MTT maps vs. 69.2% for NCCT), as well as superior specificity of CBF and CBV maps (90.9% and 92.7%, respectively, vs. 65.0% for NCCT).[110]

However, the real promise of CTP lies not in its ability to detect acute stroke, but in its ability, like that of MRP, to distinguish between infarct core and the ischemic penumbra. CTP produces maps of the same perfusion parameters that are generated by MRP, and CTP maps are interpreted in a similar manner, with one important exception: with CTP, DWI images are usually not available to identify the infarct core. Therefore, CBV maps are usually used to define the infarct core. Tissue that appears normal in CBV maps, but abnormal in CBF or MTT maps, is taken to represent the ischemic penumbra.

Several studies have validated the ability of CTP to distinguish between core and penumbra. In one study, Wintermark et al.[111] found that the volumes of early infarcts in CTP CBV maps were highly correlated with volumes of early DWI lesions, whereas volumes of lesions seen in CTP CBF maps were close to those seen in the corresponding MRP MTT maps. In another study, the volume of the CBF abnormality in an acute-stage infarct was highly correlated with final infarct volume in patients who did not exhibit recanalization after thrombolysis, consistent with extension of infarction into the penumbra. However, in patients who did exhibit recanalization after thrombolysis, final infarct volume was highly correlated with the initial CBV abnormality, consistent with failure of infarcts to extend into the ischemic penumbra.[112]

Perfusion Imaging: Arterial Spin Labeling

It should be noted that perfusion imaging of the brain can also be performed in a completely noninvasive manner, without an exogenous contrast agent, using an MRI technique called arterial spin labeling (ASL).[113,114] In ASL, an additional MRI coil is placed over the patient's neck and used to excite hydrogen nuclei ("spins") as they pass through one of the major cervical arteries en route to the brain. In this way, the spins themselves serve as an endogenous contrast agent, whose passage through the brain can be used to measure the perfusion parameters described above. This method offers major theoretical advantages. Besides being safe in patients with contrast allergies, ASL offers the possibility of performing perfusion imaging over and over again within a short period of time, without concerns of cumulative contrast dose. This could be useful, for example, in periodically assessing the effects of an ongoing recanalization procedure. Also, individual cervical arteries can be selectively labeled in ASL, so that the vascular territory of each cervical artery can be individually imaged. This is not possible with MRP or CTP.

Although ASL has been performed in the acute stroke setting,[115] this currently is seldom done, for several reasons. Current ASL pulse sequences are somewhat more time consuming than DSC, requiring 6 minutes in the study cited above, compared to approximately 1 minute for DSC or CTP. ASL perfusion maps are far noisier than DSC maps, and have less spatial resolution.

Researchers are actively at work improving both the speed of ASL sequences and the quality of the resulting images, and ASL may prove an important acute stroke imaging technique in the future.

Permeability Imaging

Cerebral ischemia injures not only neurons and glial cells, but also the cells that comprise the walls of microscopic blood vessels.[116,117] Damage to vessels may lead to rupture and likely accounts for the potential for ischemic infarcts to undergo hemorrhagic transformation, particularly after treatment with thrombolytic agents.[118] Animal studies have shown that MRI can detect vascular injury by measuring increases in vascular permeability to a gadolinium-based contrast agent and that these permeability changes can be used to predict the risk of hemorrhage.[119–121]

The utility of permeability imaging in predicting hemorrhagic transformation has also been demonstrated in a small study of 10 human acute stroke patients.[122] Three of those patients demonstrated increased vascular permeability within their acute infarcts. All three of these patients, but none of the other seven, subsequently exhibited hemorrhagic transformation. This study was performed using a specialized and relatively time-consuming MRI pulse sequence designed to measure permeability quantitatively. The authors noted that this method was more sensitive for detecting increased vascular permeability than routine postcontrast T1-weighted images, which showed enhancement in only one of the three cases.

Several studies have shown that FLAIR images can also detect increased permeability of the blood–brain barrier in acute stroke patients. FLAIR is an MRI technique that is discussed above and is commonly included as a precontrast pulse sequence in examinations of the brain. However, when performed after contrast injection, FLAIR images can demonstrate leakage of contrast through damaged blood vessels into the subarachnoid space, which is manifested by hyperintensity of sulcal CSF. This sign, which has been called the "hyperintense acute reperfusion marker" or HARM, has been associated with increased incidence of hemorrhagic transformation.[123,124]

The clinical role of permeability imaging has yet to be assessed by a large clinical trial, but these techniques continue to hold promise for the future, as intracranial hemorrhage is the most significant potential complication of what is currently the only FDA-approved treatment for acute stroke.

Sodium Imaging

Virtually every clinical MRI technique produces images based on signal arising from hydrogen nuclei. However, one group has proposed studying acute stroke patients with images that are based on the concentration of sodium in different parts of the brain. This is of interest because of the large differences in sodium concentration that normally exist between the intracellular space, where ion pumps maintain a low concentration of approximately 10 mM, and the extracellular space, where systemic autoregulation maintains a nearly constant concentration of approximately 145 mM. The intracellular space is much larger in volume than the extracellular space, occupying approximately 80% of the brain's volume under normal conditions. Therefore, when ischemic damage causes cell membranes to become permeable to sodium ions, a large potential reservoir for sodium is effectively opened and ions begin to shift from the extracellular space to the intracellular space. Provided there is at least some residual perfusion of the ischemic tissue, the lost extracellular sodium ions are replenished by the effectively infinite supply in the bloodstream, resulting in an overall increase in the amount of sodium that is present, which serves as a detectable marker of cell membrane damage.

In serial studies of acute stroke performed with sodium imaging, Thulborn and colleagues have noted that sodium concentrations may continue to increase markedly in ischemic brain tissue, even several days after stroke onset. This is in contrast to the most widely available marker of tissue damage, the ADC of water, measured with DWI, which drops quickly within minutes of stroke onset, but changes relatively little thereafter. Therefore, sodium concentration could serve as a more precise indicator of the stage of ischemic injury. Thulborn and colleagues have shown that changes in sodium concentration do not necessarily parallel those of ADC and that a sodium concentration threshold of 70 mM can identify irreversibly damaged tissue with very high specificity.

Sodium imaging is relatively time consuming and cannot be performed on standard clinical scanners without specialized hardware and software upgrades. Nevertheless, the unique physiologic information provided by sodium imaging may make this technique an important tool in acute stroke imaging in years to come.

Multiparametric Tissue Modeling

The above sections describe many different imaging techniques that provide complimentary information about the viability of different parts of an acute stroke patient's brain. Neuroradiologists and stroke neurologists mentally synthesize the information provided by these different images to arrive at decisions regarding treatment decisions. Some groups have proposed combining different kinds of images quantitatively, using computers, in order to produce composite maps showing the risk of infarction in different parts of the brain. Wu et al.[125] developed a multiparametric predictive model, incorporating DWI and MRP data, which achieved 66% sensitivity and 84% specificity in identifying individual tissue voxels destined for infarction. Rose et al.[126] used a different multiparametric model to achieve mean sensitivity of 72% and specificity of 97%.

Currently, multiparametric predictive algorithms are largely confined to the realm of research and are not generally used clinically. However, it is easy to imagine a time in the future when acute stroke patients undergo a quick imaging evaluation, using many of the methods mentioned above, the results of which are used by a multiparametric model that immediately produces composite maps showing which areas of the brain are likely to infarct if each of various therapeutic approaches are undertaken. Such a model, once empirically validated, could dramatically enhance the treatment of acute stroke patients.

CONCLUSION

This chapter has reviewed many of an increasingly wide variety of techniques that are used in imaging the acute stroke patient. The field of acute stroke imaging continues to progress rapidly, driven by the tremendous incidence of the disease, the often devastating nature of its consequences, and the opportunity to make a meaningful difference in the lives of a large number of patients by guiding judiciously the application of increasingly effective stroke therapies, the most widely available of which is intravenous thrombolysis using rt-PA. Advanced CT and MR imaging techniques that show a mismatch between "core" and "penumbra" regions have the potential to be critically important tools in selecting patients who may undergo intravenous thrombolysis outside of the currently accepted therapeutic window of 3 hours after stroke onset. Other imaging techniques that are at earlier stages of development may provide even more detailed characterization of tissue viability.

REFERENCES

1. Hand PJ, Kwan J, Lindley RI, Dennis MS, Wardlaw JM. Distinguishing between stroke and mimic at the bedside: the brain attack study. *Stroke* 2006;37:769–775.
2. Kidwell CS, Chalela JA, Saver JL, Starkman S, Hill MD, Demchuk AM, Butman JA, Patronas N, Alger JR, Latour LL, Luby ML, Baird AE, Leary MC, Tremwel M, Ovbiagele B, Fredieu A, Suzuki S, Villablanca JP, Davis S, Dunn B, Todd JW, Ezzeddine MA, Haymore J, Lynch JK, Davis L, Warach S. Comparison of MRI and CT for detection of acute intracerebral hemorrhage. *JAMA* 2004;292:1823–1830.
3. Kucinski T. Unenhanced CT and acute stroke physiology. *Neuroimaging Clin N Am* 2005;15:397–407.
4. Horowitz SH, Zito JL, Donnarumma R, Patel M, Alvir J. Computed tomographic–angiographic findings within the first five hours of cerebral infarction. *Stroke* 1991;22:1245–1253.
5. Lev MH, Farkas J, Gemmete JJ, Hossain ST, Hunter GJ, Koroshetz WJ, Gonzalez RG. Acute stroke: improved nonenhanced CT detection—benefits of soft-copy interpretation by using variable window width and center level settings. *Radiology* 1999;213:150–155.

6. Wolpert SM, Bruckmann H, Greenlee R, Wechsler L, Pessin MS, del Zoppo GJ. Neuroradiologic evaluation of patients with acute stroke treated with recombinant tissue plasminogen activator. The rt-PA Acute Stroke Study Group. *Am J Neuroradiol* 1993;14:3–13.
7. Barber PA, Demchuk AM, Hudon ME, Pexman JH, Hill MD, Buchan AM. Hyperdense Sylvian fissure MCA "dot" sign: a CT marker of acute ischemia. *Stroke* 2001;32:84–88.
8. Launes J, Ketonen L. Dense middle cerebral artery sign: an indicator of poor outcome in middle cerebral artery area infarction. *J Neurol Neurosurg Psychiatry* 1987;50: 1550–1552.
9. Zorzon M, Mase G, Pozzi-Mucelli F, Biasutti E, Antonutti L, Iona L, Cazzato G. Increased density in the middle cerebral artery by nonenhanced computed tomography. Prognostic value in acute cerebral infarction. *Eur Neurol* 1993;33:256–259.
10. von Kummer R, Holle R, Grzyska U, Hoffman H, Jansen O, Petersen D, Schumacher M, Sartor K. Interobserver agreement in assessing early CT signs of middle cerebral artery infarction. *Am J Neuroradiol* 1996;17:1743–1748.
11. Wardlaw JM, Dorman PJ, Lewis SC, Sandercock PAG. Can stroke physicians and neuroradiologists identify signs of early cerebral infarction on CT? *J Neurol Neurosurg Psychiatry* 1999;67:651–653.
12. Mullins ME, Lev MH, Schellingerhout D, Koroshetz WJ, Gonzalez RG. Influence of availability of clinical history on detection of early stroke using unenhanced CT and diffusion-weighted MR imaging. *Am J Roentgenol* 2002;179:223–228.
13. Barber PA, Demchuk AM, Zhang J, Buchan AM. Validity and reliability of a quantitative computed tomography score in predicting outcome of hyperacute stroke before thrombolytic therapy. ASPECTS Study Group. Alberta Stroke Programme Early CT Score. *Lancet* 2000;355:1670–1674.
14. Patel SC, Levine SR, Tilley BC, Grotta JC, Lu M, Frankel M, Haley EC, Jr., Brott TG, Broderick JP, Horowitz S, Lyden PD, Lewandowski CA, Marler JR, Welch KM, National Institute of Neurological D, Stroke rt PASSG. Lack of clinical significance of early ischemic changes on computed tomography in acute stroke. *JAMA* 2001;286:2830–2838.
15. Dzialowski I, Hill MD, Coutts SB, Demchuk AM, Kent DM, Wunderlich O, von Kummer R. Extent of early ischemic changes on computed tomography (CT) before thrombolysis: prognostic value of the Alberta Stroke Program Early CT Score in ECASS II. *Stroke* 2006;37:973–978.
16. NINDS rt-PA Study Group. Tissue plasminogen activator for acute ischemic stroke. The National Institute of Neurological Disorders and Stroke rt-PA Stroke Study Group. *N Engl J Med* 1995;333:1581–1587.
17. Yuh WT, Crain MR, Loes DJ, Greene GM, Ryals TJ, Sato Y. MR imaging of cerebral ischemia: findings in the first 24 hours. *Am J Neuroradiol.* 1991;12:621–629.
18. Perkins CJ, Kahya E, Roque CT, Roche PE, Newman GC. Fluid-attenuated inversion recovery and diffusion- and perfusion-weighted MRI abnormalities in 117 consecutive patients with stroke symptoms. *Stroke*. 2001;32:2774–2781.
19. Lövblad KO, Laubach HJ, Baird AE, Curtin F, Schlaug G, Edelman RR, Warach S. Clinical experience with diffusion-weighted MR in patients with acute stroke. *Am J Neuroradiol.* 1998;19:1061–1066.
20. Singer MB, Chong J, Lu D, Schonewille WJ, Tuhrim S, Atlas SW. Diffusion-weighted MRI in acute subcortical infarction. *Stroke* 1998;29:133–136.

21. van Everdingen KJ, van der Grond J, Kappelle LJ, Ramos LM, Mali WP. Diffusion-weighted magnetic resonance imaging in acute stroke. *Stroke* 1998;29:1783–1790.
22. Hacke W, Albers G, Al-Rawi Y, Bogousslavsky J, Davalos A, Eliasziw M, Fischer M, Furlan A, Kaste M, Lees KR, Soehngen M, Warach S, Group DS. The Desmoteplase in Acute Ischemic Stroke Trial (DIAS): a phase II MRI-based 9-hour window acute stroke thrombolysis trial with intravenous desmoteplase. *Stroke* 2005;36:66–73.
23. Gonzalez RG, Schaefer PW, Buonanno FS, Schwamm LH, Budzik RF, Rordorf G, Wang B, Sorensen AG, Koroshetz WJ. Diffusion-weighted MR imaging: diagnostic accuracy in patients imaged within 6 hours of stroke symptom onset. *Radiology* 1999;210: 155–162.
24. Urbach H, Flacke S, Keller E, Textor J, Berlis A, Hartmann A, Reul J, Solymosi L, Schild HH. Detectability and detection rate of acute cerebral hemisphere infarcts on CT and diffusion-weighted MRI. *Neuroradiology* 2000;42:722–727.
25. Fiebach JB, Schellinger PD, Jansen O, Meyer M, Wilde P, Bender J, Schramm P, Juttler E, Oehler J, Hartmann M, Hahnel S, Knauth M, Hacke W, Sartor K. CT and diffusion-weighted MR imaging in randomized order: diffusion- weighted imaging results in higher accuracy and lower interrater variability in the diagnosis of hyperacute ischemic stroke. *Stroke* 2002;33:2206–2210.
26. Mullins ME, Schaefer PW, Sorensen AG, Halpern EF, Ay H, He J, Koroshetz WJ, Gonzalez RG. CT and conventional and diffusion-weighted MR imaging in acute stroke: study in 691 patients at presentation to the emergency department. *Radiology* 2002;224:353–360.
27. Grant PE, He J, Halpern EF, Wu O, Schaefer PW, Schwamm LH, Budzik RF, Sorensen AG, Koroshetz WJ, Gonzalez RG. Frequency and clinical context of decreased apparent diffusion coefficient reversal in the human brain. *Radiology* 2001;221:43–50.
28. Parsons MW, Barber PA, Chalk J, Darby DG, Rose S, Desmond PM, Gerraty RP, Tress BM, Wright PM, Donnan GA, Davis SM. Diffusion- and perfusion-weighted MRI response to thrombolysis in stroke. *Ann Neurol* 2002;51:28–37.
29. Kidwell CS, Saver JL, Starkman S, Duckwiler G, Jahan R, Vespa P, Villablanca JP, Liebeskind DS, Gobin YP, Vinuela F, Alger JR. Late secondary ischemic injury in patients receiving intraarterial thrombolysis. *Ann Neurol* 2002;52:698–703.
30. Warach S, Chien D, Li W, Ronthal M, Edelman RR. Fast magnetic resonance diffusion-weighted imaging of acute human stroke. *Neurology* 1992;42:1717–1723.
31. Warach S, Gaa J, Siewert B, Wielopolski P, Edelman RR. Acute human stroke studied by whole brain echo planar diffusion-weighted magnetic resonance imaging. *Ann Neurol* 1995;37:231–241.
32. Lutsep HL, Albers GW, de Crespigny A, Kamat GN, Marks MP, Moseley ME. Clinical utility of diffusion-weighted magnetic resonance imaging in the assessment of ischemic stroke. *Ann Neurol* 1997;41:574–580.
33. Schlaug G, Siewert B, Benfield A, Edelman RR, Warach S. Time course of the apparent diffusion coefficient (ADC) abnormality in human stroke. *Neurology* 1997;49:113–119.
34. Nagesh V, Welch KM, Windham JP, Patel S, Levine SR, Hearshen D, Peck D, Robbins K, D'Olhaberriague L, Soltanian-Zadeh H, Boska MD. Time course of ADCw changes in ischemic stroke: beyond the human eye. *Stroke* 1998;29:1778–1782.
35. Schwamm LH, Koroshetz WJ, Sorensen AG, Wang B, Copen WA, Budzik R, Rordorf G, Buonanno FS, Schaefer PW, Gonzalez RG. Time course of lesion development in

patients with acute stroke: serial diffusion- and hemodynamic-weighted magnetic resonance imaging. *Stroke* 1998;29:2268–2276.

36. Yang Q, Tress BM, Barber PA, Desmond PM, Darby DG, Gerraty RP, Li T, Davis SM. Serial study of apparent diffusion coefficient and anisotropy in patients with acute stroke. *Stroke* 1999;30:2382–2390.
37. Beaulieu C, de Crespigny A, Tong DC, Moseley ME, Albers GW, Marks MP. Longitudinal magnetic resonance imaging study of perfusion and diffusion in stroke: evolution of lesion volume and correlation with clinical outcome. *Ann Neurol* 1999;46:568–578.
38. Marks MP, Tong DC, Beaulieu C, Albers GW, de Crespigny A, Moseley ME. Evaluation of early reperfusion and i.v. tPA therapy using diffusion- and perfusion-weighted MRI. *Neurology* 1999;52:1792–1798.
39. Lansberg MG, Thijs VN, O'Brien MW, Ali JO, de Crespigny AJ, Tong DC, Moseley ME, Albers GW. Evolution of apparent diffusion coefficient, diffusion-weighted, and T2-weighted signal intensity of acute stroke. *Am J Neuroradiol* 2001;22:637–644.
40. Copen WA, Schwamm LH, Gonzalez RG, Wu O, Harmath CB, Schaefer PW, Koroshetz WJ, Sorensen AG. Ischemic stroke: effects of etiology and patient age on the time course of the core apparent diffusion coefficient. *Radiology* 2001;221:27–34.
41. Fiebach JB, Jansen O, Schellinger PD, Heiland S, Hacke W, Sartor K. Serial analysis of the apparent diffusion coefficient time course in human stroke. *Neuroradiology* 2002;44:294–298.
42. Morris P. *Practical Neuroangiography*. Baltimore, MD: Lippincott, Williams, and Wilkins; 1997.
43. Lameier NH. Contrast-induced nephropathy—prevention and risk reduction. *Nephrol Dial Transplant* 2006;21:i11–i23.
44. Idée JM, Pinès E, Prigent P, Corot C. Allergy-like reactions to iodinated contrast agents. A critical analysis. *Fundam Clin Pharmacol* 2005;19:263–281.
45. Wolf GL, Mishkin MM, Roux SG, Halpern EF, Gottlieb J, Zimmerman J, Gillen J, Thellman C. Comparison of the rates of adverse drug reactions. Ionic contrast agents, ionic agents combined with steroids, and nonionic agents. *Invest Radiol* 1991;26: 404–410.
46. Katayama H, Yamaguchi K, Kozuka T, Takashima T, Seez P, Matsuura K. Adverse reactions to ionic and nonionic contrast media. A report from the Japanese Committee on the Safety of Contrast Media. *Radiology* 1990;175:621–628.
47. Pomerantz SR, Harris GJ, Desai HJ, Lev MH. Computed tomography angiograph and computed tomography perfusion in ischemic stroke: a step-by-step approach to image acquisition and three-dimensional postprocessing. *Semin Ultrasound CT MR* 2006;27:243–270.
48. Lev MH, Farkas J, Rodriguez VR, Schwamm LH, Hunter GJ, Putman CM, Rordorf GA, Buonanno FS, Budzik R, Koroshetz WJ, Gonzalez RG. CT angiography in the rapid triage of patients with hyperacute stroke to intraarterial thrombolysis: accuracy in the detection of large vessel thrombus. *J Comput Assist Tomogr* 2001;25:520–528.
49. Kucinski T, Koch C, Grzyska U, Freitag HJ, Kromer H, Zeumer H. The predictive value of early CT and angiography for fatal hemispheric swelling in acute stroke. *Am J Neuroradiol* 1998;19:839–846.

50. Smith WS, Tsao JW, Billings ME, Johnston SC, Hemphill JC, 3rd, Bonovich DC, Dillon WP. Prognostic significance of angiographically confirmed large vessel intracranial occlusion in patients presenting with acute brain ischemia. *Neurocrit Care* 2006;4:14–17.
51. Slivka A, Murphy E, Horrocks L. Cerebral edema after temporary and permanent middle cerebral artery occlusion in the rat. *Stroke* 1995;26:1061–1065.
52. Arnold M, Nedeltchev K, Brekenfeld C, Fischer U, Remonda L, Schroth G, Mattle H. Outcome of acute stroke patients without visible occlusion on early arteriography. *Stroke* 2004;35:1135–1138.
53. del Zoppo GJ, Poeck K, Pessin MS, Wolpert SM, Furlan AJ, Ferbert A, Alberts MJ, Zivin JA, Wechsler L, Busse O. Recombinant tissue plasminogen activator in acute thrombotic and embolic stroke. *Ann Neurol* 1992;32:78–86.
54. Wildermuth S, Knauth M, Brandt T, Winter R, Sartor K, Hacke W. Role of CT angiography in patient selection for thrombolytic therapy in acute hemispheric stroke. *Stroke* 1998;29:935–938 [see comment].
55. Hunter GJ, Hamberg LM, Ponzo JA, Huang-Hellinger FR, Morris PP, Rabinov J, Farkas J, Lev MH, Schaefer PW, Ogilvy CS, Schwamm LH, Buonanno FS, Koroshetz WJ, Wolf GL, Gonzalez RG. Assessment of cerebral perfusion and arterial anatomy in hyperacute stroke with three-dimensional functional CT: early clinical results. *Am J Neuroradiol* 1998;19:29–37.
56. Lev MH, Segal AZ, Farkas J, Hossain ST, Putman C, Hunter GJ, Budzik R, Harris GJ, Buonanno FS, Ezzeddine MA, Chang Y, Koroshetz WJ, Gonzalez RG, Schwamm LH. Utility of perfusion-weighted CT imaging in acute middle cerebral artery stroke treated with intra-arterial thrombolysis: prediction of final infarct volume and clinical outcome. *Stroke* 2001;32:2021–2028.
57. Schramm P, Schellinger PD, Klotz E, Kallenberg K, Fiebach JB, Kulkens S, Heiland S, Knauth M, Sartor K. Comparison of perfusion computed tomography and computed tomography angiography source images with perfusion-weighted imaging and diffusion-weighted imaging in patients with acute stroke of less than 6 hours' duration. *Stroke* 2004;35:1652–1658.
58. Coutts SB, Lev MH, Eliasziw M, Roccatagliata L, Hill MD, Schwamm LH, Pexman JH, Koroshetz WJ, Hudon ME, Buchan AM, Gonzalez RG, Demchuk AM. ASPECTS on CTA source images versus unenhanced CT: added value in predicting final infarct extent and clinical outcome. *Stroke* 2004;35:2472–2476.
59. Hamberg LM, Hunter GJ, Kierstead D, Lo EH, Gilberto Gonzalez R, Wolf GL. Measurement of cerebral blood volume with subtraction three-dimensional functional CT. *Am J Neuroradiol* 1996;17:1861–1869.
60. Remonda L, Heid O, Schroth G. Carotid artery stenosis, occlusion, and pseudo-occlusion: first-pass, gadolinium-enhanced, three-dimensional MR angiography—preliminary study. *Radiology* 1998;209:95–102 [see comment].
61. Heiserman JE, Drayer BP, Keller PJ, Fram EK. Intracranial vascular stenosis and occlusion: evaluation with three-dimensional time-of-flight MR angiography. *Radiology* 1992;185:667–673.
62. Korogi Y, Takahashi M, Mabuchi N, Miki H, Shiga H, Watabe T, O'Uchi T, Nakagawa T, Horikawa Y, Fujiwara S. Intracranial vascular stenosis and occlusion: diagnostic accuracy of three-dimensional, Fourier transform, time-of-flight MR angiography. *Radiology* 1994;193:187–193.

63. Cenic A, Nabavi DG, Craen RA, Gelb AW, Lee TY. Dynamic CT measurement of cerebral blood flow: a validation study. *Am J Neuroradiol* 1999;20:63–73.
64. Nabavi DG, Cenic A, Dool J, Smith RM, Espinosa F, Craen RA, Gelb AW, Lee TY. Quantitative assessment of cerebral hemodynamics using CT: stability, accuracy, and precision studies in dogs. *J Comput Assist Tomogr* 1999;23:506–515.
65. Wintermark M, Thiran JP, Maeder P, Schnyder P, Meuli R. Simultaneous measurement of regional cerebral blood flow by perfusion CT and stable xenon CT: a validation study. *Am J Neuroradiol* 2001;22:905–914 [see comment].
66. Gillard JH, Antoun NM, Burnet NG, Pickard JD. Reproducibility of quantitative CT perfusion imaging. *Br J Radiol* 2001;74:552–555.
67. Furukawa M, Kashiwagi S, Matsunaga N, Suzuki M, Kishimoto K, Shirao S. Evaluation of cerebral perfusion parameters measured by perfusion CT in chronic cerebral ischemia: comparison with xenon CT. *J Comput Assist Tomogr* 2002;26:272–278.
68. Rempp KA, Brix G, Wenz F, Becker CR, Guckel F, Lorenz WJ. Quantification of regional cerebral blood flow and volume with dynamic susceptibility contrast-enhanced MR imaging. *Radiology* 1994;193:637–641.
69. Østergaard L, Smith DF, Vestergaard-Poulsen P, Hansen SB, Gee AD, Gjedde A, Gyldensted C. Absolute cerebral blood flow and blood volume measured by magnetic resonance imaging bolus tracking: comparison with positron emission tomography values. *J Cereb Blood Flow Metab* 1998;18:425–432.
70. Hagen T, Bartylla K, Piepgras U. Correlation of regional cerebral blood flow measured by stable xenon CT and perfusion MRI. *J Comput Assist Tomogr* 1999;23:257–264.
71. Sakoh M, Rohl L, Gyldensted C, Gjedde A, Østergaard L. Cerebral blood flow and blood volume measured by magnetic resonance imaging bolus tracking after acute stroke in pigs: comparison with [(15)O]H(2)O positron emission tomography. *Stroke* 2000;31: 1958–1964.
72. Smith AM, Grandin CB, Duprez T, Mataigne F, Cosnard G. Whole brain quantitative CBF, CBV, and MTT measurements using MRI bolus tracking: implementation and application to data acquired from hyperacute stroke patients. *J Magn Reson Imaging* 2000;12:400–410.
73. Lin W, Celik A, Derdeyn C, An H, Lee Y, Videen T, Østergaard L, Powers WJ. Quantitative measurements of cerebral blood flow in patients with unilateral carotid artery occlusion: a PET and MR study. *J Magn Reson Imaging* 2001;14: 659–667.
74. Endo H, Inoue T, Ogasawara K, Fukuda T, Kanbara Y, Ogawa A. Quantitative assessment of cerebral hemodynamics using perfusion-weighted MRI in patients with major cerebral artery occlusive disease: comparison with positron emission tomography. *Stroke* 2006;37:388–392.
75. Sorensen AG, Buonanno FS, Gonzalez RG, Schwamm LH, Lev MH, Huang-Hellinger FR, Reese TG, Weisskoff RM, Davis TL, Suwanwela N, Can U, Moreira JA, Copen WA, Look RB, Finklestein SP, Rosen BR, Koroshetz WJ. Hyperacute stroke: evaluation with combined multisection diffusion-weighted and hemodynamically weighted echo-planar MR imaging. *Radiology* 1996;199:391–401.
76. Tong DC, Yenari MA, Albers GW, O'Brien M, Marks MP, Moseley ME. Correlation of perfusion- and diffusion-weighted MRI with NIHSS score in acute (<6.5 hour) ischemic stroke. *Neurology* 1998;50:864–870.

77. Sorensen AG, Copen WA, Østergaard L, Buonanno FS, Gonzalez RG, Rordorf G, Rosen BR, Schwamm LH, Weisskoff RM, Koroshetz WJ. Hyperacute stroke: simultaneous measurement of relative cerebral blood volume, relative cerebral blood flow, and mean tissue transit time. *Radiology* 1999;210:519–527.
78. Karonen JO, Vanninen RL, Liu Y, Østergaard L, Kuikka JT, Nuutinen J, Vanninen EJ, Partanen PL, Vainio PA, Korhonen K, Perkio J, Roivainen R, Sivenius J, Aronen HJ. Combined diffusion and perfusion MRI with correlation to single-photon emission CT in acute ischemic stroke. Ischemic penumbra predicts infarct growth. *Stroke* 1999;30:1583–1590.
79. Schaefer PW, Hunter GJ, He J, Hamberg LM, Sorensen AG, Schwamm LH, Koroshetz WJ, Gonzalez RG. Predicting cerebral ischemic infarct volume with diffusion and perfusion MR imaging. *Am J Neuroradiol* 2002;23:1785–1794.
80. Karonen JO, Liu Y, Vanninen RL, Østergaard L, Kaarina Partanen PL, Vainio PA, Vanninen EJ, Nuutinen J, Roivainen R, Soimakallio S, Kuikka JT, Aronen HJ. Combined perfusion- and diffusion-weighted MR imaging in acute ischemic stroke during the 1st week: a longitudinal study. *Radiology* 2000;217:886–894.
81. Baird AE, Benfield A, Schlaug G, Siewert B, Lovblad KO, Edelman RR, Warach S. Enlargement of human cerebral ischemic lesion volumes measured by diffusion-weighted magnetic resonance imaging. *Ann Neurol* 1997;41:581–589.
82. Barber PA, Darby DG, Desmond PM, Yang Q, Gerraty RP, Jolley D, Donnan GA, Tress BM, Davis SM. Prediction of stroke outcome with echoplanar perfusion- and diffusion-weighted MRI. *Neurology* 1998;51:418–426.
83. Schlaug G, Benfield A, Baird AE, Siewert B, Lovblad KO, Parker RA, Edelman RR, Warach S. The ischemic penumbra: operationally defined by diffusion and perfusion MRI. *Neurology* 1999;53:1528–1537.
84. Neumann-Haefelin T, Wittsack HJ, Wenserski F, Siebler M, Seitz RJ, Modder U, Freund HJ. Diffusion- and perfusion-weighted MRI. The DWI/PWI mismatch region in acute stroke. *Stroke* 1999;30:1591–1597.
85. Parsons MW, Yang Q, Barber PA, Darby DG, Desmond PM, Gerraty RP, Tress BM, Davis SM. Perfusion magnetic resonance imaging maps in hyperacute stroke: relative cerebral blood flow most accurately identifies tissue destined to infarct. *Stroke* 2001;32:1581–1587.
86. Østergaard L, Weisskoff RM, Chesler DA, Gyldensted C, Rosen BR. High resolution measurement of cerebral blood flow using intravascular tracer bolus passages. Part I: Mathematical approach and statistical analysis. *Magn Reson Med* 1996;36:715–725.
87. Wu O, Østergaard L, Sorensen AG. Technical aspects of perfusion-weighted imaging. *Neuroimaging Clin N Am* 2005;15:623–637.
88. Butcher KS, Parsons M, MacGregor L, Barber PA, Chalk J, Bladin C, Levi C, Kimber T, Schultz D, Fink J, Tress B, Donnan G, Davis S, Investigators E. Refining the perfusion–diffusion mismatch hypothesis. *Stroke* 2005;36:1153–1159.
89. Hacke W, Kaste M, Fieschi C, Toni D, Lesaffre E, von Kummer R, Boysen G, Bluhmki E, Hoxter G, Mahagne MH. Intravenous thrombolysis with recombinant tissue plasminogen activator for acute hemispheric stroke. The European Cooperative Acute Stroke Study (ECASS). *JAMA* 1995;274:1017–1025.
90. Hacke W, Kaste M, Fieschi C, von Kummer R, Davalos A, Meier D, Larrue V, Bluhmki E, Davis S, Donnan G, Schneider D, Diez-Tejedor E, Trouillas P. Randomised

double-blind placebo-controlled trial of thrombolytic therapy with intravenous alteplase in acute ischaemic stroke (ECASS II). Second European–Australasian Acute Stroke Study Investigators. *Lancet* 1998;352:1245–1251 [see comment].

91. Clark WM, Wissman S, Albers GW, Jhamandas JH, Madden KP, Hamilton S. Recombinant tissue-type plasminogen activator (Alteplase) for ischemic stroke 3 to 5 hours after symptom onset. The ATLANTIS Study: a randomized controlled trial. Alteplase Thrombolysis for Acute Noninterventional Therapy in Ischemic Stroke. *JAMA* 1999;282:2019–2026 [see comment].
92. Ribo M, Molina CA, Rovira A, Quintana M, Delgado P, Montaner J, Grive E, Arenillas JF, Alvarez-Sabin J. Safety and efficacy of intravenous tissue plasminogen activator stroke treatment in the 3- to 6-hour window using multimodal transcranial Doppler/MRI selection protocol. *Stroke* 2005;36:602–606.
93. Furlan AJ, Eyding D, Albers GW, Al-Rawi Y, Lees KR, Rowley HA, Sachara C, Soehngen M, Warach S, Hacke W, Investigators D. Dose Escalation of Desmoteplase for Acute Ischemic Stroke (DEDAS): evidence of safety and efficacy 3 to 9 hours after stroke onset. *Stroke* 2006;37:1227–1231.
94. Cho A-H, Lee DH, Kim JS, Choong GC, Kwon SU, Suh DC, Choi J, Chun S-B, Kim SJ, Kang D-W. MRI-Based thrombolysis in acute stroke patients with unclear onset time is safe and feasible *Stroke* 2006;37:634 (abstract, American Stroke Association International Stroke Conference 2006).
95. Katzan IL, Furlan AJ, Lloyd LE, Frank JI, Harper DL, Hinchey JA, Hammel JP, Qu A, Sila CA. Use of tissue-type plasminogen activator for acute ischemic stroke: the Cleveland area experience. *JAMA* 2000;283:1151–1158.
96. Barber PA, Zhang J, Demchuk AM, Hill MD, Buchan AM. Why are stroke patients excluded from TPA therapy? An analysis of patient eligibility. *Neurology* 2001;56: 1015–1020.
97. Cocho D, Belvis R, Marti-Fabregas J, Molina-Porcel L, Diaz-Manera J, Aleu A, Pagonabarraga J, Garcia-Bargo D, Mauri A, Marti-Vilalta JL. Reasons for exclusion from thrombolytic therapy following acute ischemic stroke. *Neurology* 2005;64: 719–720.
98. Smith MA, Doliszny KM, Shahar E, McGovern PG, Arnett DK, Luepker RV. Delayed hospital arrival for acute stroke: the Minnesota Stroke Survey. *Ann Intern Med* 1998;129:190–196.
99. O'Connor RE, McGraw P, Edelsohn L. Thrombolytic therapy for acute ischemic stroke: why the majority of patients remain ineligible for treatment. *Ann Emerg Med* 1999;33: 9–14.
100. Darby DG, Barber PA, Gerraty RP, Desmond PM, Yang Q, Parsons M, Li T, Tress BM, Davis SM. Pathophysiological topography of acute ischemia by combined diffusion-weighted and perfusion MRI. *Stroke* 1999;30:2043–2052.
101. Fiebach JB, Schellinger PD, Gass A, Kucinski T, Siebler M, Villringer A, Olkers P, Hirsch JG, Heiland S, Wilde P, Jansen O, Rother J, Hacke W, Sartor K. Stroke magnetic resonance imaging is accurate in hyperacute intracerebral hemorrhage: a multicenter study on the validity of stroke imaging. *Stroke* 2004;35:502–506.
102. Cohnen M, Wittsack HJ, Assadi S, Muskalla K, Ringelstein A, Poll LW, Saleh A, Modder U. Radiation exposure of patients in comprehensive computed tomography of the head in acute stroke. *Am J Neuroradiol* 2006;27:1741–1745.

103. Grubb RL, Jr., Phelps ME, Ter-Pogossian MM. Regional cerebral blood volume in humans. X-ray fluorescence studies. *Arch Neurol* 1973;28:38–44.

104. Sakai F, Nakazawa K, Tazaki Y, Ishii K, Hino H, Igarashi H, Kanda T. Regional cerebral blood volume and hematocrit measured in normal human volunteers by single-photon emission computed tomography. *J Cereb Blood Flow Metab* 1985;5:207–213.

105. Perlmutter JS, Powers WJ, Herscovitch P, Fox PT, Raichle ME. Regional asymmetries of cerebral blood flow, blood volume, and oxygen utilization and extraction in normal subjects. *J Cereb Blood Flow Metab* 1987;7:64–67.

106. Leggett RW, Williams LR. Suggested reference values for regional blood volumes in humans. *Health Phys* 1991;60:139–154.

107. Boxerman JL, Hamberg LM, Rosen BR, Weisskoff RM. MR contrast due to intravascular magnetic susceptibility perturbations. *Magn Reson Med* 1995;34:555–566.

108. Speck O, Chang L, DeSilva NM, Ernst T. Perfusion MRI of the human brain with dynamic susceptibility contrast: gradient-echo versus spin-echo techniques. *J Magn Reson Imaging* 2000;12:381–387.

109. Donahue KM, Krouwer HG, Rand SD, Pathak AP, Marszalkowski CS, Censky SC, Prost RW. Utility of simultaneously acquired gradient-echo and spin-echo cerebral blood volume and morphology maps in brain tumor patients. *Magn Reson Med* 2000;43:845–853.

110. Wintermark M, Fischbein NJ, Smith WS, Ko NU, Quist M, Dillon WP. Accuracy of dynamic perfusion CT with deconvolution in detecting acute hemispheric stroke. *Am J Neuroradiol* 2005;26:765104–765112.

111. Wintermark M, Reichhart M, Cuisenaire O, Maeder P, Thiran JP, Schnyder P, Bogousslavsky J, Meuli R. Comparison of admission perfusion computed tomography and qualitative diffusion- and perfusion-weighted magnetic resonance imaging in acute stroke patients. *Stroke* 2002;33:2025–2031.

112. Wintermark M, Reichhart M, Thiran JP, Maeder P, Chalaron M, Schnyder P, Bogousslavsky J, Meuli R. Prognostic accuracy of cerebral blood flow measurement by perfusion computed tomography, at the time of emergency room admission, in acute stroke patients. *Ann Neurol* 2002;51:417–432.

113. Edelman RR, Siewert B, Darby DG, Thangaraj V, Nobre AC, Mesulam MM, Warach S. Qualitative mapping of cerebral blood flow and functional localization with echo-planar MR imaging and signal targeting with alternating radio frequency. *Radiology* 1994;192:513–520.

114. Zaharchuk G, Ledden PJ, Kwong KK, Reese TG, Rosen BR, Wald LL. Multislice perfusion and perfusion territory imaging in humans with separate label and image coils. *Magn Reson Med* 1999;41:1093–1098.

115. Chalela JA, Alsop DC, Gonzalez-Atvales JB, Maldjian JA, Kasner SE, Detre JA. Magnetic resonance perfusion imaging in acute ischemic stroke using continuous arterial spin labeling. *Stroke* 2000;31:680–687.

116. del Zoppo GJ, von Kummer R, Hamann GF. Ischaemic damage of brain microvessels: inherent risks for thrombolytic treatment in stroke. *J Neurol Neurosurg Psychiatry* 1998;65:1–9.

117. del Zoppo GJ, Mabuchi T. Cerebral microvessel responses to focal ischemia. *J Cereb Blood Flow Metab* 2003;23:879–894.

118. Anonymous. Intracerebral hemorrhage after intravenous t-PA therapy for ischemic stroke. The NINDS t-PA Stroke Study Group. *Stroke* 1997;28:2109–2118.

119. Knight RA, Barker PB, Fagan SC, Li Y, Jacobs MA, Welch KM. Prediction of impending hemorrhagic transformation in ischemic stroke using magnetic resonance imaging in rats. *Stroke* 1998;29:144–151.

120. Neumann-Haefelin C, Brinker G, Uhlenkuken U, Pillekamp F, Hossmann KA, Hocehn M. Prediction of hemorrhagic transformation after thrombolytic therapy of clot embolism: an MRI investigation in rat brain. *Stroke* 2002;33:1392–1398.

121. Vo KD, Santiago F, Lin W, Hsu CY, Lee Y, Lee JM. MR imaging enhancement patterns as predictors of hemorrhagic transformation in acute ischemic stroke. *Am J Neuroradiol* 2003;24:674–679.

122. Kassner A, Roberts T, Taylor K, Silver F, Mikulis D. Prediction of hemorrhage in acute ischemic stroke using permeability MR imaging. *Am J Neuroradiol* 2005;26:2213–2217.

123. Latour LL, Kang DW, Ezzeddine MA, Chalela JA, Warach S. Early blood–brain barrier disruption in human focal brain ischemia. *Ann Neurol* 2004;56:468–477.

124. Warach S, Latour LL. Evidence of reperfusion injury, exacerbated by thrombolytic therapy, in human focal brain ischemia using a novel imaging marker of early blood–brain barrier disruption. *Stroke* 2004;35:2659–2661.

125. Wu O, Koroshetz WJ, Østergaard L, Buonanno FS, Copen WA, Gonzalez RG, Rordorf G, Rosen BR, Schwamm LH, Weisskoff RM, Sorensen AG. Predicting tissue outcome in acute human cerebral ischemia using combined diffusion- and perfusion-weighted MR imaging. *Stroke* 2001;32:933–942.

126. Rose SE, Chalk JB, Griffin MP, Janke AL, Chen F, McLachan GJ, Peel D, Zelaya FO, Markus HS, Jones DK, Simmons A, O'Sullivan M, Jarosz JM, Strugnell W, Doddrell DM, Semple J. MRI based diffusion and perfusion predictive model to estimate stroke evolution. *Magn Reson Imaging* 2001;19:1043–1053.

3

INTRAVENOUS THROMBOLYSIS

SHERRY H.-Y. CHOU AND ERIC E. SMITH

INTRODUCTION

Stroke is the leading cause of major long-term disability in adults and the third leading cause of death in the United States.[1] On average, a new stroke occurs every 45 seconds.[1] Thrombolytic therapy with intravenous recombinant tissue-plasminogen activator (IV rt-PA) is the most effective treatment for acute ischemic stroke. In this chapter, we review the rationale for thrombolysis in acute ischemic stroke, clinical evidence supporting the use of thrombolytics, and the application of thrombolysis in practice.

RATIONALE FOR THERAPY

Ischemic stroke has numerous causes. Cerebral infarction may result from large artery atherosclerosis, cardiac embolism, small artery lipohyalinosis, cryptogenic embolism, or, more rarely, from other diverse conditions such as arterial dissection, infective endocarditis, and sickle cell disease.[2] Arterial occlusion is the cause of at least 80% of acute cerebral infarctions.[3,4]

Decreased cerebral blood flow, resulting from acute arterial occlusion, reduces oxygen and glucose delivery to brain tissue with subsequent lactic acid production, blood–brain barrier breakdown, inflammation, sodium and calcium pump dysfunction, glutamate release, intracellular calcium influx, free-radical generation, and finally membrane and nucleic acid breakdown and cell death.[5] The degree of cerebral blood flow reduction following arterial occlusion is not uniform. Tissue at the

Acute Ischemic Stroke: An Evidence-based Approach, Edited by David M. Greer.

center of the zone of hypoperfusion is typically exposed to lower blood flow than tissue at the periphery. Animal studies suggest that brain tissue with cerebral blood flow <8–10 mL/100 g/min will almost certainly not survive, while brain tissue with cerebral blood flow 18–20 mL/100 g/min is nonfunctional, but may recover if perfusion is re-established.[6] This forms the basis of the concept of the ischemic "penumbra"—viable but dysfunctional brain tissue, often surrounding a zone of irreversible damage that is destined for infarction in the absence of perfusion.[6] Restoration of blood flow to the penumbra is the goal of thrombolytic therapy.[7–9] As time passes, more and more of the hypoperfusion zone goes on to infarction, and the relative size of the penumbra decreases.[10] Late reperfusion, in contrast to early reperfusion, may be associated with reperfusion injury and hemorrhagic transformation of the infarction, with worse outcomes than those observed in the absence of reperfusion.[11]

Preclinical studies have suggested that early thrombolysis, within 3.5 hours of arterial occlusion, resulted in neurological improvement with an acceptable risk of secondary central nervous system hemorrhage.[3,12–21]

INTRAVENOUS THROMBOLYTICS

Thrombolytic agents cause the breakdown or dissolution of thrombi. Many of these agents work by converting inactive plasminogen into plasmin, a serine protease, which then cleaves fibrin within the thrombus (Fig. 3.1). Agents that have been studied in acute ischemic stroke include human rt-PA, urokinase, streptokinase, and desmoteplase. Systemic administration of these agents may also cause systemic fibrinogen degradation, reduction in circulating plasminogen and $\alpha 2$-antiplasmin, inactivation of factors V and VIII, platelet disaggregation, and possibly platelet

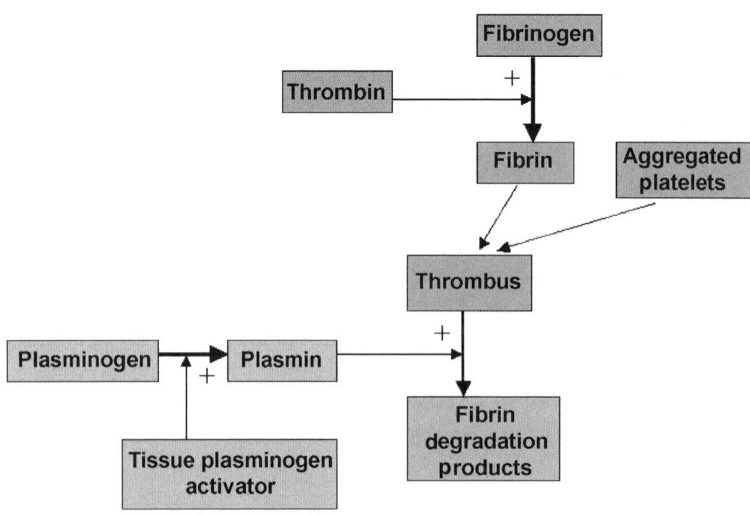

FIGURE 3.1 Fibrinolysis.

dysfunction.[22,23] This may lead to systemic hypofibrinogenemia, prolongation of the activated partial thromboplastin time (aPTT), and coagulopathy.

This section will review the phase III clinical trials of IV thrombolytic agents for acute ischemic stroke, organized by the type of agent and the time window from stroke onset to study drug delivery (Table 3.1). The 1995 National Institute of Neurological Disorders and Stroke (NINDS) rt-PA trial is presented first because it showed that IV rt-PA, given within 3 hours of stroke onset, reduced stroke-related disability. This trial was the basis for the United States Food and Drug Administration (FDA) approval for rt-PA for use in acute ischemic stroke.

TABLE 3.1 Large Randomized Controlled Trials of Intravenous Thrombolysis for Acute Ischemic Stroke.

Drug	Study	*N*	Dose	Time from Symptom Onset (h)	Result	Symptomatic ICH (Treatment vs. Placebo)
rt-PA	NINDS I[24]	291	0.9 mg/kg	≤3	No improvement in 24-h NIHSS	5.6% vs. 0%
rt-PA	NINDS II[24]	333	0.9 mg/kg	≤3	Better global outcome at 90 days	7.1% vs. 1.2%
rt-PA	NINDS I + II[24]	624	0.9 mg/kg	≤3	Better global outcome at 90 days	6.4% vs. 0.6%
rt-PA	ATLANTIS A[31]	142	0.9 mg/kg	0–6	No benefit	11.3% vs. 0%
rt-PA	ATLANTIS B[32]	613	0.9 mg/kg	3–5	No benefit	6.7% vs. 1.3%
rt-PA	ECASS-I[28]	620	1.1 mg/kg	≤6	No benefit	19.8% vs. 6.8%
rt-PA	ECASS-II[30]	800	0.9 mg/kg	≤6	No benefit	8.8% vs. 3.4%
Streptokinase	ASK[42]	340	1.5 mU	≤4	No benefit, excess mortality	13.2% vs. 3%
Streptokinase	MAST-E[44]	310	1.5 mU	≤6	No benefit, excess mortality	21.2% vs. 2.6%
Streptokinase	MAST-I[43]	622	1.5 mU	≤6	No benefit	6.0% vs. 0.6%
Ancrod	STAT[45]	500	0.082–0.167 IU/kg/h × 72 h	≤3	Better outcome at 90 days	5.2% vs 2.0%

rt-PA, tissue plasminogen activator; ICH, intracranial hemorrhage.

Intravenous rt-PA: 0–3 Hours After Stroke Onset

The current use of IV rt-PA for acute stroke thrombolysis is based on the NINDS rt-PA study, a two-part randomized, double blind, placebo-controlled trial.[24] This trial was preceded by two open-label, dose-escalation safety studies that suggested that treatment within 180 minutes of stroke onset, and rt-PA dosages no higher than 0.95 mg/kg, was safe and effective.[25,26]

The NINDS rt-PA study was divided into two parts. NINDS part I included 291 patients and NINDS part II included 333 patients. In both parts, acute ischemic stroke patients presenting within 3 hours of symptom onset were randomized to placebo versus treatment with the human rt-PA Alteplase (Activase). The dose was 0.9 mg/kg (maximum dose 90 mg), with 10% of the total dose given as a bolus and the remaining 90% infused over 60 minutes. Inclusion and exclusion criteria for both parts are listed in Table 3.2. These criteria are now the standard clinical criteria used to determine IV rt-PA eligibility in acute stroke patients.

The primary outcome of NINDS part I was early clinical improvement by 24 hours, defined as complete resolution of the stroke symptoms or an improvement in the National Institute of Health Stroke Scale (NIHSS) score by 4 or more points. There was no difference in early clinical improvement in the rt-PA group compared to the placebo group (relative risk 1.2, 95% CI 0.9–1.6, $p = 0.21$).

The primary outcome of NINDS part II was a favorable outcome at 3 months, as assessed by four commonly used assessment scales: the Barthel Index (BI), modified Rankin Scale (mRS), Glasgow Outcome Scale (GOS), and NIHSS. A

TABLE 3.2 Inclusion and Exclusion Criteria for Treatment with Intravenous Tissue Plasminogen Activator[a].

Inclusion Criteria	Exclusion Criteria
Clearly defined time of onset <3 h	Stroke or head trauma within 3 months
Measurable stroke-related deficit	Major surgery within 14 days
No intracranial hemorrhage on CT	History of intracranial hemorrhage
	SBP > 185 mm Hg or DBP >110 mm Hg
	Rapidly improving or minor symptoms
	Symptoms suggestive of subarachnoid hemorrhage
	Gastrointestinal hemorrhage or urinary tract hemorrhage within the previous 21 days
	Arterial puncture at a noncompressible site within the previous 7 days
	Seizure at stroke onset
	Anticoagulant or heparin use <48 h before onset with elevated partial-thromboplastin time
	Prothrombin time >15 s
	Platelet count <100,000/mm^3
	Glucose concentration <50 mg/dL or >400 mg/dL

[a]Based primarily on the study protocol of the 1995 NINDS rt-PA study.[24] Many centers would also exclude patients with known documented endocarditis or aortic dissection, and those with CT hypoattenuation in more than one third of the middle cerebral artery territory.[39] There are insufficient data to support the use of rt-PA for ischemic stroke in pregnancy or in the pediatric population (age <18 years).

global endpoint was derived from the individual scales with the use of scale-specific cut-points that were defined as a favorable outcome. NINDS part II found that IV rt-PA-treated patients were more likely to have a favorable outcome on each of the assessment scales ($p = 0.02$–0.03, Fig. 3.2). When the results from the four scales were combined into the global test statistic, the odds ratio (OR) for a favorable outcome in the rt-PA group, compared to the placebo group, was 1.7 (95% CI 1.2–2.6, $p = 0.0008$). The absolute percent differences between rt-PA and placebo across the four assessment scales ranged from 11% to 13% (Fig. 3.2), There was a 12% absolute increase in the number of patients with minimal or no disability in the rt-PA group, using the global statistic, which corresponds to a number needed to treat (NNT) of 8.3.

Combined analysis of parts I and II of the NINDS study confirmed the effect of IV rt-PA on favorable outcome at 3 months. There was no difference in mortality (17% for rt-PA group vs. 21% for placebo, $p = 0.30$). There was, however, an increase in symptomatic intracerebral hemorrhage (sICH) in the rt-PA-treated group (6% vs. 0.6% in the placebo group, $p < 0.0001$) during the first 36 hours poststroke. Among those with sICH, the 3-month mortality rate was 61%. Therefore, the improvement in 3-month stroke outcomes in the rt-PA group and the overall lack of increased mortality compared to placebo occurred despite the excess mortality from sICH in the rt-PA group. A secondary analysis showed that a group difference in favorable outcome, favoring the IV rt-PA group, was still present at 1 year.[27]

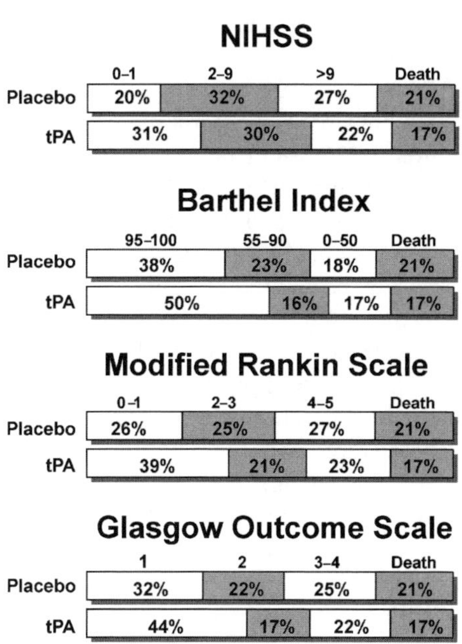

FIGURE 3.2 Differences between IV rt-PA and placebo-treated patients on four assessment scales using data taken from part II of the 1995 NINDS trial.[24] Values do not total 100% because of rounding. The odds ratio for a global favorable outcome with intravenous rt-PA was 1.7 (95% CI 1.2–2.6, $p = 0.008$). The global favorable outcome was defined as NIHSS, 0–1; Barthel Index, 95–100; modified Rankin Scale, 0–1; and Glasgow Outcome Scale, 5.

Intravenous rt-PA: More Than 3 Hours Beyond Stroke Onset

Three large randomized trials, the European Cooperative Acute Stroke Study (ECASS) parts I and II, and the Alteplase Thrombolysis for Acute Noninterventional Therapy in Ischemic Stroke (ATLANTIS), have investigated the efficacy of IV rt-PA in acute stroke beyond the 3-hour window. All three studies showed high rates of sICH complicating rt-PA treatment, and no overall efficacy of rt-PA.

ECASS-I, reported in 1995, was the first large randomized controlled trial of IV thromblysis.[28] Patients with acute ischemic hemispheric stroke and moderate-to-severe clinical deficits, presenting within 6 hours of stroke onset, were randomized to rt-PA ($n = 313$) or placebo ($n = 307$). The rt-PA dose was 1.1 mg/kg, with 10% given as a bolus and the remaining 90% infused over 60 minutes. Patients with very severe stroke signs (hemiplegia, impaired consciousness, or forced head or eye deviation), or signs of infarction involving more than one-third of the middle cerebral artery (MCA) territory on the initial computed tomography (CT) scan were excluded because of preliminary studies showing little evidence for a beneficial effect of thrombolysis in those groups.[29] A post hoc analysis, including a centralized blinded re-review of the initial CT scans, showed a high proportion of protocol violations (18%). Most violations were because the initial CT showed more extensive infarction than allowed by the trial protocol.

The primary hypotheses of ECASS-I were that rt-PA-treated patients, compared to placebo, would have a $\geq$15-point difference in BI score and $\geq$1 grade difference in mRS score at 90 days. Intent-to-treat analyses showed no difference in either the BI scores ($p = 0.99$) or the mRS scores ($p = 0.41$). Parenchymal hematoma on post-treatment CT was seen in 20% of rt-PA-treated patients and 7% of placebo controls ($p < 0.001$). There was a higher 90-day mortality in the rt-PA-treated group compared to the placebo group (22% vs. 16%, $p = 0.04$), partly because there were more deaths attributed to intracranial hemorrhage (6% vs. 2%, $p = 0.02$). When the data were reanalyzed, excluding patients with protocol violations, there was no difference in the BI-scores ($p = 0.14$) but there was a difference in the mRS scores (median 90-day mRS was 2 in the rt-PA group and 3 in the placebo group, $p = 0.04$).

ECASS-II was designed to test a lower dose of rt-PA (0.9 mg/kg) during the same 0–6-hours time period after stroke onset, using similar inclusion criteria as in ECASS-I.[30] The primary endpoint was the proportion with a favorable outcome on the mRS scale (defined as a score of 0 or 1). There was no difference in this outcome between rt-PA-treated and placebo controls (40% vs. 37%, $p = 0.28$). A separate analysis of the 158 subjects enrolled within 3 hours of stroke onset also showed no difference in the proportion with a favorable outcome (42% vs. 38%, $p = 0.63$); this result, however, must be treated with caution because in ECASS-II there was a substantially lower number of patients treated within 3 hours of stroke onset, compared to the 1995 NINDS rt-PA study. Parenchymal hematoma on post-treatment CT was seen in 12% of rt-PA-treated and 3% of placebo patients ($p < 0.001$). The 90-day mortality rate was 11% for the rt-PA group and 11% for the placebo group ($p = 0.54$). Protocol violations were much less frequent in ECASS-II compared to ECASS-I (9% vs. 18%), probably because of standardized training in CT interpretation at the study sites.

The ATLANTIS trial was designed to test the hypothesis that rt-PA, at a dose of 0.9 mg/kg, would result in better outcomes when given to patients within 6 hours of stroke onset.[31] The trial was stopped early, after 142 patients were enrolled, because of a high rate of sICH in patients enrolled 5–6 hours after stroke symptom onset (4/22 rt-PA compared to 0/24 placebo, $p = 0.03$).[31] It was decided to start a new trial, enrolling patients 0–5 hours after stroke (ATLANTIS Part B).[32] However, the time window for ATLANTIS Part B was changed to 3–5 hours after the first 31 patients were enrolled because of FDA approval for IV rt-PA use within 3 hours of stroke onset. Acute ischemic stroke patients were randomized to 0.9 mg/kg rt-PA ($n = 307$) or placebo ($n = 306$).[32] The primary outcome was the proportion with an excellent recovery, defined as an NIHSS score of 0 or 1 at 90 days. There was no difference in the primary outcome (35% of rt-PA-treated patients and 34% of placebo patients had an excellent recovery, $p = 0.89$). In the rt-PA-treated group, there was a higher rate of sICH (7% vs. 1%, $p < 0.001$) and a trend toward higher mortality (11% vs. 7%, $p = 0.08$).

The combined experience with IV rt-PA treatment beyond 3 hours, therefore, suggests reduced effectiveness compared to treatment within 3 hours. A pooled analysis of the ATLANTIS, ECASS, and NINDS rt-PA studies confirmed that the odds of a favorable 3-month outcome, defined as minimal or no poststroke disability on the BI, mRS, and NIHSS, decreased with increasing stroke onset to start of treatment time (OTT) ($p = 0.005$).[33] The odds ratios for favorable outcome with rt-PA treatment were 2.8 (95% CI 1.8–4.5) for OTT 0–90 minutes, 1.6 (95% CI 1.1–2.2) for 91–180 minutes, 1.4 (95% CI 1.1–1.9) for 181–270 minutes, and 1.2 (95% CI 0.9–1.5) for 271–360 minutes. This finding, that earlier treatment is associated with more therapeutic efficacy, supports the adage that in the delivery of acute stroke therapy "time is brain."[34] The rate of sICH was not associated with OTT.[33]

rt-PA-RELATED HEMORRHAGE

Posttreatment sICH is the most feared complication of IV rt-PA treatment. The independent risk factors for sICH in the NINDS rt-PA study were rt-PA treatment, severity of the neurological deficit, and evidence of brain edema or mass effect on the pretreatment CT.[35] Increased age was a risk factor in the univariate analysis ($p = 0.05$), but was no longer significant after controlling for the other factors. The regression model showed relatively low sensitivity and specificity for age as a predictor of sICH, suggesting that it is not clinically useful for patient selection. Moreover, there was no convincing evidence that rt-PA was ineffective in the patients at highest risk of sICH. Those with mass effect or edema on pretreatment CT had a nonsignificantly increased odds of favorable outcome with rt-PA (OR 3.4, 95% CI 0.6–20.7); the wide confidence intervals reflect the small number of rt-PA-treated patients with mass effect or edema ($n = 16$). Patients with NIHSS > 20 had an increased odds of favorable outcome with rt-PA treatment (OR 4.3, 95% CI 1.6–11.9). Therefore, there is little justification for withholding rt-PA treatment because of high stroke severity.

Risk factors for rt-PA-related hemorrhage have also been determined from the ECASS-I and ECASS-II data. In those studies, the hemorrhages were divided into hemorrhagic infarction, consisting of small petechiae without mass effect, and parenchymal hematoma, consisting of a blood clot sometimes accompanied by mass effect.[35] Most sICH was caused by parenchymal hematoma rather than hemorrhagic infarction.[36] For analysis, the extent of hypoattenuation on the pretreatment CT scan was categorized into 0%, ≤33%, and >33% of the MCA territory. In ECASS-I, risk factors for parenchymal hematoma were rt-PA and age; risk factors for sICH were not reported.[35] In ECASS-II, the independent risk factors for parenchymal hematoma were rt-PA, extent of hypoattenuation on the pretreatment CT scan, history of congestive heart failure, increasing age, and baseline systolic blood pressure.[37] In the rt-PA-treated group, treatment with aspirin was an additional risk factor.[37] The risk factors for sICH were the same, with the exception that baseline systolic blood pressure was no longer significant.[37] Similar to the NINDS data, there was no combination of factors that predicted the future occurrence of sICH with high sensitivity and specificity.

These data therefore suggest that rt-PA should not be withheld for fear of sICH, even when risk factors for sICH are present. The possible exception, based on the ECASS-II data, is when extensive hypoattenuation, greater than one third of the MCA territory, is present.[37] An American Academy of Chest Physicians guideline statement recommends against treatment with rt-PA when there are CT signs of infarction in greater than one third of the MCA territory, although it is acknowledged that there is insufficient evidence to make definite conclusions about the degree of risk.[38] There has been a concern that the elderly, particularly those >80 years old, may be at special risk of rt-PA-related sICH. Among the rt-PA trials, >80 year-olds were only enrolled in the 1995 NINDS rt-PA study and separate outcomes were not reported among this fairly small subgroup. Nonrandomized studies, however, suggest that rt-PA may be safe and effective in >80-year-olds.[39,40] Control of elevated blood pressure to <185/110[41] and avoidance of concurrent administration of antiplatelet agents for 24 hours are reasonable steps to minimize the risk of sICH in all rt-PA-treated patients.

OTHER THROMBOLYTICS

There have been three large randomized trials of streptokinase in acute ischemic stroke treatment, all of which were terminated early because of increased sICH and mortality in the treatment group (Table 3.1).[42–44]

There has been a single large randomized trial of the defibrinogenating agent ancrod in acute ischemic stroke. The Stroke Treatment with Ancrod Trial (STAT)[45] randomized acute ischemic stroke patients, presenting within 3 hours of symptom onset, to ancrod ($n = 248$) or placebo ($n = 252$). Ancrod is a purified fraction of Malaysian pit viper venom, which induces rapid defibrinogenation by splitting fibrinopeptide A from fibrinogen. It was given as a 72-hour infusion with a rate of 0.082–0.167 IU/kg, depending on the pretreatment fibrinogen level, targeting a plasma fibrinogen level of 1.18–2.03 μmol/L. The primary endpoint was favorable outcome at 90 days, defined as BI $\geq$95. More patients in the ancrod group, compared to placebo, had a favorable outcome (42% vs. 34%, $p = 0.04$). There was a trend toward more sICH in the ancrod group (5.2% vs. 2.0%, $p = 0.06$). Mortality was not different between the groups (25% for the ancrod group and 23% for the placebo group, $p = 0.62$). Ancrod has, however, not been adopted for routine use in acute ischemic stroke therapy in the United States.

SUBGROUP ANALYSES: WHO BENEFITS THE MOST FROM rt-PA TREATMENT?

The NINDS rt-PA Stroke Study Group performed analyses, combining the data from parts I and II of the study, to identify specific patient subgroups that may have a higher likelihood of benefit or harm from IV rt-PA.[46] The hypotheses tested, using interaction terms within a logistic regression model, were whether there was a significant difference in the magnitude of the rt-PA effect within the subgroups. In the final model, the independent predictors of outcome were rt-PA treatment, increased age, NIHSS score, diabetes, admission mean arterial blood pressure, and pretreatment CT findings of hypodensity or a hyperdense vessel sign (suggesting the presence of intravascular thrombus). Interactions were found between age, NIHSS, and mean arterial pressure, such that increased age and higher NIHSS, and increased age and higher mean arterial pressure were associated with reduced odds of a favorable outcome. rt-PA treatment remained strongly and independently associated with increased odds of a favorable outcome (OR 2.02, 95% CI 1.45–2.81, $p < 0.001$). Importantly, there were no subgroups in which there was statistical evidence of a differential treatment effect of rt-PA. The subgroups tested included age, sex, race, stroke severity (measured by NIHSS), stroke subtype (categorized as cardioembolic, large artery disease, or small vessel disease), admission mean arterial blood pressure, history of diabetes, history of hypertension, history of previous stroke, and pretreatment CT findings of hypodensity or hyperdense vessel sign. An apparent lack of benefit for rt-PA in the 49 subjects aged more than 75 years with NIHSS >20 proved, on review, to be caused by a ceiling effect; none of the subjects in this group had a favorable outcome as defined by the trial protocol. When the data were inspected it was, however, apparent that rt-PA treatment in the subjects aged more than 75 years with NIHSS >20 was associated with better outcomes on the stroke-rating scales. For example, 30% of rt-PA-treated patients had a 90-day mRS $\leq$3, compared to 14% of placebo-treated patients.

A combined analysis of the ATLANTIS, ECASS-II, and NINDS rt-PA study data found that females had a greater benefit from rt-PA than males ($p = 0.04$), despite similar initial stroke severity and rates of sICH.[47] This finding may not be relevant to the clinical, FDA-approved use of rt-PA, because most of the analyzed subjects from ATLANTIS and ECASS-II were randomized greater than 3 hours after stroke onset. Therefore, sex should not be a criterion for patient selection for thrombolysis.

The relevant subgroup analyses therefore provide no additional criteria for patient selection for IV rt-PA. Subgroup analyses, however, must be interpreted with caution because of the possibility of either type I error, resulting from multiple hypothesis testing due to the large number of subgroups, or type II error, resulting from testing hypotheses on subsets of the study data, in a study sample that was designed to have adequate power only for testing the main trial endpoint.

The Stroke-Thrombolytic Predictive Instrument (Stroke-TPI) has recently been developed in order to provide patient-specific estimates of the probability of a more favorable outcome with rt-PA, and has been proposed as a decision-making aid to patient selection for rt-PA.[48] The estimates from this tool should, however, be treated with caution. The prediction rule is dependent on *post hoc* mathematical modeling, uses clinical trial data from subjects randomized beyond 3 hours who are not rt-PA-eligible according to FDA labeling and current best practice, and has not been externally validated. It is, therefore, not appropriate to exclude patients from rt-PA treatment based solely on Stroke-TPI predictions.

IV rt-PA USE IN THE COMMUNITY

rt-PA in the United States: Prevalence and Outcomes

In 1996, the United States FDA approved the use of rt-PA for acute ischemic stroke of less than 3 hours duration. An early observational study raised concerns that rt-PA therapy, when given outside the context of a research trial, may be associated with worse outcomes than in the NINDS trial.[49] In this study, involving several Cleveland hospitals, the sICH rate of 15.7% compared unfavorably with the rate of 6.4% from the NINDS trial. Although neurologists were directly involved in 96% of IV rt-PA treatment decisions in this patient cohort, in 50% of the cases, there were deviations from national treatment guidelines. The most frequent deviations were the use of antiplatelet drugs or anticoagulants within 24 hours of rt-PA administration, and treatment beyond 3 hours after stroke onset. In contrast, other cohort studies have, for the most part, shown rates of sICH that are similar to the trial data.[50, 51] A follow-up study from the Cleveland group showed that, after the initiation of a stroke quality improvement program, the rate of sICH decreased to 6.4%.[52] In order to obtain a valid nationally representative estimate of the prevalence of rt-PA use, and the risk of rt-PA-associated sICH, the United States Centers for Disease Control (CDC) has sponsored the Paul Coverdell National Acute Stroke Registry.[53] Data collected as part of the pilot prototype, involving multiple centers within four states (Georgia, Massachusetts, Michigan, and Ohio), showed an sICH rate of 0–6.1%.[53] Therefore, the preponderance of the data suggests that rt-PA may be used safely in clinical practice, with rates of sICH similar to that in the NINDS clinical trial.

Despite being listed in the official recommendation and guidelines for stroke management by the American Stroke Association, the American Heart Association, the American Academy of Neurology, and the American College of Chest Physicians,[38,54,55] the rate of IV rt-PA use in the community has been disappointingly low. Several single-center and multicenter convenience samples have reported that 1.6–9% of acute ischemic stroke patients received treatment.[49,52,56–62] Studies using a nationally representative administrative database suggest the true treatment rate is even lower, in the range of 1–2% of all ischemic strokes.[63, 64] There is probably hospital and geographic variation in the use of rt-PA,[65] although little is known about the causes of this variability. In the pilot prototype of the CDC-sponsored Paul Coverdell National Acute Stroke Registry, the treatment rate varied from 3% in Georgia to 8.5% in Massachusetts.[53] This was despite the fact that 20–25% of ischemic stroke patients arrived within 3 hours of symptom onset and had no documented contraindications to rt-PA.[53] Only 10–20% of treated patients received the drug within 60 minutes of presentation to the ER,[53] as recommended by guidelines.[66]

There is a strong suspicion that stroke systems of care are one of the factors that influence the safety and efficacy of delivery of IV rt-PA therapy.[67,68] In 2000, the Brain Attack Coalition recommended criteria, based for the most part on consensus opinion rather than scientific evidence, for the establishment of primary stroke centers.[66] These criteria, summarized in Table 3.3, have formed the basis for a voluntary stroke certification program offered by the Joint Commission on the Accreditation of Healthcare Organizations.[69] The departments of public health of several states, including New York, have incorporated similar criteria in state-based stroke certification programs. The initial experience in New York suggests that hospital compliance with certification is likely to be associated with improvements in care delivery, such as shortened door-to-CT time.[70]

The most common reason for lack of rt-PA use in otherwise eligible patients remains, however, delay in presentation to the hospital. The California Acute Stroke Pilot Registry (CASPR) investigators examined the effect of various hypothetical interventions on the rate of rt-PA use.[71] Their data suggested that if all patients with a known time of onset presented to medical attention immediately, the expected overall rate of thrombolytic treatment within 3 hours would have increased from 4.3% to 28.6%. By comparison, the expected rate of treatment that would result from instantaneous prehospital response was 5.5%, from perfect hospital care was 11.5%, and from extension of time window to 6 hours was 8.3%.

TABLE 3.3 Brain Attack Coalition—Recommended Major Elements of a Primary Stroke Center.

Patient care areas
Acute stroke teams
Written care protocols
Emergency medical services
Emergency department
Stroke unit
Neurosurgical services
Support services
Stroke center director with support of medical organization
Neuroimaging services
Laboratory services
Outcome and quality improvement activities
Continuing medical education

The authors concluded that campaigns to educate patients to seek treatment sooner should be major components of system-wide interventions to increase the rate of thrombolysis for acute ischemic stroke. There is some evidence that public education may help to increase the rate of rt-PA utilization by encouraging earlier presentation when stroke symptoms occur.[68]

Cost-Effectiveness of IV rt-PA

IV rt-PA may be associated with a net cost savings to the health care system. Data from the NINDS rt-PA trial[24] showed that hospital length-of-stay was shorter in the rt-PA-treated group (10.9 days vs. 12.4 days, $p = 0.02$) and more rt-PA patients were discharged to home than to inpatient rehabilitation or a nursing home (48% vs. 36% $p = 0.002$). A 1998 analysis used the NINDS rt-PA trial data and Medicare data to estimate, using Markov regression models, the costs associated with rt-PA therapy.[72] Per 1000 treated patients, rt-PA use was associated with a model-predicted increase in hospitalization costs of $1.7 million United States dollars, a decrease in rehabilitation costs of $1.4 million, and a decrease in nursing home costs of $4.8 million. Multiway sensitivity analysis revealed a greater than 90% probability of cost savings. The estimated impact on long-term health outcomes was 564 (95% CI 3–850) quality-adjusted life-years saved, over 30 years, per 1000 patients.

IMPLEMENTATION OF AN ACUTE STROKE TEAM AND ACUTE STROKE PROTOCOLS

The overwhelming prerogative, in thrombolysis for acute ischemic stroke, is the need for rapid, yet complete, evaluation of potential therapeutic candidates within the 3-hour treatment window. Time is the acute stroke clinician's worst enemy.[33]

The acute stroke protocol should begin at the first of point of contact with the healthcare system: the call to an ambulance dispatcher. Stroke symptoms should be recognized and given high priority for dispatch. Emergency medical technicians (EMTs) should be trained to identify potential thrombolysis candidates in the field by recognizing signs of stroke,[73,74] and several simple scales have been created for this purpose.[75–78] Prenotification by the EMTs, before hospital arrival, allows time for notification of the acute stroke team and preparation of the CT scanner before patient arrival, and has been associated with fewer in-hospital delays in treatment.[79,80]

The initial evaluation, after arrival in the emergency department, should include a rapid assessment of vital signs, placement of a peripheral intravenous catheter, venous sampling for laboratory studies, and an electrocardiogram. Serum laboratories of critical importance are the complete blood count, partial thromboplastin time, PTT, and serum chemistries, including glucose. A focused history should be obtained in order to determine the stroke symptoms, time of symptom onset, presence of allergies, use of warfarin, and the presence or absence of diabetes or epilepsy (both of which may be associated with conditions such as hypoglycemia or seizure that may mimic acute stroke). An abbreviated neurological exam, designed to identify major neurological deficits that would likely result in permanent disability if left untreated, should be performed; the NIHSS is adequate for this purpose. To minimize time delays, portions of the evaluation may be performed while the patient is being transported to the CT, or after the CT is done.

An important part of the evaluation, sometimes overlooked by inexperienced clinicians, is to obtain not only the time that the symptoms were discovered, *but also the time when the patient was last known to be free of stroke symptoms.* In cases where the onset was not witnessed, it is the latter time that, for practical purposes, must be assumed to be the time of symptom onset. A frequently encountered scenario is one in which a family member reports that the patient's stroke occurred early in the morning, for example, at 7 AM. Specific questioning often reveals that the last time the patient was known to be symptom free was the previous evening, for example, at 10 PM; the actual time of stroke onset is therefore unknown but could have been up to 9 hours before discovery, making the patient ineligible for IV rt-PA therapy.

The goal of the initial evaluation is to identify potential treatment candidates and obtain a CT scan within 25 minutes of arrival to the emergency department. This may be enhanced by placement of the CT scanner in the emergency department.[79] The CT scan should be evaluated for the presence of intracranial hemorrhage (Fig. 3.3) or early signs of infarction (Fig. 3.4). There are no signs or symptoms that reliably distinguish between brain infarction and brain hemorrhage, making CT a mandatory part of the evalutation.[81] Interpretation by experienced personnel is critical because the radiographic signs may be subtle.[82] Some tertiary care centers have incorporated more advanced imaging into their acute stroke protocols, including CT angiography, MRI, and perfusion imaging.[83,84] The benefits of these advanced imaging protocols are uncertain because they have not been evaluated in randomized trials. In centers with MRI-based

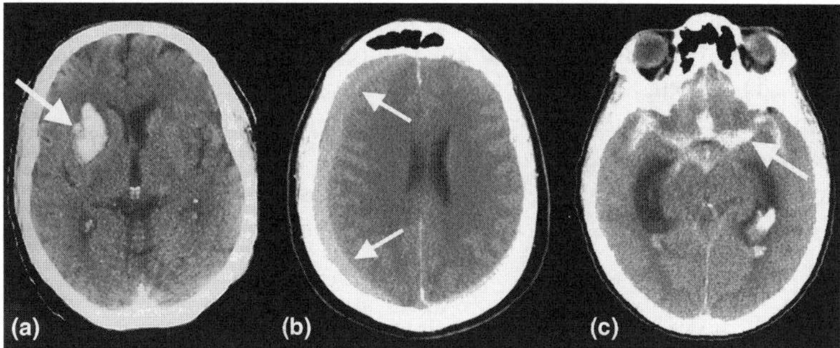

FIGURE 3.3 Intracranial hemorrhage on CT is a contraindication to intravenous rt-PA treatment. There are no clinical signs or symptoms that can reliably distinguish between ischemic and hemorrhagic stroke, making CT a mandatory part of the patient assessment. (**a**) Intraparenchymal hemorrhage centered in the right putamen (arrow). (**b**) Subdural hematoma. (**c**) Subarachnoid hemorrhage layering in the basal cisterns (arrow), causing hydrocephalus. The most common clinical findings in subarachnoid hemorrhage are headache and impaired consciousness, although focal neurological signs and symptoms may also occur.

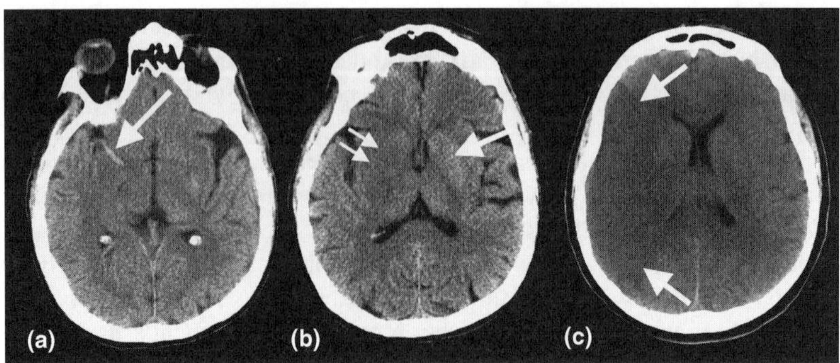

FIGURE 3.4 Early CT signs of infarction. (**a**) Hyperdense right middle cerebral artery, suggesting intravascular occlusion by thromboembolism. (**b**) Loss of differentiation between gray and white matter. The left lentiform nucleus is visible, as normal, as a slightly hyperdense structure (single arrow), but is absent on the right (double arrow) because of edema from infarction. (**c**) Large area of hypoattenuation (arrows), with sulcal effacement and mild mass effect in the entire right middle cerebral artery territory. This patient was not treated with intravenous rt-PA because of hypoattentuation in more than one third of the middle cerebral artery territory, in accordance with a guideline statement from the American Academy of Chest Physicians.

protocols, there has been a concern that MRI evidence of past silent brain hemorrhages ("microbleeds") may indicate a propensity for rt-PA-related sICH.[85] However, the current best evidence, albeit limited, suggests that rt-PA for acute ischemic stroke may be safe even in those with MRI microbleeds.[86,87]

The list of contraindications to rt-PA should be reviewed (Table 3.2) and, if none are present, then rt-PA should be given, with a goal of administering the drug within 60 minutes of presentation to the emergency department. Other neurological diseases may, uncommonly, mimic stroke (Table 3.4) and should be excluded based on the available data. The most common contraindication to rt-PA, however, is the time elapsed. Among time-eligible patients the most frequent contraindication, present in 30–40%, is mild or improving stroke symptoms.[88–92] There is, however, evidence that outcomes are not uniformly good in this group, with short-term disability or death in about 30%.[88,89] It is therefore reasonable to recommend rt-PA in all circumstances where the expected neurological deficit, at the time of evaluation,

TABLE 3.4 Common Disorders, Other than Stroke, that May Present with an Acute Neurological Deficit.

Seizure with postictal Todd's paresis
Migraine with aura
Hypoglycemia or hyperglycemia
Hyponatremia
Delirium (may be mistaken for aphasia)
Psychiatric (conversion, factitious disorder, malingering)

would result in a permanent disability. In patients with recent improvement in symptoms, it may not be warranted to assume that additional future short-term improvement will occur.

IV rt-PA has been safely given in patients with cervical arterial dissection.[93] There are four reports of IV rt-PA use in pregnancy, with one case complicated by intrauterine hematoma,[94,95] rt-PA should be used in this setting only after careful assessment of the risks and benefits. There is insufficient data to determine the benefit of rt-PA in the pediatric population,[96–98] with no randomized trials.

As is evident from the preceding paragraphs, the delivery of acute stroke treatment involves a number of specialists, including ambulance dispatchers, EMTs, nurses, emergency department physicians, pharmacists, neurologists, and radiologists, and timely access to CT scanning. The coordination of acute stroke care is a challenge, given the number of involved personnel, and greatly benefits from a team approach, with written protocols and an identified stroke team. There is evidence that written protocols, and reorganization of the emergency department to facilitate the acute stroke evaluation, result in faster evaluation times and treatment.[79,99] Many smaller hospitals may find it challenging to maintain 24-hour access to an acute stroke team.[100] Preliminary data suggest that telemedicine consultation with an off-site stroke specialist may increase rt-PA treatment rates, with an acceptable risk of sICH.[101,102]

FUTURE DIRECTIONS

Although IV rt-PA is an effective drug for the treatment of acute ischemic stroke, its impact on public health is limited because of the small number of patients eligible for treatment. In order to find more effective therapies and expand the pool of eligible patients, future research on IV thrombolysis for acute ischemic stroke is therefore warranted and has proceeded along the following main directions: (1) finding alternative, more effective, IV thrombolytics; (2) improving patient selection using advanced imaging to define a radiological surrogate for the core infarct and ischemic penumbra; (3) adjunct therapy with other antiplatelet or antithrombotic agents; (4) adjunct therapy with mechanical devices, such as ultrasound energy by transcranial Doppler ultrasound, or catheter-based clot retrieval; and (5) adjunct therapy with neuroprotective agents.

Desmoteplase, a recombinant plasminogen activator, derived from the *Desmodus* vampire bat salivary plasminogen activator, was evaluated in a phase III randomized placebo-controlled trial for ischemic stroke of 3–9 hours duration, with patient selection based on the presence of a radiological surrogate of the ischemic penumbra. Desmoteplase has theoretical advantages over recombinant human rt-PA: it is more fibrin-specific, has a longer half-life (allowing it to be given as a single bolus), and may exhibit less neurotoxicity than rt-PA.[103] Phase II randomized trials showed better clinical outcomes with desmoteplase, and acceptable rates of sICH.[104,105] The phase III trial failed, however, to show benefit over placebo (unpublished data).

The Combined Lysis of Thrombus in Brain Ischemia Using Transcranial Ultrasound and Systemic rt-PA (CLOTBUST) study was a phase II randomized trial which compared continuous transcranial Doppler ultrasound insonation, in subjects with ultrasound evidence of MCA occlusion being given IV rt-PA, to sham insonation.[106] There was an increased rate of arterial recanalization with the continuous insonation (49% vs. 30%, $p = 0.03$) and no increased risk of sICH.

The effectiveness of catheter-based intra-arterial therapy to remove residual thrombus after IV rt-PA treatment is being tested in the Interventional Management of Stroke study (IMS-III). This study will randomize patients to 0.6 mg/kg IV rt-PA, followed by angiography with additional intra-arterial therapy as indicated, or IV full-dose rt-PA (0.9 mg/kg). A nonrandomized safety study suggested that intra-arterial therapy, after 0.6 mg/kg IV rt-PA, could be accomplished with acceptable rates of sICH.[107]

Pharmacologic neuroprotection, which might be expected to prevent tissue necrosis or apoptosis until tissue reperfusion can be achieved with rt-PA, is a theoretically attractive adjunct to rt-PA treatment. Despite positive studies in animals,[108] all evaluations of neuroprotective agents in humans have failed.[109] Most recently, the promising initial results for intravenous NXY-059,[110] a free-radical-trapping agent, were not replicated in a confirmatory phase III trial (unpublished data).

CONCLUSIONS

Acute ischemic stroke remains an important public health concern with limited therapeutic options at this time. Intravenous rt-PA has been shown to improve acute stroke outcomes if given within 3 hours of symptom onset. Intravenous thrombolysis beyond 3 hours in unselected patients has been shown to be ineffective. Rt-PA-associated sICH is the most important complication of treatment; unfortunately, there are no clinical features that predict sICH with high sensitivity or specificity. There are no patient subgroups in which rt-PA is proven to be of extra benefit, or risk, although it is a common practice, supported by a guideline statements, to withhold therapy from patients with CT evidence of established infarction in more than one third of the MCA territory. Observational studies of rt-PA therapy in community practice suggest that it has a similar safety profile as that seen in the 1995 NINDS trial. The proportion of all United States ischemic stroke patients who receive rt-PA is low, mostly because of the restrictive time window for treatment, and also because of inadequate stroke systems of care. Written clinical protocols, an identified acute stroke team, and reorganization of the emergency department to prioritize the stroke evaluation are essential for providing quality acute stroke care. Clinical management should focus on rapid evaluation and transport to the CT scanner. Newer thrombolytic agents such as desmoteplase, as well as adjunct therapies for enhanced thrombolysis or neuroprotection, are currently under investigation and may, in the future, allow the use of thrombolysis to be expanded to a larger group of patients.

ACKNOWLEDGMENT

Dr. Smith is supported by grant funding from the National Institute of Neurological Disorders and Stroke (K23 NS-046327).

REFERENCES

1. Thom T, Haase N, Rosamond W, Howard VJ, Rumsfeld J, Manolio T, Zheng ZJ, Flegal K, O'Donnell C, Kittner S, Lloyd-Jones D, Goff DC, Jr., Hong Y, Adams R, Friday G, Furie K, Gorelick P, Kissela B, Marler J, Meigs J, Roger V, Sidney S, Sorlie P, Steinberger J, Wasserthiel-Smoller S, Wilson M, Wolf P. Heart disease and stroke statistics–2006 update: A report from the American Heart Association statistics committee and stroke statistics subcommittee. *Circulation.* 2006;113:e85–151.
2. Adams HP, Jr., Bendixen BH, Kappelle LJ, Biller J, Love BB, Gordon DL, Marsh EE, 3rd. Classification of subtype of acute ischemic stroke. Definitions for use in a multicenter clinical trial. TOAST. Trial of Org 10172 in Acute Stroke Treatment. *Stroke.* 1993;24:35–41.
3. Del Zoppo GJ, Poeck K, Pessin MS, Wolpert SM, Furlan AJ, Ferbert A, Alberts MJ, Zivin JA, Wechsler L, Busse O. Recombinant tissue plasminogen activator in acute thrombotic and embolic stroke. *Ann Neurol.* 1992;32:78–86.
4. Fieschi C, Argentino C, Lenzi GL, Sacchetti ML, Toni D, Bozzao L. Clinical and instrumental evaluation of patients with ischemic stroke within the first six hours. *J Neurol Sci.* 1989;91:311–321.
5. Lo EH, Moskowitz MA, Jacobs TP. Exciting, radical, suicidal: How brain cells die after stroke. *Stroke.* 2005;36:189–192.
6. Astrup J, Siesjo BK, Symon L. Thresholds in cerebral ischemia - the ischemic penumbra. *Stroke.* 1981;12:723–725.
7. Liu Y, Karonen JO, Vanninen RL, Ostergaard L, Roivainen R, Nuutinen J, Perkio J, Kononen M, Hamalainen A, Vanninen EJ, Soimakallio S, Kuikka JT, Aronen HJ. Cerebral hemodynamics in human acute ischemic stroke: A study with diffusion- and perfusion-weighted magnetic resonance imaging and spect. *J Cereb Blood Flow Metab.* 2000;20:910–920.
8. Furlan M, Marchal G, Viader F, Derlon JM, Baron JC. Spontaneous neurological recovery after stroke and the fate of the ischemic penumbra. *Ann Neurol.* 1996;40: 216–226.
9. Grandin CB, Duprez TP, Smith AM, Mataigne F, Peeters A, Oppenheim C, Cosnard G. Usefulness of magnetic resonance-derived quantitative measurements of cerebral blood flow and volume in prediction of infarct growth in hyperacute stroke. *Stroke.* 2001;32:1147–1153.
10. Shen Q, Ren H, Fisher M, Bouley J, Duong TQ. Dynamic tracking of acute ischemic tissue fates using improved unsupervised isodata analysis of high-resolution quantitative perfusion and diffusion data. *J Cereb Blood Flow Metab.* 2004;24: 887–897.
11. Dijkhuizen RM, Asahi M, Wu O, Rosen BR, Lo EH. Delayed rt-PA treatment in a rat embolic stroke model: Diagnosis and prognosis of ischemic injury and hemorrhagic transformation with magnetic resonance imaging. *J Cereb Blood Flow Metab.* 2001;21:964–971.

12. Zivin JA, Fisher M, DeGirolami U, Hemenway CC, Stashak JA. Tissue plasminogen activator reduces neurological damage after cerebral embolism. *Science*. 1985;230: 1289–1292.

13. Zivin JA, Lyden PD, DeGirolami U, Kochhar A, Mazzarella V, Hemenway CC, Johnston P. Tissue plasminogen activator. Reduction of neurologic damage after experimental embolic stroke. *Arch Neurol*. 1988;45:387–391.

14. Del Zoppo GJ, Copeland BR, Anderchek K, Hacke W, Koziol JA. Hemorrhagic transformation following tissue plasminogen activator in experimental cerebral infarction. *Stroke*. 1990;21:596–601.

15. Slivka A, Pulsinelli W. Hemorrhagic complications of thrombolytic therapy in experimental stroke. *Stroke*. 1987;18:1148–1156.

16. Lyden PD, Zivin JA, Clark WA, Madden K, Sasse KC, Mazzarella VA, Terry RD, Press GA. Tissue plasminogen activator-mediated thrombolysis of cerebral emboli and its effect on hemorrhagic infarction in rabbits. *Neurology*. 1989;39:703–708.

17. Del Zoppo GJ, Copeland BR, Waltz TA, Zyroff J, Plow EF, Harker LA. The beneficial effect of intracarotid urokinase on acute stroke in a baboon model. *Stroke*. 1986;17:638–643.

18. Phillips DA, Fisher M, Smith TW, Davis MA. The safety and angiographic efficacy of tissue plasminogen activator in a cerebral embolization model. *Ann Neurol*. 1988;23:391–394.

19. Phillips DA, Davis MA, Fisher M. Selective embolization and clot dissolution with tPA in the internal carotid artery circulation of the rabbit. *AJNR Am J Neuroradiol*. 1988;9:899–902.

20. Kissel P, Chehrazi B, Seibert JA, Wagner FC, Jr. Digital angiographic quantification of blood flow dynamics in embolic stroke treated with tissue-type plasminogen activator. *J Neurosurg*. 1987;67:399–405.

21. Papadopoulos SM, Chandler WF, Salamat MS, Topol EJ, Sackellares JC. Recombinant human tissue-type plasminogen activator therapy in acute thromboembolic stroke. *J Neurosurg*. 1987;67:394–398.

22. Marder VJ, Sherry S. Thrombolytic therapy: Current status. *N Engl J Med*. 1988;318:1512–1520.

23. Loscalzo J, Vaughan DE. Tissue plasminogen activator promotes platelet disaggregation in plasma. *J Clin Invest*. 1987;79:1749–1755.

24. The National Institute of Neurological Disorders and Stroke rt-PA Stroke Study Group. Tissue plasminogen activator for acute ischemic stroke. *N Engl J Med*. 1995;333:1581–1587.

25. Brott TG, Haley EC, Jr., Levy DE, Barsan W, Broderick J, Sheppard GL, Spilker J, Kongable GL, Massey S, Reed R, et al. Urgent therapy for stroke. Part i. Pilot study of tissue plasminogen activator administered within 90 minutes. *Stroke*. 1992;23:632–640.

26. Haley EC, Jr., Levy DE, Brott TG, Sheppard GL, Wong MC, Kongable GL, Torner JC, Marler JR. Urgent therapy for stroke. Part II. Pilot study of tissue plasminogen activator administered 91-180 minutes from onset. *Stroke*. 1992;23:641–645.

27. Kwiatkowski TG, Libman RB, Frankel M, Tilley BC, Morgenstern LB, Lu M, Broderick JP, Lewandowski CA, Marler JR, Levine SR, Brott T. Effects of tissue plasminogen activator for acute ischemic stroke at one year. National Institute of Neurological Disorders and Stroke Recombinant Tissue Plasminogen Activator Stroke Study Group. *New England Journal of Medicine*. 1999;340:1781–1787.

28. Hacke W, Kaste M, Fieschi C, Toni D, Lesaffre E, von Kummer R, Boysen G, Bluhmki E, Hoxter G, Mahagne MH, et al. Intravenous thrombolysis with recombinant tissue plasminogen activator for acute hemispheric stroke. The european cooperative acute stroke study (ECASS). *JAMA*. 1995;274:1017–1025.
29. von Kummer R, Hacke W. Safety and efficacy of intravenous tissue plasminogen activator and heparin in acute middle cerebral artery stroke. *Stroke*. 1992;23:646–652.
30. Hacke W, Kaste M, Fieschi C, von Kummer R, Davalos A, Meier D, Larrue V, Bluhmki E, Davis S, Donnan G, Schneider D, Diez-Tejedor E, Trouillas P. Randomised double-blind placebo-controlled trial of thrombolytic therapy with intravenous alteplase in acute ischaemic stroke (ECASS II). Second European-Australasian Acute Stroke Study Investigators. *Lancet*. 1998;352:1245–1251.
31. Clark WM, Albers GW, Madden KP, Hamilton S. The rtPA (alteplase) 0- to 6-hour acute stroke trial, part a (a0276g): results of a double-blind, placebo-controlled, multicenter study. Thrombolytic Therapy in Acute Ischemic Stroke Study Investigators. *Stroke*. 2000;31:811–816.
32. Clark WM, Wissman S, Albers GW, Jhamandas JH, Madden KP, Hamilton S. Recombinant tissue-type plasminogen activator (alteplase) for ischemic stroke 3 to 5 hours after symptom onset. The ATLANTIS study: A randomized controlled trial. Alteplase Thrombolysis for Acute Noninterventional Therapy in Ischemic Stroke. *JAMA*. 1999;282:2019–2026.
33. Hacke W, Donnan G, Fieschi C, Kaste M, von Kummer R, Broderick JP, Brott T, Frankel M, Grotta JC, Haley EC, Jr., Kwiatkowski T, Levine SR, Lewandowski C, Lu M, Lyden P, Marler JR, Patel S, Tilley BC, Albers G, Bluhmki E, Wilhelm M, Hamilton S. Association of outcome with early stroke treatment: Pooled analysis of ATLANTIS, ECASS, and NINDS rt-PA stroke trials. *Lancet*. 2004;363:768–774.
34. Saver JL. Time is brain–quantified. *Stroke*. 2006;37:263–266.
35. Intracerebral hemorrhage after intravenous t-pa therapy for ischemic stroke. The NINDS t-pa stroke study group. *Stroke*. 1997;28:2109–2118.
36. Larrue V, von Kummer R, del Zoppo G, Bluhmki E. Hemorrhagic transformation in acute ischemic stroke. Potential contributing factors in the European Cooperative Acute Stroke Study. *Stroke*. 1997;28:957–960.
37. Fiorelli M, Bastianello S, von Kummer R, del Zoppo GJ, Larrue V, Lesaffre E, Ringleb AP, Lorenzano S, Manelfe C, Bozzao L. Hemorrhagic transformation within 36 hours of a cerebral infarct: Relationships with early clinical deterioration and 3-month outcome in the european cooperative acute stroke study i (ECASS i) cohort. *Stroke*. 1999; 30:2280–2284.
38. Larrue V, von Kummer RR, Muller A, Bluhmki E. Risk factors for severe hemorrhagic transformation in ischemic stroke patients treated with recombinant tissue plasminogen activator: A secondary analysis of the european-australasian acute stroke study (ECASS II). *Stroke*. 2001;32:438–441.
39. Albers GW, Amarenco P, Easton JD, Sacco RL, Teal P. Antithrombotic and thrombolytic therapy for ischemic stroke: The seventh ACCP Conference on Antithrombotic and Thrombolytic Therapy. *Chest*. 2004;126:483S-512S.
40. Engelter ST, Reichhart M, Sekoranja L, Georgiadis D, Baumann A, Weder B, Muller F, Luthy R, Arnold M, Michel P, Mattle HP, Tettenborn B, Hungerbuhler HJ, Baumgartner RW, Sztajzel R, Bogousslavsky J, Lyrer PA. Thrombolysis in stroke

patients aged 80 years and older: Swiss survey of IV thrombolysis. *Neurology*. 2005; 65:1795–1798.

41. Tanne D, Gorman MJ, Bates VE, Kasner SE, Scott P, Verro P, Binder JR, Dayno JM, Schultz LR, Levine SR. Intravenous tissue plasminogen activator for acute ischemic stroke in patients aged 80 years and older: The tPA stroke survey experience. *Stroke*. 2000;31:370–375.
42. Tanne D, Kasner SE, Demchuk AM, Koren-Morag N, Hanson S, Grond M, Levine SR. Markers of increased risk of intracerebral hemorrhage after intravenous recombinant tissue plasminogen activator therapy for acute ischemic stroke in clinical practice: The Multicenter rt-PA Stroke Survey. *Circulation*. 2002;105:1679–1685.
43. Donnan GA, Davis SM, Chambers BR, Gates PC, Hankey GJ, McNeil JJ, Rosen D, Stewart-Wynne EG, Tuck RR. Streptokinase for acute ischemic stroke with relationship to time of administration: Australian Streptokinase (ASK) trial study group. *JAMA*. 1996;276:961–966.
44. Randomised controlled trial of streptokinase, aspirin, and combination of both in treatment of acute ischaemic stroke. Multicentre Acute Stroke Trial–Italy (MAST-I) group. *Lancet*. 1995;346:1509–1514.
45. Thrombolytic therapy with streptokinase in acute ischemic stroke. The Multicenter Acute Stroke Trial–Europe study group. *N Engl J Med*. 1996;335:145–150.
46. Sherman DG, Atkinson RP, Chippendale T, Levin KA, Ng K, Futrell N, Hsu CY, Levy DE. Intravenous ancrod for treatment of acute ischemic stroke: The STAT study: A randomized controlled trial. Stroke Treatment with Ancrod Trial. *JAMA*. 2000;283: 2395–2403.
47. Generalized efficacy of t-pa for acute stroke. Subgroup analysis of the NINDS t-pa stroke trial. *Stroke*. 1997;28:2119–2125.
48. Kent DM, Price LL, Ringleb P, Hill MD, Selker HP. Sex-based differences in response to recombinant tissue plasminogen activator in acute ischemic stroke: A pooled analysis of randomized clinical trials. *Stroke*. 2005;36:62–65.
49. Kent DM, Selker HP, Ruthazer R, Bluhmki E, Hacke W. The Stroke-Thrombolytic Predictive Instrument. A predictive instrument for intravenous thrombolysis in acute ischemic stroke. *Stroke*. 2006;37:2957–2962.
50. Katzan IL, Furlan AJ, Lloyd LE, Frank JI, Harper DL, Hinchey JA, Hammel JP, Qu A, Sila CA. Use of tissue-type plasminogen activator for acute ischemic stroke: The Cleveland area experience. *JAMA*. 2000;283:1151–1158.
51. Albers GW, Bates VE, Clark WM, Bell R, Verro P, Hamilton SA. Intravenous tissue-type plasminogen activator for treatment of acute stroke: The Standard Treatment with Alteplase to Reverse stroke (STARS) study. *JAMA*. 2000;283:1145–1150.
52. Tanne D, Bates VE, Verro P, Kasner SE, Binder JR, Patel SC, Mansbach HH, Daley S, Schultz LR, Karanjia PN, Scott P, Dayno JM, Vereczkey-Porter K, Benesch C, Book D, Coplin WM, Dulli D, Levine SR. Initial clinical experience with IV tissue plasminogen activator for acute ischemic stroke: A multicenter survey. The t-PA Stroke Survey Group. *Neurology*. 1999;53:424–427.
53. Katzan IL, Hammer MD, Furlan AJ, Hixson ED, Nadzam DM. Quality improvement and tissue-type plasminogen activator for acute ischemic stroke: A Cleveland update. *Stroke*. 2003;34:799–800.
54. The Paul Coverdell Prototype Registries Writing Group. Acute stroke care in the US: results from 4 pilot prototypes of the Paul Coverdell National Acute Stroke Registry. *Stroke*. 2005;36:1232–1240.

55. Adams HP, Jr., Adams RJ, Brott T, del Zoppo GJ, Furlan A, Goldstein LB, Grubb RL, Higashida R, Kidwell C, Kwiatkowski TG, Marler JR, Hademenos GJ. Guidelines for the early management of patients with ischemic stroke: A scientific statement from the Stroke Council of the American Stroke Association. *Stroke*. 2003;34:1056–1083.

56. Practice advisory: Thrombolytic therapy for acute ischemic stroke–summary statement. Report of the quality standards subcommittee of the American Academy of Neurology. *Neurology*. 1996;47:835–839.

57. Chiu D, Krieger D, Villar-Cordova C, Kasner SE, Morgenstern LB, Bratina PL, Yatsu FM, Grotta JC. Intravenous tissue plasminogen activator for acute ischemic stroke: Feasibility, safety, and efficacy in the first year of clinical practice. *Stroke*. 1998;29: 18–22.

58. Wang DZ, Rose JA, Honings DS, Garwacki DJ, Milbrandt JC. Treating acute stroke patients with intravenous tPA. The OSF stroke network experience. *Stroke*. 2000;31:77–81.

59. Reed SD, Cramer SC, Blough DK, Meyer K, Jarvik JG. Treatment with tissue plasminogen activator and inpatient mortality rates for patients with ischemic stroke treated in community hospitals. *Stroke*. 2001;32:1832–1840.

60. Grotta JC, Burgin WS, El-Mitwalli A, Long M, Campbell M, Morgenstern LB, Malkoff M, Alexandrov AV. Intravenous tissue-type plasminogen activator therapy for ischemic stroke: Houston experience 1996 to 2000. *Arch Neurol*. 2001;58:2009–2013.

61. Heuschmann PU, Berger K, Misselwitz B, Hermanek P, Leffmann C, Adelmann M, Buecker-Nott HJ, Rother J, Neundoerfer B, Kolominsky-Rabas PL. Frequency of thrombolytic therapy in patients with acute ischemic stroke and the risk of in-hospital mortality: The German Stroke Registers Study Group. *Stroke*. 2003;34:1106–1113.

62. Kissela B, Schneider A, Kleindorfer D, Khoury J, Miller R, Alwell K, Woo D, Szaflarski J, Gebel J, Moomaw C, Pancioli A, Jauch E, Shukla R, Broderick J. Stroke in a biracial population: The excess burden of stroke among blacks. *Stroke*. 2004;35:426–431.

63. Schenkel J, Weimar C, Knoll T, Haberl RL, Busse O, Hamann GF, Koennecke HC, Diener HC, German Stroke Data Bank C. Systemic thrombolysis in German stroke units–the experience from the German Stroke Data Bank. *Journal of Neurology*. 2003;250: 320–324.

64. Bateman BT, Schumacher HC, Boden-Albala B, Berman MF, Mohr JP, Sacco RL, Pile-Spellman J. Factors associated with in-hospital mortality after administration of thrombolysis in acute ischemic stroke patients: An analysis of the nationwide inpatient sample 1999 to 2002. *Stroke*. 2006;37:440–446.

65. Dubinsky R, Lai SM. Mortality of stroke patients treated with thrombolysis: Analysis of nationwide inpatient sample. *Neurology*. 2006;66:1742–1744.

66. Deng YZ, Reeves MJ, Jacobs BS, Birbeck GL, Kothari RU, Hickenbottom SL, Mullard AJ, Wehner S, Maddox K, Majid A. IV tissue plasminogen activator use in acute stroke: experience from a statewide registry. *Neurology*. 2006;66:306–312.

67. Alberts MJ, Hademenos G, Latchaw RE, Jagoda A, Marler JR, Mayberg MR, Starke RD, Todd HW, Viste KM, Girgus M, Shephard T, Emr M, Shwayder P, Walker MD. Recommendations for the establishment of primary stroke centers. Brain Attack Coalition. *JAMA*. 2000;283:3102–3109.

68. Schwamm LH, Pancioli A, Acker JE, 3rd, Goldstein LB, Zorowitz RD, Shephard TJ, Moyer P, Gorman M, Johnston SC, Duncan PW, Gorelick P, Frank J, Stranne SK, Smith R, Federspiel W, Horton KB, Magnis E, Adams RJ. Recommendations for the establishment of stroke systems of care: recommendations from the American

Stroke Association's task force on the development of stroke systems. *Stroke*. 2005;36:690–703.

69. Morgenstern LB, Staub L, Chan W, Wein TH, Bartholomew LK, King M, Felberg RA, Burgin WS, Groff J, Hickenbottom SL, Saldin K, Demchuk AM, Kalra A, Dhingra A, Grotta JC. Improving delivery of acute stroke therapy: The TLL Temple Foundation Stroke Project. *Stroke*. 2002;33:160–166.
70. *Primary stroke center certification guide*. Oakbrook, IL: Joint Commission on Accreditation of Healthcare Organizations; 2005.
71. Gropen TI, Gagliano PJ, Blake CA, Sacco RL, Kwiatkowski T, Richmond NJ, Leifer D, Libman R, Azhar S, Daley MB. Quality improvement in acute stroke: The New York State Stroke Center Designation Project. *Neurology*. 2006;67:88–93.
72. California Acute Stroke Pilot Registry (CASPR) Investigators. Prioritizing interventions to improve rates of thrombolysis for ischemic stroke. *Neurology*. 2005;64: 654–659.
73. Fagan SC, Morgenstern LB, Petitta A, Ward RE, Tilley BC, Marler JR, Levine SR, Broderick JP, Kwiatkowski TG, Frankel M, Brott TG, Walker MD. Cost-effectiveness of tissue plasminogen activator for acute ischemic stroke. NINDS rt-PA Stroke Study Group. *Neurology*. 1998;50:883–890.
74. Wojner-Alexandrov AW, Alexandrov AV, Rodriguez D, Persse D, Grotta JC. Houston Paramedic and Emergency Stroke Treatment and Outcomes Study (HoPSTO). *Stroke*. 2005;36:1512–1518.
75. Bray JE, Martin J, Cooper G, Barger B, Bernard S, Bladin C. An interventional study to improve paramedic diagnosis of stroke. *Prehosp Emerg Care*. 2005;9: 297–302.
76. Kidwell CS, Saver JL, Schubert GB, Eckstein M, Starkman S. Design and retrospective analysis of the Los Angeles Prehospital Stroke Screen (LAPSS). *Prehosp Emerg Care*. 1998;2:267–273.
77. Llanes JN, Kidwell CS, Starkman S, Leary MC, Eckstein M, Saver JL. The Los Angeles Motor Scale (LAMS): A new measure to characterize stroke severity in the field. *Prehosp Emerg Care*. 2004;8:46–50.
78. Kothari RU, Pancioli A, Liu T, Brott T, Broderick J. Cincinnati Prehospital Stroke Scale: reproducibility and validity. *Ann Emerg Med*. 1999;33:373–378.
79. Bray JE, Martin J, Cooper G, Barger B, Bernard S, Bladin C. Paramedic identification of stroke: Community validation of the Melbourne Ambulance Stroke Screen. *Cerebrovasc Dis*. 2005;20:28–33.
80. Lindsberg PJ, Happola O, Kallela M, Valanne L, Kuisma M, Kaste M. Door to thrombolysis: ER reorganization and reduced delays to acute stroke treatment. *Neurology*. 2006;67:334–336.
81. Goodacre S, Kelly AM, Kerr D. Potential impact of interventions to reduce times to thrombolysis. *Emerg Med J*. 2004;21:625–629.
82. Mohr JP, Caplan LR, Melski JW, Goldstein RJ, Duncan GW, Kistler JP, Pessin MS, Bleich HL. The Harvard Cooperative Stroke Registry: a prospective registry. *Neurology*. 1978;28:754–762.
83. Schriger DL, Kalafut M, Starkman S, Krueger M, Saver JL. Cranial computed tomography interpretation in acute stroke: physician accuracy in determining eligibility for thrombolytic therapy. *JAMA*. 1998;279:1293–1297.

84. Lev MH, Segal AZ, Farkas J, Hossain ST, Putman C, Hunter GJ, Budzik R, Harris GJ, Buonanno FS, Ezzeddine MA, Chang Y, Koroshetz WJ, Gonzalez RG, Schwamm LH. Utility of perfusion-weighted CT imaging in acute middle cerebral artery stroke treated with intra-arterial thrombolysis: Prediction of final infarct volume and clinical outcome. *Stroke*. 2001;32:2021–2028.

85. Kidwell CS, Chalela JA, Saver JL, Starkman S, Hill MD, Demchuk AM, Butman JA, Patronas N, Alger JR, Latour LL, Luby ML, Baird AE, Leary MC, Tremwel M, Ovbiagele B, Fredieu A, Suzuki S, Villablanca JP, Davis S, Dunn B, Todd JW, Ezzeddine MA, Haymore J, Lynch JK, Davis L, Warach S. Comparison of MRI and CT for detection of acute intracerebral hemorrhage. *JAMA*. 2004;292:1823–1830.

86. Kidwell CS, Saver JL, Villablanca JP, Duckwiler G, Fredieu A, Gough K, Leary MC, Starkman S, Gobin YP, Jahan R, Vespa P, Liebeskind DS, Alger JR, Vinuela F. Magnetic resonance imaging detection of microbleeds before thrombolysis: An emerging application. *Stroke*. 2002;33:95–98.

87. Kakuda W, Thijs VN, Lansberg MG, Bammer R, Wechsler L, Kemp S, Moseley ME, Marks MP, Albers GW, Investigators D. Clinical importance of microbleeds in patients receiving IV thrombolysis. *Neurology*. 2005;65:1175–1178.

88. Derex L, Nighoghossian N, Hermier M, Adeleine P, Philippeau F, Honnorat J, Yilmaz H, Dardel P, Froment JC, Trouillas P. Thrombolysis for ischemic stroke in patients with old microbleeds on pretreatment MRI. *Cerebrovasc Dis*. 2004;17: 238–241.

89. Barber PA, Zhang J, Demchuk AM, Hill MD, Buchan AM. Why are stroke patients excluded from tPA therapy? An analysis of patient eligibility. *Neurology*. 2001;56:1015–1020.

90. Smith EE, Abdullah AR, Petkovska I, Rosenthal E, Koroshetz WJ, Schwamm LH. Poor outcomes in patients who do not receive intravenous tissue plasminogen activator because of mild or improving ischemic stroke. *Stroke*. 2005;36:2497–2499.

91. Katzan IL, Hammer MD, Hixson ED, Furlan AJ, Abou-Chebl A, Nadzam DM. Utilization of intravenous tissue plasminogen activator for acute ischemic stroke. *Arch Neurol*. 2004;61:346–350.

92. Kleindorfer D, Kissela B, Schneider A, Woo D, Khoury J, Miller R, Alwell K, Gebel J, Szaflarski J, Pancioli A, Jauch E, Moomaw C, Shukla R, Broderick JP. Eligibility for recombinant tissue plasminogen activator in acute ischemic stroke: a population-based study. *Stroke*. 2004;35:e27–29.

93. Cocho D, Belvis R, Marti-Fabregas J, Molina-Porcel L, Diaz-Manera J, Aleu A, Pagonabarraga J, Garcia-Bargo D, Mauri A, Marti-Vilalta JL. Reasons for exclusion from thrombolytic therapy following acute ischemic stroke. *Neurology*. 2005;64:719–720.

94. Georgiadis D, Lanczik O, Schwab S, Engelter S, Sztajzel R, Arnold M, Siebler M, Schwarz S, Lyrer P, Baumgartner RW. IV thrombolysis in patients with acute stroke due to spontaneous carotid dissection. *Neurology*. 2005;64:1612–1614.

95. Murugappan A, Coplin WM, Al-Sadat AN, McAllen KJ, Schwamm LH, Wechsler LR, Kidwell CS, Saver JL, Starkman S, Gobin YP, Duckwiler G, Krueger M, Rordorf G, Broderick JP, Tietjen GE, Levine SR. Thrombolytic therapy of acute ischemic stroke during pregnancy. *Neurology*. 2006;66:768–770.

96. Wiese KM, Talkad A, Mathews M, Wang D. Intravenous recombinant tissue plasminogen activator in a pregnant woman with cardioembolic stroke. *Stroke*. 2006;37:2168–2169.

97. Carlson MD, Leber S, Deveikis J, Silverstein FS. Successful use of rt-PA in pediatric stroke. *Neurology.* 2001;57:157–158.

98. Shuayto MI, Lopez JI, Greiner F. Administration of intravenous tissue plasminogen activator in a pediatric patient with acute ischemic stroke. *J Child Neurol.* 2006;21:604–606.

99. Thirumalai SS, Shubin RA. Successful treatment for stroke in a child using recombinant tissue plasminogen activator. *J Child Neurol.* 2000;15:558.

100. Douglas VC, Tong DC, Gillum LA, Zhao S, Brass LM, Dostal J, Johnston SC. Do the Brain Attack Coalition's criteria for stroke centers improve care for ischemic stroke? *Neurology.* 2005;64:422–427.

101. Schwamm LH, Smith EE, Abdullah AR, Palmeri G, Prvu J, Goyette L, McElligott C, Dreyer P. Hospital characteristics associated with successful state-based licensure for acute stroke services: The Massachusetts experience. *Stroke.* 2006;37:719.

102. Audebert HJ, Kukla C, Vatankhah B, Gotzler B, Schenkel J, Hofer S, Furst A, Haberl RL. Comparison of tissue plasminogen activator administration management between telestroke network hospitals and academic stroke centers: The Telemedical Pilot Project for Integrative Stroke Care in Bavaria/Germany. *Stroke.* 2006;37:1822–1827.

103. Schwamm LH, Rosenthal ES, Hirshberg A, Schaefer PW, Little EA, Kvedar JC, Petkovska I, Koroshetz WJ, Levine SR. Virtual Telestroke support for the emergency department evaluation of acute stroke. *Acad Emerg Med.* 2004;11:1193–1197.

104. Liberatore GT, Samson A, Bladin C, Schleuning WD, Medcalf RL. Vampire bat salivary plasminogen activator (desmoteplase): A unique fibrinolytic enzyme that does not promote neurodegeneration. *Stroke.* 2003;34:537–543.

105. Hacke W, Albers G, Al-Rawi Y, Bogousslavsky J, Davalos A, Eliasziw M, Fischer M, Furlan A, Kaste M, Lees KR, Soehngen M, Warach S. The Desmoteplase in Acute Ischemic Stroke trial (DIAS): A phase II MRI-based 9-hour window acute stroke thrombolysis trial with intravenous desmoteplase. *Stroke.* 2005;36:66–73.

106. Furlan AJ, Eyding D, Albers GW, Al-Rawi Y, Lees KR, Rowley HA, Sachara C, Soehngen M, Warach S, Hacke W. Dose Escalation of Desmoteplase for Acute Ischemic Stroke (DEDAS): Evidence of safety and efficacy 3 to 9 hours after stroke onset. *Stroke.* 2006;37:1227–1231.

107. Alexandrov AV, Molina CA, Grotta JC, Garami Z, Ford SR, Alvarez-Sabin J, Montaner J, Saqqur M, Demchuk AM, Moye LA, Hill MD, Wojner AW. Ultrasound-enhanced systemic thrombolysis for acute ischemic stroke. *N Engl J Med.* 2004;351:2170–2178.

108. IMS Study Investigators. Combined intravenous and intra-arterial recanalization for acute ischemic stroke: the Interventional Management of Stroke study. *Stroke.* 2004;35:904–911.

109. O'Collins VE, Macleod MR, Donnan GA, Horky LL, van der Worp BH, Howells DW. 1,026 experimental treatments in acute stroke. *Ann Neurol.* 2006;59:467–477.

110. Martinez-Vila E, Irimia P. Challenges of neuroprotection and neurorestoration in ischemic stroke treatment. *Cerebrovasc Dis.* 2005;20 Suppl 2:148–158.

111. Lees KR, Zivin JA, Ashwood T, Davalos A, Davis SM, Diener HC, Grotta J, Lyden P, Shuaib A, Hardemark HG, Wasiewski WW. NXY-059 for acute ischemic stroke. *N Engl J Med.* 2006;354:588–600.

4

ENDOVASCULAR APPROACHES TO ACUTE STROKE

Raul G. Nogueira, Guilherme C. Dabus, Joshua A. Hirsch, and Lee H. Schwamm

INTRODUCTION

Stroke remains the third most common cause of death in industrialized nations, after myocardial infarction and cancer, and the single most common reason for permanent disability.[1] In 1996, the Food and Drug Administration (FDA) approved intravenous (IV) thrombolysis with recombinant tissue-plasminogen activator (rt-PA, Alteplase) for the treatment of acute ischemic stroke within 3 hours of onset after reviewing the results of the National Institute of Neurological Disorders and Stroke (NINDS) and rt-PA Stroke Study Group trial.[2] IV rt-PA thrombolysis was the first approved treatment for acute stroke that effectively treats the causative vascular occlusion. This strategy has the advantage of being relatively easy and rapid to initiate, and it does not require specialized equipment or technical expertise. Even though IV thrombolysis was initially a matter of relative controversy, it has now been endorsed as a Class IA level of evidence intervention by the major national guideline development organizations.[3,4] A Cochrane Database Review including 18 trials (16 double-blind) with a total of 5727 patients who received thrombolytics (IV urokinase, streptokinase, rt-PA, or recombinant intra-arterial prourokinase) up to 6 hours after ischemic stroke showed a significant reduction in the proportion of patients who were dead or dependent (modified Rankin Scale (mRS) score 3–6) at follow-up at 3–6 months (odds ratio (OR) 0.84, 95% CI 0.75–0.95), despite a significant increase in the odds of death within the first 10 days

Acute Ischemic Stroke: An Evidence-based Approach, Edited by David M. Greer.

(OR 1.81, 95% CI 1.46–2.24), most of which were related to symptomatic intracranial hemorrhage (OR 3.37, 95% CI 2.68–4.22).[5] In addition, a pooled analysis of six major randomized placebo-controlled IV rt-PA stroke trials (Alteplase Thrombolysis for Acute Noninterventional Therapy in Ischemic Stroke (ATLANTIS) I and II, European Cooperative Acute Stroke Study (ECASS) I and II, and NINDS I and II), including 2775 patients who were treated with IV rt-PA or placebo within 360 minutes of stroke onset, confirmed the benefit up to 3 hours and suggested a potential benefit beyond 3 hours for some patients. The pattern of a decreasing chance of a favorable 3-month outcome as the time interval from stroke onset to start of treatment increased was consistent with the findings of the original NINDS study.[6]

To extend the window of benefit for initiating IV rt-PA, it has been proposed that patient selection be based on mismatch between areas of abnormal perfusion-weighted imaging (PWI) compared with diffusion-weighted imaging (DWI) on magnetic resonance imaging (MRI). This idea that advanced neuroimaging and better-engineered thrombolytic agents may allow for an extension of the treatment window for thrombolysis and improved outcomes has been supported by the recent joint analysis of the phase II desmoteplase in acute stroke (DIAS) and desmoteplase in acute ischemic stroke (DEDAS) trials. This analysis included 94 patients with PWI/DWI mismatch on MRI who were treated with placebo (90 μg/kg) or 125 μg/kg of IV desmoteplase within 3–9 hours of stroke onset. Intention-to-treat analysis revealed reperfusion rates of 23.5%, 34.6%, and 62.1%, and good outcome rates of 22.9%, 37.9%, and 60%, respectively. The combined rate of intracerebral hemorrhage (ICH) in the desmoteplase group was only 1.7%.[7]

However, IV thrombolysis is not a panacea for acute stroke. The recanalization rates of IV rt-PA for proximal arterial occlusions range from only 10% for internal carotid artery (ICA) occlusions to 30% for proximal middle cerebral artery (MCA) occlusions.[8] Analysis of the NINDS trial data shows a 12% absolute increase in good outcomes between the placebo and rt-PA groups at 3 months.[9] In other words, eight stroke patients must be treated with rt-PA to achieve one additional good outcome. However, this analysis understates the impact of rt-PA on stroke patients because it fails to include the patients who partially improved.[10] Indeed, an analysis based on the shift in mRS scores suggests a number needed to treat of only 3 for any improvement with IV rt-PA.[11] Even when considering this argument, rates of improvement are far from ideal, and given the prevalence and impact of ischemic stroke, it is imperative to devise strategies that can be more effective. This is based on the implicit assumption that faster and more complete recanalization will translate into better long-term patient outcomes.

Local intra-arterial thrombolysis (IAT) has several theoretical advantages over IV thrombolysis. For instance, by using coaxial microcatheter techniques, the occluded intracranial vessel is directly accessible and the fibrinolytic agent can be infused directly into the thrombus. This permits a smaller dose of fibrinolytic agent to reach a higher local concentration than that reached by systemic infusion, and ideally it allows for more complete recanalization with lower total doses of thrombolytic. With the smaller dose, complications from systemic fibrinolytic effects, including ICH, can theoretically be reduced.

For these reasons, the treatment window for IAT can be extended beyond the typical IV window of 3 hours. Another major advantage is the combination of thrombolytic treatment with mechanical manipulation of the clot, which may improve recanalization rates.[12] Indeed, mechanical thrombolysis with the use of little or no chemical thrombolysis has emerged as a key option for patients who either have a contraindication to chemical thrombolysis (e.g., recent surgery) or are late in their presentation.[13,14] Furthermore, adjunctive endovascular treatment may be essential for the accomplishment of successful thrombolysis, for example, through stenting of a dissected vessel, or through angioplasty with or without stenting of a proximal occlusive lesion.[15–17]

The major disadvantages to endovascular strategies include the complexity of the procedure, the level of required technical expertise, delays in initiating endovascular treatment, and the additional risks and expense of an invasive procedure compared with IV rt-PA.

INTRA-ARTERIAL THROMBOLYSIS TRIALS

Background

Much like the experience with IV thrombolysis, the majority of the early work in IAT has been reported in nonrandomized case series. Reports of successful IAT go back to the late 1950s, when Sussmann and Fitch[18] described the recanalization of an acutely occluded ICA with an intra-arterial injection of plasmin. Nonetheless, it was not until the early 1990s that this approach was studied in a more systematic manner.

Lisboa et al.[19] analyzed the safety and efficacy of IAT on the basis of current published data. They found a total of 27 studies (10 patients minimum) with a total of 852 patients who received IAT and 100 control subjects. There were more favorable outcomes in the IAT than in the control group (41.5% vs. 23%), with a lower mortality rate for IAT (27.2% vs. 40%). The IAT group had an OR of 2.4 for favorable outcomes, despite a higher frequency of symptomatic ICH (9.5% vs. 3%). In addition, they found a trend toward better outcomes with combined IV rt-PA and IAT than with IAT alone. They also remarked that IAT-treated supratentorial strokes are more likely to have favorable outcomes than infratentorial ones (42.2% vs. 25.6%).

A recent study compared 144 patients treated within 6 hours of symptom onset with IAT using urokinase versus 147 patients treated with aspirin who were matched for age and stroke severity according to National Institutes of Health Stroke Scale (NIHSS) (median 14). The study demonstrated superiority of IAT to aspirin in patients achieving an mRS score of 0–2 (56% vs. 42%, $p = 0.037$) and in patients achieving an mRS score of 0–1 at 2 years (40% vs. 24%, $p = 0.008$) with no difference in mortality (23% vs. 24%).[20]

A single-center review of 350 acute stroke patients treated with IAT using urokinase showed recanalization rates greater than 75% when additional endovascular techniques (such as mechanical fragmentation of the thrombus, thromboaspiration, percutaneous transluminal angioplasty (PTA), and implantation of stents) were used. These authors also found that low NIHSS at admission ($p < 0.001$), good collateral circulation ($p < 0.001$), and successful endovascular recanalization ($p < 0.001$) predicted favorable outcomes, whereas diabetes mellitus ($p < 0.001$) and symptomatic ICH ($p < 0.001$) predicted unfavorable outcomes.[21]

Anterior Circulation Thrombolysis

Middle Cerebral Artery Occlusion and the PROACT Trial The safety and efficacy of IAT in the anterior circulation have been evaluated in two randomized, multicenter, placebo-controlled trials. In the Prolyse in Acute Cerebral Thromboembolism (PROACT) I and II trials, patients with proximal MCA (M1 or M2 segment) occlusions within 6 hours of symptom onset were treated with recombinant prourokinase (r-pro-UK) or placebo.[22,23]

In the PROACT-I trial, 26 patients with a median NIHSS of 17 were treated with r-pro-UK and 14 patients with a median NIHSS of 19 were treated with placebo at a median of 5.5 hours from symptom onset.[22] Patients in the treatment group received 6 mg of IA r-pro-UK over 2 hours, and all patients received high- or low-dose IV heparin given as a bolus followed by a 4-hour infusion at the time of the angiogram. Mechanical disruption of the clot was not allowed. Both the recanalization rates (TIMI 2 or 3 flow: 57.7% vs. 14.3%) and the incidence of symptomatic ICH (15.4% vs. 7.1%) were higher in the r-pro-UK than in the placebo group. Of note, all patients in the r-pro-UK group with early CT changes involving >33% of the MCA territory suffered ICH. In the r-pro-UK group, the rates of recanalization were dependent upon the administered dose of heparin. At the end of the 2-hour r-pro-UK infusion, 81.8% of the patients treated with high-dose heparin (100 IU/kg bolus followed by 1000 IU/h infusion for 4 hours) demonstrated recanalization, whereas only 40% recanalized in the low-dose heparin subgroup (2000 IU bolus, followed by a 500 IU/h infusion for 4 hours). However, the rate of symptomatic ICH at 24 hours was also higher in the high-dose heparin group (27.3% vs. 6.7%). The overall 90-day cumulative mortality was 26.9% in the r-pro-UK group and 42.9% in the placebo group. While the number of patients in this study was too low to allow any definite conclusions regarding efficacy, its results led to the larger PROACT-II trial.

The PROACT-II trial was designed to assess the clinical efficacy and safety of IA r-pro-UK. In this study, 180 patients were enrolled in a 2:1 randomization scheme to receive either 9 mg IA r-pro-UK plus 4 hours of low-dose IV heparin, or low-dose IV heparin alone.[23] The primary clinical outcome, the proportion of patients with slight or no disability at 90 days (mRS of ≤ 2), was achieved in 40% of the 121 patients in the r-pro-UK treatment group, compared to 25% of the 59 patients in the control group (absolute benefit 15%, relative benefit 58%, number need to treat = 7; $p = 0.04$). The recanalization rate (TIMI 2 and 3) was 66% for the r-pro-UK group and 18% for the control group ($p < 0.001$). Symptomatic ICH within 24 hours occurred in 10% of r-pro-UK patients and 2% of control patients ($p = 0.06$). All symptomatic ICHs occurred in patients with a baseline NIHSS score of 11 or higher (NIHSS 11–20, 11%; NIHSS >20, 13%). Mortality after symptomatic ICH was 83% (10/12 patients). Elevated serum glucose was significantly associated with symptomatic ICH in the r-pro-UK-treated patients (patients with a baseline serum glucose >200 mg/dL experienced a 36% risk of symptomatic ICH compared with 9% for those with ≤ 200 mg/dL).[24]

Mortality was 25% for the r-pro-UK, group and 27% for the control group ($p = \text{NS}$) despite the higher incidence of ICH in the r-pro-UK, patients. Secondary clinical outcomes at 90 days included the percentage of patients with an NIHSS score of <1, a $\geq 50\%$ reduction from baseline NIHSS, and a Barthel Index (BI) score ≥ 60 or ≥ 90. Despite a trend in favor of the r-pro-UK, group, none of these secondary functional or neurological outcome measures achieved statistical significance. Interestingly, a recent analysis of the PROACT-II suggests that women may benefit more from IAT than men.[25] Although encouraging, the results of PROACT-II were not enough for the FDA to grant approval of IA r-pro-UK, likely secondary to the increased risk of hemorrhage, and another larger trial was requested.

Internal Carotid Artery Occlusion Acute stroke due to a distal ICA "T" (T = terminus) occlusion carry a much worse prognosis than MCA occlusions. In a recent analysis of 24 consecutive patients (median NIHSS 19) presenting with T occlusions of the ICA who were treated by IAT using urokinase at an average of 237 minutes from symptom onset, only four patients (16.6%) had a favorable outcome at 3 months. Partial recanalization of the intracranial ICA was achieved in 15 (63%), of the MCA in 4 (17%), and of the ACA in 8 patients (33%). Complete recanalization did not occur. The presence of good leptomeningeal collaterals and age <60 years were the only predictors of a favorable clinical outcome.[26] New treatment strategies, such as the combination of IV rt-PA and IAT[27], or the use of new mechanical devices[13] may improve the outcome in these patients.

Posterior Circulation Thrombolysis

No randomized, placebo-controlled studies of IAT for vertebrobasilar occlusion have been reported thus far, and most of the rationale for its use is based on the favorable reports of uncontrolled case series. Since the first series of IAT for basilar artery occlusions was published by Zeumer et al.,[28] approximately 278 cases have been reported with an overall recanalization rate of 60% and a mortality rate of 90% in non-recanalized patients versus 31% in at least partially recanalized patients.[29] In general, distal occlusions, which are usually of embolic origin, have higher recanalization rates than proximal occlusions, which are more commonly caused by atherothrombosis. Most stroke experts agree that the time window for IAT in the posterior circulation should be longer than the 6–8 hours for strokes in the carotid circulation, although no consensus guidelines exist to define this interval. The underlying rationale for the longer time window in basilar occlusion cases includes not only the dire prognosis of untreated lesions (mortality rates as high as 90%) but also a *lower* rate of hemorrhagic transformation with IAT in this vascular territory. In our institution, we typically treat basilar occlusion up to 12 hours after the onset of symptoms if neither coma at onset nor a large area of infarction is present on neuroimaging. We consider an extension of this window to up to 24 or even 48 hours for patients with fluctuating symptoms and small infarcts on diffusion-weighted MRI. This is clearly an area that requires further study, however, and can be considered only as an investigational or a salvage therapy at this time.

Lindsberg and Mattle[30] recently analyzed published case series reporting on the outcome of basilar artery occlusion (BAO) after IAT or IV thrombolysis. In 420 BAO patients treated with IV thrombolysis (76) and IAT (344), death or dependency was equally common: 78% (59 of 76) and 76% (260 of 344). Recanalization was achieved more frequently with IAT (225 of 344; 65%) than with IV thrombolysis (40 of 76; 53%; $p = 0.05$), but survival rates after IV thrombolysis (38 of 76; 50%) and IAT (154 of 344; 45%) were equal ($p = 0.48$). A total of 24% of patients treated with IAT and 22% treated with IV thrombolysis reached good outcomes ($p = 0.82$). Without recanalization, the likelihood of achieving a good outcome was close to nil (2%). The authors conclude that recanalization occurs in more than half of BAO patients treated with IAT or IV thrombolysis, and 45–55% of survivors regain functional independence. They advised that hospitals not equipped for IAT should consider setting up IV thrombolysis protocols for BAO since the effect of IVT did not appear to be much different from the effect of IAT.

Combined Intravenous and Intra-Arterial Thrombolysis

Some studies have evaluated the feasibility, safety, and efficacy of combined IV rt-PA at a dose of 0.6 mg/kg with IAT in patients presenting with acute strokes within 3 hours of symptom onset.[31–34] This approach has the potential of combining the advantages of IV rt-PA (fast and easy to use) with the advantages of IAT (directed therapy, titrated dosing, mechanical aids to recanalization, and higher rates of recanalization), thus improving the speed and frequency of recanalization.

The Emergency Management of Stroke (EMS) Bridging Trial was a double-blind, randomized, placebo-controlled, multicenter phase I study of IV rt-PA or IV placebo followed by immediate IAT with rt-PA.[31] Seventeen patients were randomly assigned to the IV/IA group and 18 to the placebo/IA group. Clot was found in 22 of 34 patients. TIMI 3 flow recanalization occurred in 6 of 11 IV/IA patients versus 1 of 10 placebo/IA patients ($p = 0.03$), and correlated with the total dose of rt-PA ($p = 0.05$). However, no difference in the 7- to 10-day or 3-month outcomes was found, and there were more deaths in the IV/IA group. Eight intraparenchymal hemorrhages occurred. Symptomatic ICH occurred in one placebo/IA patient and two IV/IA patients. Life-threatening bleeding complications occurred in two patients, both in the IV/IA group.

Ernst et al.[32] performed a retrospective analysis of 20 consecutive patients (median NIHSS 21) who presented within 3 hours of stroke symptoms and were treated using IV rt-PA (0.6 mg/kg) followed by IA rt-PA (up to 0.3 mg/kg or 24 mg, whichever was less, over a maximum period of 2 hours) in 16 of the 20 patients. Despite a high number of ICA occlusions (8/16), TIMI 2 and 3 recanalization rates were obtained in 50% (8/16) and 19% (3/16) of the patients, respectively. One patient (5%) developed a fatal ICH. Ten patients (50%) recovered to an mRS score of 0–1, three patients (15%) to an mRS score of 2, and five patients (25%) to an mRS score of 4–5.

Suarez et al.[33] studied "bridging" therapy in 45 patients using IV rt-PA at 0.6 mg/kg within 3 hours of stroke onset. Patients exhibiting evidence of PWI/DWI mismatch on MRI underwent subsequent IAT. Eleven patients received IAT with rt-PA (maximum dose 0.3 mg/kg) and 13 patients received IAT with urokinase (maximum dose 750,000 units). Symptomatic ICH occurred in 2 of the 21 patients in the IV rt-PA-only group but in none of the patients in the IV rt-PA/IAT group. Of the 24 patients in the IV rt-PA/IAT group, 21 had MCA occlusions, 2 had ACA occlusions, and 1 had a PCA occlusion. Complete recanalization occurred in 5 of the 13 IV rt-PA/IA urokinase-treated patients, and in 4 of the 11 IV rt-PA/IA rt-PA-treated patients. Partial recanalization also occurred in 5 of the 13 IV rt-PA/IA urokinase-treated patients and 4 of the 11 IV rt-PA/IA rt-PA-treated patients. Favorable outcomes (BI $\geq$ 95) were seen in 92%, 64%, and 66% of the IV rt-PA/IA urokinase, IV rt-PA/IA rt-PA, and IV rt-PA-only-treated patients, respectively.

A "reversed bridging" approach has been proposed by Keris et al.[35] In this study, 12 patients (three ICA occlusions and nine MCA occlusions) out of the 45 enrolled (all with an NIHSS score >20) were randomized to receive an initial IA infusion of 25 mg of rt-PA over 5–10 minutes, followed by IV infusion of another 25 mg over 60 minutes, within 6 hours of stroke onset (total combined dose 50 mg with a maximum dose of 0.7 mg/kg). The remaining 33 patients were assigned to a control group and did not undergo any thrombolysis. TIMI 2 and 3 recanalization occurred in 1 of 12 and 5 of 12 of the patients, respectively. There were no symptomatic ICHs. At 12 months, 83% of the patients in the thrombolysis group were functionally independent, whereas only 33% of the control subjects had a good outcome.

In a prospective, open-label study, Hill et al.[36] assessed the feasibility of a "bridging" approach using full-dose IV rt-PA. Following IV infusion of 0.9 mg/kg rt-PA, six patients underwent IAT with rt-PA (maximum dose 20 mg) and one underwent intracranial angioplasty. TIMI 2 or 3 recanalization was achieved in three of these patients. There were no symptomatic ICHs.

The Interventional Management of Stroke (IMS I) Study was a multicenter, open-labeled, single-arm pilot study in which 80 patients (median NIHSS 18) were enrolled to receive IV rt-PA (0.6 mg/kg, 60 mg maximum, 15% of the dose as a bolus with the remainder administered over 30 minutes) within 3 hours of stroke onset (median time to initiation 140 minutes).[34] Additional rt-PA was subsequently administered via a microcatheter at the site of the thrombus in 62 of the 80 patients, up to a total dose of 22 mg over 2 hours of infusion or until complete recanalization. Primary comparisons were with similar subsets of the placebo and rt-PA-treated subjects from the NINDS rt-PA Stroke Trial. The 3-month mortality in IMS I subjects (16%) was numerically lower but not statistically different than the mortality of the placebo (24%) or rt-PA-treated subjects (21%) in the NINDS rt-PA Stroke Trial. The rate of symptomatic ICH (6.3%) in IMS I subjects was similar to that of the rt-PA-treated subjects (6.6%) but higher than the rate in the placebo-treated subjects (1.0%, $p = 0.018$) in the NINDS rt-PA Stroke Trial. IMS I subjects had a significantly better outcome at 3 months than NINDS placebo-treated subjects for all outcome measures (OR ≥ 2). For the 62 subjects who received IA rt-PA in addition to IV rt-PA, the rate of complete recanalization (TIMI 3 flow) was 11% (7/62), and the rate of partial or complete recanalization (TIMI 2 or 3 flow) was 56% (35/62).

The IMS II objective was to continue investigating the feasibility of the combined IV and IA approach to restore cerebral blood flow in acute stroke patients.[37] The difference between IMS I and IMS II is that IMS II used the EKOS microcatheter to deliver the rt-PA into the clot, using microcatheter ultrasound technology. The rationale is that the ultrasound energy delivered in the clot loosens the fibrin strands, increasing the permeability and penetration of the thrombolytic agents. In IMS II, patients aged 18–80 years with a baseline NIHSS $\geq$10 were given IV rt-PA (0.6 mg/kg, 60 mg maximum over 30 minutes) within 3 hours of stroke onset. Patients with eligible clot in extra- or intracranial cerebral vessels were subsequently administered up to 22 mg IA rt-PA, as well as low-energy ultrasound energy at the clot site using the EKOS ultrasound catheter for a maximum period of 2 hours of infusion or until thrombolysis was achieved. If the EKOS catheter could not access the clot, standard microcatheters were used as per the IMS I protocol. Primary comparisons were made with similar subsets of placebo and rt-PA-treated subjects from the NINDS rt-PA Stroke Trial, as well as subjects from IMS I. Seventy-three subjects were enrolled with a median baseline NIHSS score of 19 and a median time from symptom onset to initiation of IV rt-PA of 141 minutes. In IMS II, 45% of patients had an mRS score of 0–2 at 90 days, compared to 43% in the IMS I and 39% in the NINDS IV rt-PA Stroke Trial. After adjustment for baseline NIHSS, age, and time-to-treatment, the OR of IMS II subjects attaining an mRS of 0–2 at 3 months was 1.65 (95% CI 0.88, 3.07) compared to rt-PA-treated subjects in the NINDS rt-PA Stroke Trial. Compared to the IMS I, the IMS II trial demonstrated a higher rate of recanalization (69%). The mortality and the symptomatic ICH rates in IMS II were 16% and 11%, respectively.

The ongoing IMS III trial is a randomized, multicenter, phase III trial continuing the investigation into the efficacy of the combined IV and IA approach to treat acute stroke. Patients are being randomized to IV/IA therapy and IV rt-PA alone in a 2:1 ratio. In the group allocated to combination IV/IA therapy, the physician will select either the EKOS microcatheter or a standard microcatheter to infuse rt-PA, or select the Mechanical Embolus Removal in Cerebral Ischemia (MERCI) clot retrieval device. The primary outcome is the percentage of patients with an mRS score of 0–2 at 90 days.[38]

The MERCI and Multi-MERCI Trials

The MERCI trial was a prospective single-arm, multicenter trial designed to test the safety and efficacy of the MERCI clot retrieval device to restore the patency of intracranial arteries in the first 8 hours of an acute stroke. All patients were ineligible for IV rt-PA. The occlusion sites were the intracranial vertebral artery, basilar artery, ICA, ICA terminus, or proximal MCA branches (M1 or M2). Primary outcomes were of recanalization and safety, and secondary outcomes were neurological outcomes at 90 days in recanalized versus non-recanalized patients. TIMI 2 or 3 recanalization was achieved in 46% (69/151) of patients in the intention-to-treat analysis and in 48% (68/141) of patients in whom the device was deployed. This rate is significantly higher than that expected using the control arm of the PROACT-II trial (18%) as a historical control ($p < 0.0001$). After adjunctive therapy (IA rt-PA/UK, angioplasty, snare), the rate of recanalization increased to 60.3%. Clinically significant procedural complications occurred in 10 of 141 (7.1%) patients. Symptomatic ICH was observed in 11 of 141 (7.8%) patients. Good neurological outcomes (mRS ≤ 2) at 90 days were more frequent (46% vs. 10%; relative risk (RR) 4.4) and mortality was less (32% vs. 54%; RR 0.59) with successful compared with unsuccessful recanalization.[13]

The Multi-MERCI trial was an international multicenter, single-arm trial with three objectives: to gain greater experience with the first-generation MERCI retrieval device (X5 and X6) in patients ineligible for IV rt-PA; to explore the safety and technical efficacy of the MERCI retriever in patients treated with IV rt-PA who failed to recanalize; and to collect safety and technical efficacy data on a second-generation MERCI retrieval device (L5). The primary outcome was vascular recanalization and safety. One hundred and eleven patients received the thrombectomy procedure. Mean age was 66.2 ± 17.0 years, and baseline NIHSS score was 19 ± 6.3. Thirty patients (27%) received IV rt-PA before intervention. Treatment with the retriever alone resulted in successful (TIMI 2 or 3) recanalization in 60 of 111 (54%) treatable vessels and in 77 of 111 (69%) after adjunctive therapy (IA rt-PA, mechanical). Symptomatic ICH occurred in 10 of 111 (9.0%) patients: 2 of 30 (6.7%) patients pretreated with IV rt-PA and 8 of 81 (9.9%) without IV rt-PA ($p > 0.99$). Clinically significant procedural complications occurred in 5 of 111 (4.5%) patients. The authors concluded that mechanical thrombectomy after IV rt-PA seems as safe as mechanical thrombectomy alone. Mechanical thrombectomy with both first- and second-generation MERCI devices is efficacious in opening intracranial vessels during acute ischemic strokes in patients who either are ineligible for IV rt-PA or have failed to recanalize with IV rt-PA.[39]

INITIAL ASSESSMENT

A detailed clinical history, past medical and surgical history, medications, allergies, laboratory work-up, physical examination, and NIHSS should be obtained as quickly as possible for assessment of inclusion and exclusion criteria for IAT. Table 4.1 lists the criteria for catheter-based reperfusion therapy currently in place at the Massachusetts General Hospital (Table 4.1; see also www.acutestroke.com for updated criteria).

After the clinical and imaging evaluation suggests the need for IAT, the anesthesia team is contacted and informed of the estimated time of arrival of the patient to the interventional neuroradiology suite. Qualifying patients referred from other

TABLE 4.1 Criteria for Catheter-based Reperfusion Therapy Currently in Place at the Massachusetts General Hospital.

IA inclusion criteria

A significant neurologic deficit expected to result in long-term disability, and attributable to large vessel occlusion (basilar, vertebral, internal carotid, or middle cerebral artery M1 or M2 branches).

Noncontrast CT scan without hemorrhage or well-established infarct.

Acute ischemic stroke symptoms with onset or last known well, clearly defined. Treatment within 6 h of established, nonfluctuating deficits due to Anterior Circulation (carotid/MCA) stroke, between 6 and 8 h mechanical treatment (e.g., Concentric Retriever) should be considered. The window of opportunity for treatment is less well defined in posterior circulation (vertebral/basilar) ischemia, and patients may have fluctuating, reversible ischemic symptoms over many hours or even days and still be appropriate candidates for therapy.

Absolute contraindications

Hemorrhage or well-established acute infarct on CT involving greater than one third of the affected vascular territory.

CNS lesion with high likelihood of hemorrhage s/p chemical thrombolytic agents (e.g., brain tumors, abscess, vascular malformation, aneurysm, contusion)

Established bacterial endocarditis.

Relative contraindications

Mild or rapidly improving deficits

Significant trauma within 3 months*

CPR with chest compressions within past 10 days*

Stroke within 3 months

History of intracranial hemorrhage; or symptoms suspicious for subarachnoid hemorrhage

Major surgery within past 14 days*

Minor surgery within past 10 days, including liver and kidney biopsy, thoracocentesis, lumbar puncture*

Arterial puncture at a noncompressible site within past 14 days*

Pregnant (up to 10 days postpartum) or nursing woman*

Suspected bacterial endocarditis

Gastrointestinal, urologic, or respiratory hemorrhage within past 21 days*

Known bleeding diathesis (includes renal and hepatic insufficiency)*

Life expectancy < 1 year from other causes

Peritoneal dialysis or hemodialysis*

PTT > 40 s; platelet count $< 100{,}000$*

INR > 1.7 (PT > 15 if no INR available) with or without chronic oral anticoagulant use*

Seizure at onset of stroke (This relative contraindication is intended to prevent treatment of patients with a deficit due to postictal "Todd's" paralysis or with seizure due to some other CNS lesion that precludes thrombolytic therapy. If rapid diagnosis of vascular occlusion can be made, treatment may be given.)

Glucose < 50 or > 400 (This relative contraindication is intended to prevent treatment of patients with focal deficits due to hypo- or hyperglycemia. If the deficit persists after correction of the serum glucose, or if rapid diagnosis of vascular occlusion can be made, treatment may be given.)

Items marked with an asterisk may not be exclusions for mechanical thrombolysis with or without limited dose chemical agents.

institutions may receive IV rt-PA before transfer and while *en route* as part of a "bridging" approach.[34] If a noncontrast brain CT does not identify any contradictions (e.g., advanced infarction, other nonstroke etiology, brain hemorrhage), and CT angiography (CTA) confirms the presence of a large vessel occlusion (ICA, M1 or 2, A1, basilar or P1 segments), the patient is brought emergently to angiography. Soft-copy review of noncontrast CT with variable window width and center level settings to accentuate the contrast between normal and edematous tissue (e.g., width ~30, level ~30) may optimize the recognition of early ischemic changes.[40] We consider the presence of a readily visible hypodensity on noncontrast CT involving greater than one third of the affected vascular territory a contraindication to thrombolysis.[41]

Review of postcontrast CTA source images might provide a good estimate of whole-brain perfusion.[42] If time allows, MR or CT perfusion maps are obtained to characterize more accurately the ischemic penumbra.[43] Careful but expedited preprocedural analysis of the CTA, done in parallel with transport of the patient to the treatment area, may be extremely helpful in establishing the presence of anatomic variants (e.g., bovine aortic arch) or pathological states (e.g., vessel origin or carotid bifurcation disease) prior to the catheterization procedure.

MRI with MRA as well as DWI and PWI has the advantage of providing more complete information on brain parenchymal injury and penumbral tissue at risk. MRI can be particularly helpful in selected difficult cases. Patients who present with seizures at stroke onset (which was a contraindication to IV rt-PA treament in the NINDS trial) should undergo MRI to exclude the possibility of postictal Todd's paralysis, unless a vascular occlusion compatible with the patient's clinical syndrome is clearly seen on CTA.[44] Similarly, in other situations (such as complex migraine, functional disorder, transient global amnesia, acute demyelination, cerebral amyloid angiopathy, or brain neoplasm), the diagnostic abilities of MRI can be useful in distinguishing a stroke mimic from an acute ischemic stroke.[45] It should be noted, however, that prolonged seizures and acute demyelination can also cause restricted diffusion.[46] Of particular importance is the fact that DWI lesions can be reversed to some extent by IAT in as many as 19% of the cases.[47,48] The application of DWI and PWI in the extension of the therapeutic time window for thrombolysis in acute stroke is currently under investigation in several clinical trials.[7,49,50]

CHEMICAL THROMBOLYSIS

Basic Concepts

After a baseline angiogram confirms the presence and location of the vascular occlusion, a microcatheter is navigated over a microwire into the occluded vessel, traversing the thrombus. Once the microcatheter is positioned immediately distal to the clot, thrombolytic infusion begins; the microcatheter is then pulled back through the clot while drug is infused. Dose adjustments and total dose calculations are made depending on the clinical circumstances, pretreatment dose of rt-PA received, degree of recanalization, and relative size and function of the territory at risk.

The neurointerventionalist should limit the number of microcatheter injections performed during the exam, as there is growing evidence that this may increase the chances of hemorrhagic transformation of the infarcted tissue.[51] Direct injection of contrast into stagnant vessels, which contains injured glial cells and thus breakdown of the blood–brain barrier, allows for contrast extravasation. Contrast is readily visualized on the immediate post-thrombolysis CT as an area of high attenuation in the parenchyma. In some instances, MRI with susceptibility-weighted sequences may be useful to differentiate contrast extravasation from ICH.[52] Such a distinction may be essential in order to establish the optimal postprocedural antithrombotic regimen and blood pressure goals. Successful recanalization should therefore be based on guide catheter injections. The infusion is terminated when adequate antegrade flow is restored, or the predetermined time limit or maximal dose limit is reached. Ominous signs, such as contrast extravasation, should prompt immediate termination of drug infusion, followed by the appropriate management steps as outlined in Table 4.2.

Fibrinolytic agents have several disadvantages. First, although direct infusion maximizes local drug concentrations, dissolution of clot takes an extended period of time, and time is critical in preserving the ischemic penumbra. Second, fibrinolytics increase the risk of hemorrhage both intracranially and systemically. Lastly, not all thromboembolic occlusions can be adequately treated with thrombolytic drugs. The resistance to enzymatic degradation may be related to excessive cross-linking in mature embolic clots, or to emboli composed of cholesterol, calcium, or other debris from atherosclerotic lesions. In others, the lack of flow may result in decreased delivery of circulating plasminogen, allowing the high concentration of fibrinolytic to quickly deplete the available plasminogen. This local plasminogen deficiency would result in impaired fibrinolytic activity.[53]

TABLE 4.2 Management of Symptomatic Intracerebral Hemorrhage after Intra-arterial Thrombolysis.

STAT head CT
STAT neurosurgery consult
Check CBC, PT, PTT, platelets, fibrinogen and D-dimer. Repeat every 2 hours until bleeding is controlled
Give FFP 2 units every 6 hours for 24 hours after dose
Give cryoprecipitate 20 units. If fibrinogen level < 200 mg/dL at 1 hour, repeat cryoprecipitate dose.
Give platelets 4 units
Give protamine sulfate 1 mg/100 U heparin received in last 3 hours (give initial 10 mg test dose by slow IVP over 10 minutes and observe for anaphylaxis; if stable give entire calculated dose by slow IVP; maximum dose 100 mg)
Institute frequent neuro checks and therapy of acutely elevated ICP, as needed
May give aminocaproic acid (Amicar) 5 g in 250 cm^3 NS IV over 1 hour as a last resort

Thrombolytic Agents

Plasminogen Activators These drugs act by converting the inactive proenzyme, plasminogen, into the active enzyme, plasmin. Plasmin can digest fibrinogen, fibrin monomers, and cross-linked fibrin (as found in a thrombus) into fibrin degradation products. These agents vary in stability, half-life, and fibrin selectivity. The thrombolytics that have been reported for use in stroke IAT include urokinase (UK), alteplase, reteplase, pro-urokinase, and streptokinase (SK).[19,54] In general, the nonfibrin-selective drugs (e.g., UK and SK) can result in systemic hypofibrinogenemia, whereas the fibrin-selective agents (e.g., rt-PA and r-pro-UK) are mostly active at the site of thrombosis.

First-Generation Agents: Streptokinase, a protein derived from group C β-hemolytic streptococci, has a half-life of 16–90 minutes and low fibrin specificity. This drug proved to have a very narrow therapeutic window and significant rates of intracerebral and systemic hemorrhage[55]; it is no longer used for stroke IAT. *Urokinase* is a serine protease with a plasma half-life of 14 minutes and low fibrin specificity. The UK dose used in cerebral IAT has ranged from 0.02 to 2×10^6 units (Figure 4.1).[19]

Second-Generation Agents: Alteplase (rt-PA) is a serine protease with a plasma half-life of 3.5 minutes and a high degree of fibrin affinity and specificity. The rt-PA dose used in cerebral IAT has ranged between 20 and 60 mg.[19] The theoretical disadvantages of Alteplase include its relative short half-life and limited penetration into the clot matrix because of strong binding with surface fibrin, which could delay recanalization and increase the risk of recurrent occlusion. Additionally, rt-PA appears to have some neurotoxic properties, including activation of metalloproteinases, which may result in increased blood–brain barrier permeability leading to cerebral hemorrhage and edema, as well as amplification of calcium currents through the NMDA receptor leading to excitotoxicity and neuronal death.[56] *Prourokinase* (r-pro-UK) is the proenzyme precursor of UK. It has a plasma half-life of 7 minutes and high fibrin specificity. Despite the favorable results of the PROACT-I and -II trials,[22,23] the FDA did not approve r-pro-UK for use in stroke IAT.

Third-Generation Agents: Reteplase is a structurally modified form of *alteplase*, with a longer half-life (15–18 minutes). In addition, it does not bind as highly to fibrin; thus, unbound reteplase can theoretically better penetrate the clot and potentially improve *in vivo* fibrinolytic activity. Qureshi et al. have reported the use of low-dose IA reteplase (up to 4 units) in conjunction with mechanical thrombolysis.[54] TIMI 2 and 3 recanalization was achieved in 16 out of 19 patients, with no symptomatic ICHs. *Tenecteplase* is another modified form of rt-PA with a longer half-life (17 minutes), greater fibrin specificity, and greater resistance to PAI-1. Pilot clinical trial data of IV tenecteplase in acute ischemic stroke suggest the drug is safe and promising.[57]

New-Generation Agents: Desmoteplase is a genetically engineered version of the clot-dissolving factor found in the saliva of the vampire bat *Desmodus rotundus.*

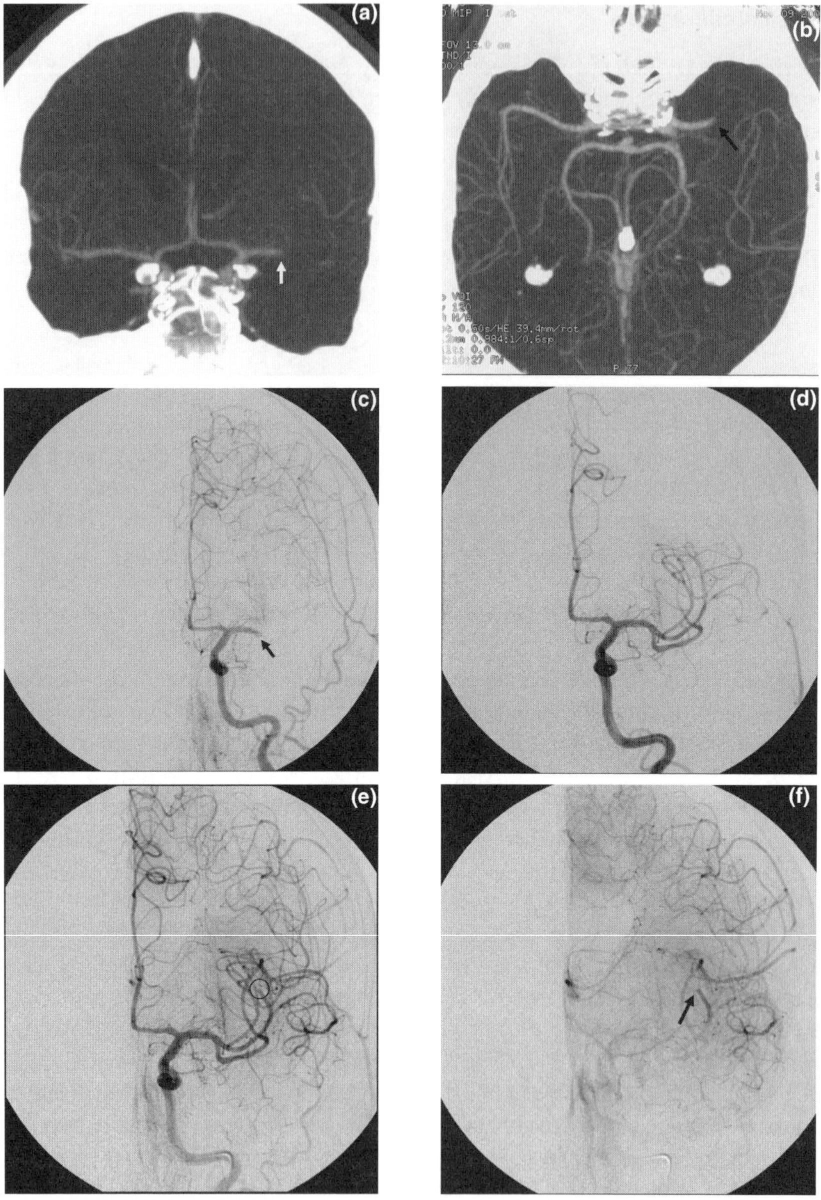

FIGURE 4.1 Eighty-four-year-old man found unresponsive, nonverbal to stimulation, with right hemiparesis, facial droop, and left gaze deviation. He was last seen normal approximately 4 hours before his presentation to the Emergency Department (ED). A CTA was performed in the ED demonstrating occlusion of the left M1 segment (**a** and **b**). A cerebral angiogram was then performed. Left internal carotid artery (LICA) angiogram confirmed the CTA findings (**c**). LICA angiogram after 150,000 units of urokinase was infused through a microcatheter within the clot demonstrating successful recanalization of the left M1 segment (**d** and **e**). Note a distal M2 clot that did not recanalize after IA urokinase treatment (circle—**e** and arrow—**f**).

This drug is more potent and more selective for fibrin-bound plasminogen than any other known plasminogen activator. Unlike t-PA, desmoteplase is not activated by fibrinogen or β-amyloid proteins, factors that may exacerbate the risk for ICH. Moreover, desmoteplase inhibits t-PA-induced potentiation of excitotoxic injury. The effect of IV administration of desmoteplase 3–9 hours after symptom onset in stroke patients who demonstrate a mismatch on PWI/DWI MRI is currently being investigated.[7]

No direct comparison trials have been reported between the different thrombolytic agents in acute ischemic stroke. In a retrospective review of the results for acute stroke IAT performed at our center, we have found significantly higher rates of recanalization and good clinical outcome in the era in which IA UK was used versus the era in which UK was not available and IAT with rt-PA was the primary treatment.[58] Conversely, in another retrospective study, Eckert et al.[59] found no major difference between the recanalization rates of UK and rt-PA.

Alternatives to Plasminogen Activation: Other Thrombolytics Thrombolytics currently in the market are plasminogen activators. Therefore, their activity is impacted by the amount of plasminogen in the thrombus. New drugs that do not depend on the availably of plasminogen are currently being evaluated for stroke therapy.

Direct Fibrinolytics: Alfimeprase is a recombinant truncated form of fibrolase, a fibrinolytic zinc metalloproteinase isolated from the venom of the Southern copperhead snake. It degrades fibrin directly and achieves thrombolysis independent of plasmin formation. This may result in faster recanalization and a decreased risk of hemorrhagic conversion. The initial data on the safety and efficacy of alfimeprase in peripheral arterial occlusion disease appeared very promising,[60] but recent communication from the sponsor revealed that the phase III trials of the drug in peripheral arterial disease and catheter obstruction (NAPA-2 and SONOMA-2) failed to meet their primary and key secondary endpoints of revascularization. A trial for IAT in acute stroke (CARNEROS-1) is planned to begin soon.

Microplasmin is a truncated form of plasmin that is more resistant to the effects of antiplasmin. In a rabbit stroke model, intravenous microplasmin infusion resulted in a high rate of clot lysis without increasing the rate of ICH. In addition, there was significant improvement in the behavioral rating scores, suggesting a neuroprotective effect.[61] The ongoing MITI-IV trial is a 40-patient multicenter, double-blind, placebo-controlled trial using three different intravenous doses of microplasmin to treat acute ischemic stroke (NIHSS >6 and <22) within 12 hours of symptom onset.

Defibrinogenating Agents *Ancrod* is the purified fraction of Malayan pit viper venom. It acts by directly cleaving and thus inactivating fibrinogen, and therefore indirectly inducing anticoagulation. In the Stroke Treatment with Ancrod Trial, 500 stroke patients presenting within 3 hours of symptom onset were randomized to receive ancrod ($n = 248$) or placebo ($n = 252$). Good outcome (BI $\geq$ 95–100 at 3 months) was achieved in 42.21% and 34.4% of the patients, respectively ($p = 0.04$). There was no significant difference in mortality but a trend toward more symptomatic ICH with ancrod (5.2% vs. 2%, $p = 0.06$).[62] The ASP-II Trial is currently enrolling patients with an NIHSS score between 5 and 25 who present within 6 hours of stroke onset for treatment with ancrod or placebo.

Adjunctive Therapy

Fibrinolytic agents have prothrombotic properties as well. The plasmin generated by thrombolysis leads to the production of thrombin, which is a potent platelet activator and converts fibrinogen to fibrin. Indeed, studies have shown early reocclusion in as many as 17% of the patients treated with IAT [17] and 34% of the patients treated with IV rt-PA.[63] Therefore, a strong rationale exists for the adjuvant use of antithrombotic agents.

Systemic anticoagulation with IV heparin during the periprocedural phase of IAT has several potential advantages, including augmentation of the thrombolytic effect,[22] prevention of acute reocclusion, and reduction in the risk of catheter-related embolism. However, these benefits must be weighed against the potentially increased risk of ICH when heparin is combined with a thrombolytic agent.

Argatroban, lepirudin, and bivalirudin are all direct thrombin inhibitors. These agents should replace heparin in cases in which the diagnosis of heparin-induced thrombocytopenia (HIT) type II is confirmed or even suspected. HIT type II is an immune-mediated disorder characterized by the formation of antibodies against the heparin–platelet factor 4 complex, resulting in thrombocytopenia, platelet aggregation, and the potential for arterial and venous thrombosis. The possibility of HIT type II should be raised in patients who demonstrate a platelet count drop to less than 100,000, or by greater than 50% from baseline, in the setting of heparin therapy (usually 5–12 days after initial exposure). Unexplained thrombotic events should also evoke this diagnosis, even in the setting of a normal platelet count. Impaired renal function must be taken into account when selecting the appropriate agent; argatroban is the only direct thrombin inhibitor that is hepatically cleared.

The use of glycoprotein (GP) IIb/IIIa antagonists, such as *Reopro* (abciximab), *Integrilin* (eptifibatide), or *Aggrastat* (tirofiban) in ischemic stroke is still investigational. No cases of major intracranial hemorrhage were seen in a pilot randomized, double-blind, placebo-controlled study in which 54 patients presenting within 24 hours after ischemic stroke onset were randomly allocated to receive escalating doses of abciximab.[64] Conversely, the AbESTT-II trial, a phase III, multicenter, randomized, double-blind, placebo-controlled study evaluating the safety and efficacy of abciximab in acute ischemic stroke treated within 6 hours after stroke onset or within 3 hours of awakening with stroke symptoms, was stopped early due to high rates of ICH. The NIH is currently sponsoring a phase II trial (ROSIE) looking at intravenous reteplase in combination with abciximab for the treatment of ischemic stroke within 3–24 hours from onset. Preliminary analysis of the first 21 patients enrolled has revealed no symptomatic ICH or major hemorrhage. The CLEAR trial is studying the combination of low-dose rt-PA and eptifibatide in patients with NIHSS scores greater than 5 who present within 3 hours from stroke onset.

The data for the use of GP IIb/IIIa inhibitors in conjunction with IAT are even more scant, and are limited to case reports. Intravenous abciximab has been successfully used as adjunctive therapy to IA rt-PA or UK in cases of acute stroke.[65–67] Deshmukh et al.[67] reported on 21 patients with large vessel occlusion refractory to IAT with rt-PA who were treated with IV and/or IA abciximab, eptifibatide, or tirofiban. Twelve patients also received IV rt-PA and 18 patients underwent balloon angioplasty. Complete or partial recanalization was achieved in 17 of 21 patients. Three patients (14%) had asymptomatic ICH, but there were no cases of symptomatic ICH. Mangiafico et al.[68] described 21 stroke patients treated with an intravenous bolus of tirofiban and heparin followed by IA urokinase. Nineteen of these patients also underwent balloon angioplasty. TIMI 2–3 flow was achieved in 17 of 21 patients. ICH occurred in 5 of 21 patients (3 symptomatic ICH and 2 SAH), and was fatal in 3 patients.[68] Qureshi et al.[69] described the use of IA reteplase and intravenous abciximab on 20 stroke patients. There was one symptomatic ICH. Partial or complete recanalization occurred in 13 of the 20 patients. Conversely, the use of abciximab was predictive of asymptomatic SAH (OR 19.2) in nine patients who received this drug as a study protocol violation in the Multi-MERCI part 1 trial.[39]

INTRA-ARTERIAL MECHANICAL TREATMENT OF STROKE

Mechanical thrombolysis (or "thromborrhexis" or "thrombectomy") has several advantages over chemical thrombolysis and may be used as a primary or adjunctive strategy. First, it lessens and may even preclude the use of chemical thrombolytics, in this manner likely reducing the risk of ICH. Second, by avoiding the use of chemical thrombolytics it may be possible to extend the treatment window beyond 6 hours. Third, mechanically fragmenting a clot increases the surface area accessible to fibrinolytic agents and allows inflow of fresh plasminogen, which in turn may increase the speed of thrombolysis. Finally, clot retrieval devices may provide faster recanalization and may be more efficient at coping with material resistant to enzymatic degradation.

The disadvantages of mechanical thrombolysis include the technical difficulty of navigating mechanical devices into the intracranial circulation, excessive trauma to the vasculature (possibly leading to vasospasm, vessel dissection, perforation, or rupture), and fragmented thrombus causing distal embolization into previously unaffected territories. Nonetheless, the advantages of mechanical thrombolysis appear significant, and this approach is being evaluated in a phase III clinical trial (MR RESCUE), which evaluates the efficacy of mechanical thrombectomy in patients with or without territory at risk as measured by MRI PWI–DWI mismatch.

IA mechanical interventions to treat acute stroke may be classified into six different categories: (1) mechanical clot disruption, (2) endovascular thrombectomy, (3) augmented fibrinolysis, (4) clot entrapment, (5) thromboaspiration, and (6) flow augmentation.

Mechanical Clot Disruption

There are several techniques available for mechanical thrombolysis. The most common is probing the thrombus with a microguidewire. This technique appears to be useful in facilitating chemical thrombolysis.[12] Alternatively, a snare (e.g., Amplatz Goose-Neck Microsnare, Microvena, White Bear Lake, MN) can be used for multiple passes through the occlusion to disrupt the thrombus.[54, 70] A snare can also be used for clot retrieval, mostly in situations in which the clot has a firm consistency or contains solid material.[71]

Studies have shown the feasibility and efficacy of percutaneous transluminal angioplasty (PTA) in acute stroke.[68,72–74] This strategy appears to result in higher recanalization rates than other current modalities (Fig. 4.2). Nakano et al.[73] performed a retrospective comparison of 34 patients with acute MCA trunk occlusions who were treated with direct PTA (with subsequent thrombolytic therapy in 21 cases) versus 36 similar patients who were treated with thrombolytic therapy alone. Partial or complete recanalization was achieved in 91.2% versus 63.9%, symptomatic ICH was seen in 2.9% versus 19.4%, and good outcome (mRS score $\leq$ 2) occurred in 73.5% versus 50% of the patients, respectively. PTA may be particularly useful in cases of atherothrombotic disease in which the residual stenosis may reduce flow sufficiently to

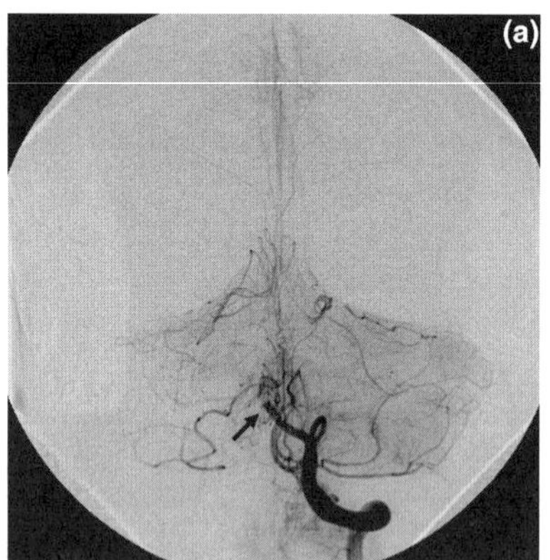

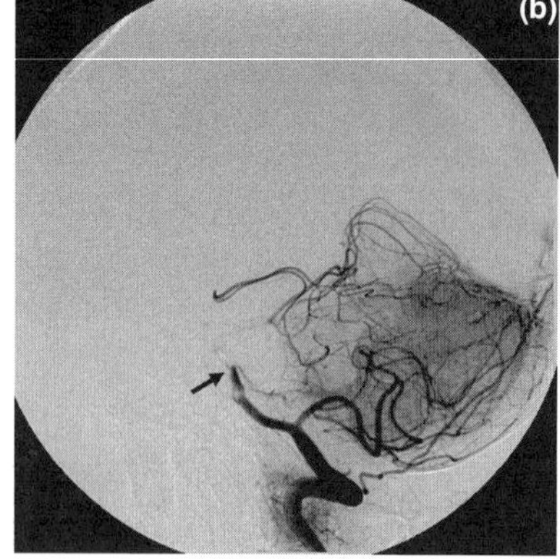

FIGURE 4.2 Seventy-three-year-old female with sudden right hemiparesis, left facial weakness, dysarthria, nausea, and downbeat nystagmus. Posterior circulation angioplasty demonstrated occlusion of the proximal basilar artery (arrows— **a** and **b**). Note the retrograde opacification of the superior cerebellar arteries through postero-inferior cerebellar to superior cerebellar arteries collaterals (**b**).

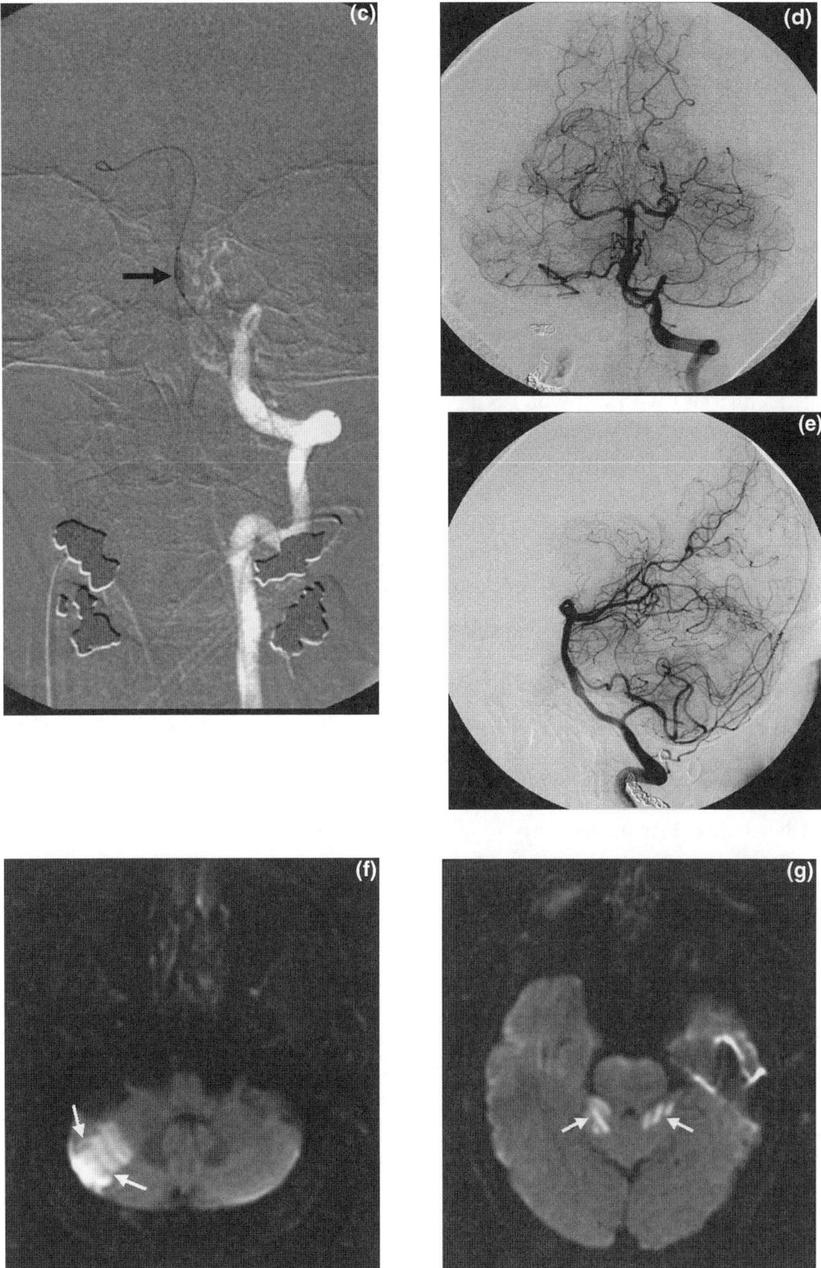

FIGURE 4.2 (*Continued*) A compliant balloon was used to perform angioplasty (**c**). Postangioplasty angiogram demonstrated complete recanalization of the basilar artery and its major branches (**d** and **e**). MRI performed 2 days later demonstrated only small areas of infarction in the cerebellar hemispheres (arrows—**f** and **g**) but no brainstem or occipital infarcts.

lead to rethrombosis.[17] Given the risks of procedural complications, such as vessel rupture and distal embolization, we tend to reserve this technique as salvage therapy for patients whose flow cannot be restored by more conservative methods. However, this technique has probably become safer with the use of low-pressure, more compliant balloons.[68,75]

Two devices that use different laser technologies have been used to disrupt intracranial clots. The Endovascular Photoacoustic Recanalization (EPAR; Endovasix Inc., Belmont, CA) is a mechanical clot fragmentation device based on laser technology. However, the emulsification of the thrombus is due to mechanical thrombolysis and not a direct laser-induced ablation. The photonic energy is converted to acoustic energy at the fiberoptic tip through creation of microcavitation bubbles. In a recent study, in which 34 patients (10 ICA, 12 MCA, 1 PCA, and 11 vertebrobasilar occlusions) with a median NIHSS of 19 were treated with EPAR, the overall intention-to-treat recanalization rate was 41.1% (14/34). Vessel recanalization occurred in 11 of 18 patients (61.1%) in whom complete EPAR treatment was possible. Additional treatment with IA rt-PA occurred in 13 patients. One patient had a vessel rupture resulting in fatality. Symptomatic intracerebral hemorrhages occurred in two patients (5.9%). The overall mortality rate was 38.2%.[76]

The LaTIS laser device (LaTIS, Minneapolis, MN) uses the slow injection of contrast material as a "light pipe" to carry the energy from the catheter to the embolus.[77] The device was evaluated in a safety and feasibility trial at two U.S. centers. A preliminary account reported that the device could not be deployed to the level of the occlusion in 2 of the first 5 patients, and enrollment stopped at 12 patients. Although the catheter design was changed, an efficacy trial has not been pursued.[78]

Endovascular Thrombectomy

Mechanical thrombectomy is a promising novel technique in interventional stroke treatment. The devices differ with regard to where they apply force on the thrombus, taking either a proximal approach with aspiration devices (see section on thromboaspiration below) or a distal approach with basket- or snare-like devices. A study comparing the effectiveness of these two approaches (Vasco35 vs. Catch device) in a swine stroke model demonstrated that the proximal device allowed fast repeated applications with a low risk of thromboembolic events (3% vs. 26%; OR 11.3, 95% CI 1.35–101.6) and vasospasm, but significantly lower success rates in retrieving thrombus than the distal device (39.4% vs. 82.6%; OR 7.3, 95% CI 2.0–26.4). The rate of embolic events with the distal device could be significantly reduced by employing the use of a proximal balloon occlusion.[79] Balloon occlusion with aspiration to promote flow reversal also facilitates clot extraction.[14]

The *Concentric Retriever* (Concentric Medical Inc., Mountain View, CA), a flexible, nitinol wire with helical tapering coil loops (X5 and X6) that is used in conjunction with a balloon guide catheter (8 or 9 French) and a microcatheter, is the only device currently approved by the FDA for the endovascular treatment of stroke patients (Fig. 4.3).[13] The second-generation devices (L5 and L6) differ from the X devices by the inclusion of a system of arcading filaments attached to a nontapering

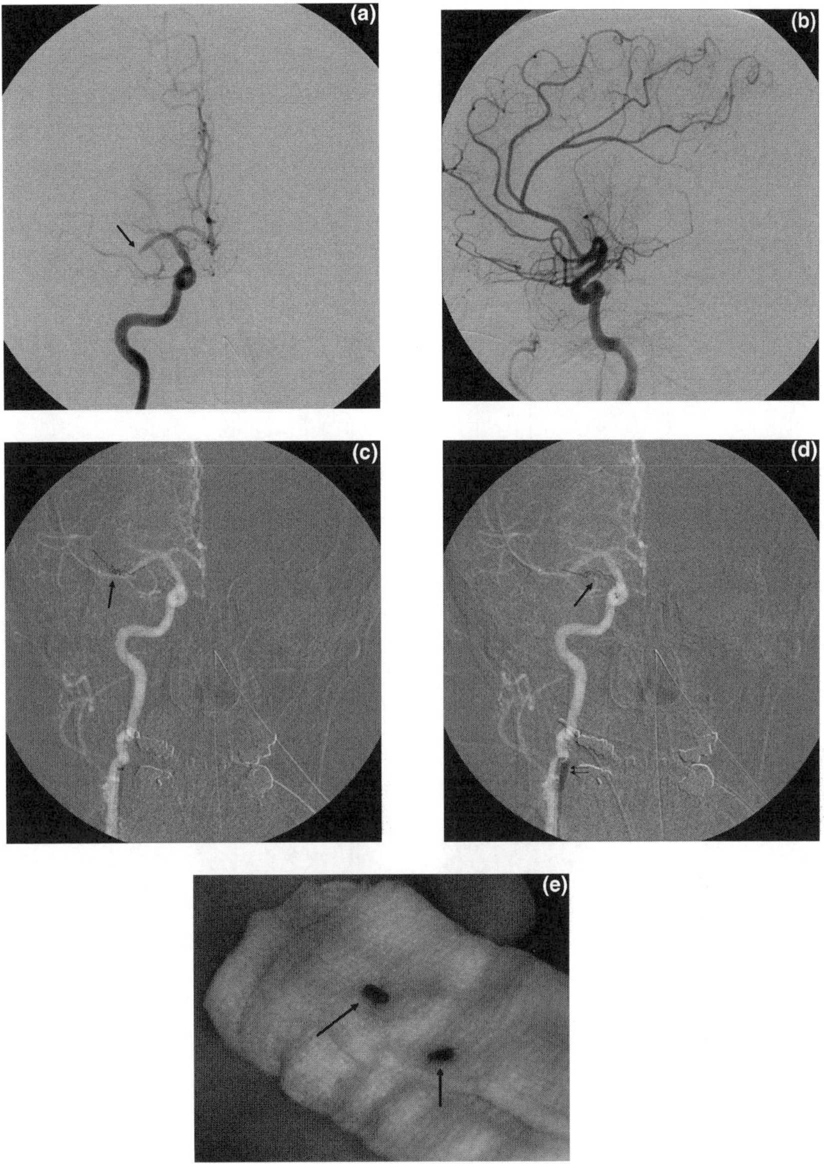

FIGURE 4.3 Sixty-two-year-old left-handed female who presented with left hemiplegia, right gaze deviation, and aphasia 5 hours after an elective thyroidectomy. Right internal carotid artery (RICA) angiogram demonstrated occlusion of the right M1 segment just distal to the origin of the anterior temporal artery (**a** and **b**). RICA roadmap images demonstrating successful deployment of the Concentric Retriever within the clot (arrow **c**). Note the torque in the system when the clot is pulled back (arrow **d**) and the guide catheter balloon inflated (double arrows **d**). Small fragments of clot are shown (**e**).

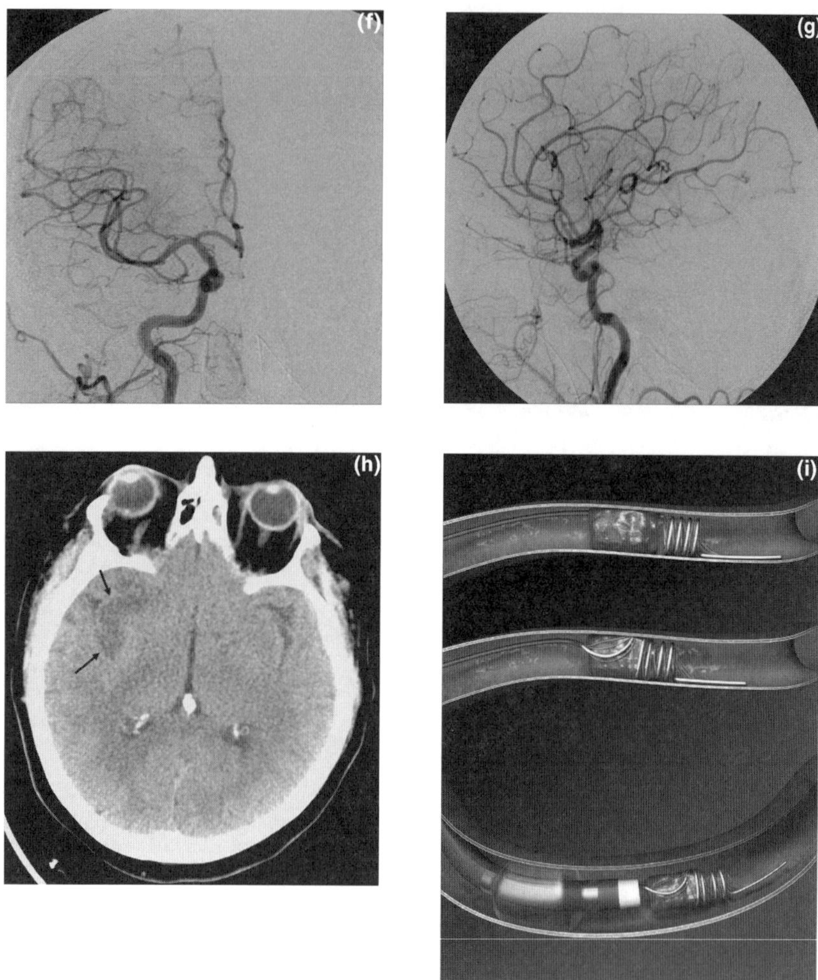

FIGURE 4.3 (*Continued*) Final RICA angiogram demonstrated complete recanalization of the M1 segment of the right middle cerebral artery (**f** and **g**). CT performed 24 hours after the procedure demonstrated only a small area of hypoattenuation in the right insular region (**h**). Schematic drawing demonstrating how the Concentric Retriever engages and retrieves the intraluminal clot (**i**).

helical nitinol coil that has a 90° angle in relation to the proximal wire component. Third-generation devices (K devices), with a smaller profile that may allow for clot retrieval from more distal vessels, are currently being tested. This embolectomy system has been systematically studied in the MERCI and Multi-MERCI trials, which were discussed above.

The *Neuronet device* (Guidant Corp., Santa Clara, CA) is a microguidewire-based laser-cut nitinol basket open proximally with the crisscrossing basket portion tapering to a shapeable platinum-tipped wire. This device has been successfully used to retrieve intracranial clots,[14,70,77] and is currently being tested in a European trial. The *Catch device* (Balt Extrusion, Montmorency, France) is a distally closed, self-expanding nitinol cage that has also been used for thrombectomy with promising results.[80]

The *Phenox Clot Retriever* consists of a metallic core made from a wire compound surrounded by a dense palisade of perpendicularly-oriented stiff polyamide microfilaments trimmed in a conical shape, which have an increasing diameter distally and are resistant to unraveling. The device is molded to the body of a 0.010-inch microguidewire. It is introduced into the target vessel through a 0.021-inch or 0.027-inch microcatheter, deployed distally to the thrombus, and slowly pulled back under continuous aspiration via the guiding catheter. Only two cases using this device have been reported thus far, including a case demonstrating recanalization of a Rolandic MCA branch.[81] The *Attracter-18 device* (Target Therapeutics, Fremont, CA) is another fiber-based retriever device that has been successfully used to recanalize an occluded superior division branch of the left MCA refractory to IA thrombolytic treatment.[82]

The *In-Time Retriever* (Boston Scientific, Natick, MA) has four to six wire loops and tends to bow when opened but has no specific opening to capture the embolus. This device has been successfully used in a case of an MCA occlusion resistant to thrombolytics and balloon angioplasty,[83] as well as in cases of basilar occlusion.[70] The *TriSpan* (Boston Scientific, Natick, MA), a neck bridge device consisting of three nitinol loops originally designed to treat wide-necked aneurysms, has also been used to treat basilar occlusions.[70]

Other snare devices that potentially can be used for embolectomy include (1) the *Alligator Retrieval Device*, which is a retriever with grasping jaws attached to the tip of a flexible wire designed to be used in conjunction with 0.21-inch microcatheter[84]; and (2) the *EnSnare* device, which has a tulip-shaped, three-loop design that opens distally. These devices, which are approved for foreign body removal/coil retrieval, have not been reported in embolectomy for stroke treatment.

Augmented Fibrinolysis

The *EKOS MicroLys US Infusion Catheter* (EKOS Corporation, Bothell, WA) is a 3 French single lumen end-hole design microcatheter with a 2-mm, 2.1-MHz piezoelectric ultrasound element (average power 0.21–0.45 W) at its distal tip that creates a microenvironment of ultrasonic vibration to facilitate thrombolysis. This is achieved by a combination of a noncavitating ultrasound, which reversibly separates fibrin strands, and acoustic streaming, which increases fluid permeation, resulting in increased drug–thrombus surface interaction (Fig. 4.4). The net result is enhanced clot dissolution without creating fragmentation emboli. In a pilot study, in which 10 anterior circulation occlusion (mean NIHSS score of 18.2) and four

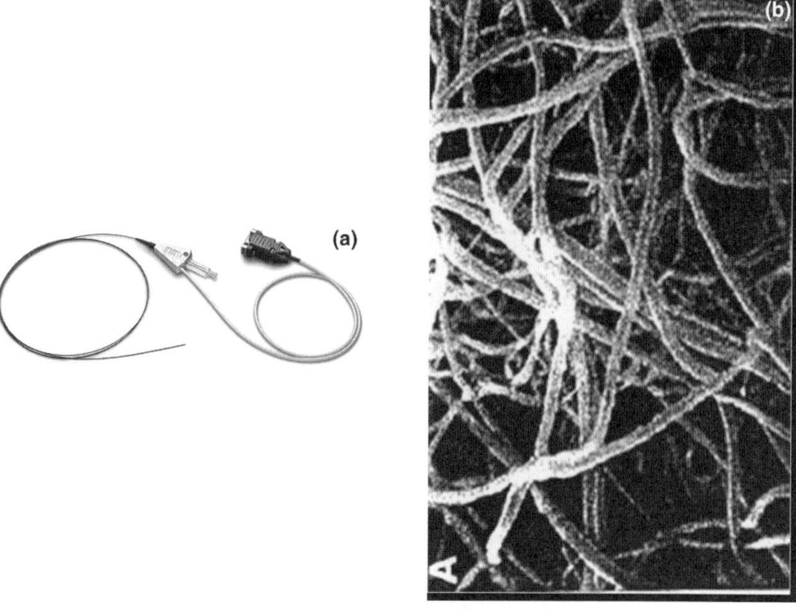

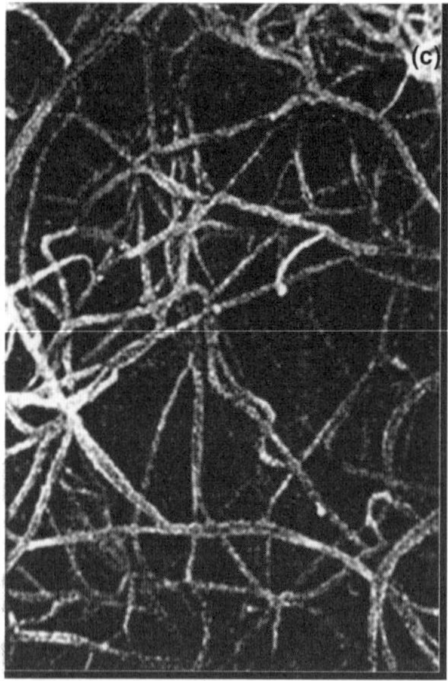

FIGURE 4.4 Picture of the EKOS MicroLys US infusion catheter (**a**). Fibrin strands of a clot before (**b**) and after (**c**) ultrasound treatment. Note the reversible loosening of fibrin strands after ultrasound treatment (**c**).

posterior circulation occlusion (mean NIHSS score of 18.75) patients were treated with this device, TIMI 2–3 flow was achieved in 8 of 14 patients in the first hour. Average time to recanalization was 46 minutes, and no catheter-related adverse events occurred.[85] The device was subsequently used in 26 of the 73 patients enrolled in the IMS II trial. A comparison between IMS I patients ($n = 80$) and IMS II patients treated with EKOS ($n = 26$) revealed a trend toward higher rates of complete recanalization in the later group (50.8% vs. 69%, $p = 0.08$).[86] Similarly, enhanced fibrinolysis with intravenous rt-PA can be achieved with the use of continuous 2-MHz transcranial Doppler ultrasonography (CLOTBUST trial).[87]

Clot Entrapment

Stenting of an acutely occluded intracranial vessel may provide fast recanalization by entrapping the thrombus between the stent and the vessel wall. A recent study in which 19 patients with acute occlusions at the ICA terminus ($n = 8$), M1/M2 ($n = 7$), or basilar artery ($n = 4$) were treated with balloon-expandable stents showed a TIMI 2 and 3 recanalization rate of 79% and no symptomatic intracranial hemorrhages (Fig. 4.5).[88]

Self-expanding stents are easier to navigate into the intracranial circulation. Moreover, higher rates of recanalization and lower rates of vasospasm and side-branch occlusion were noticed with self-expanding stents than with balloon-mounted stents in a canine model of acutely occluded vessels with clot emboli.[89] Successful recanalization after deployment of the self-expanding Neuroform stent (Boston Scientific Corp., Natick, MA) was recently reported in five acute stroke patients with clots resistant to chemical thrombolytics, balloon angioplasty, GP IIb/IIIa inhibitors, and the MERCI retriever.[90] Isolated case reports of successful intracranial recanalization with the Neuroform stent have also been reported.[91,92]

Self-expanding stents with a higher radial force (e.g., WingSpan, Boston Scientific Corp.) will probably play a key role in acute stroke cases related to intracranial atherosclerotic disease.[93] Antegrade flow is essential for the maintenance of vascular patency, as particularly evident in patients with severe proximal stenoses who commonly develop rethrombosis after vessel recanalization. Furthermore, stenting of the proximal vessels may be required in order to gain access to the intracranial thrombus with other mechanical devices or catheters. In a recent series, 23 of 25 patients (92%) with acute ($n = 15$) or subacute ($n = 10$) ICA occlusions were successfully revascularized with this technique.[94]

Thromboaspiration

Suction thrombectomy or thromboaspiration through either a microcatheter[21,95] or a guiding catheter[96] may be an option for fresh nonadhesive clot. As discussed above, aspiration devices have the advantage of causing less embolic events and vasospasm; however, the more complex design of these devices makes them more difficult to navigate into the intracranial circulation.

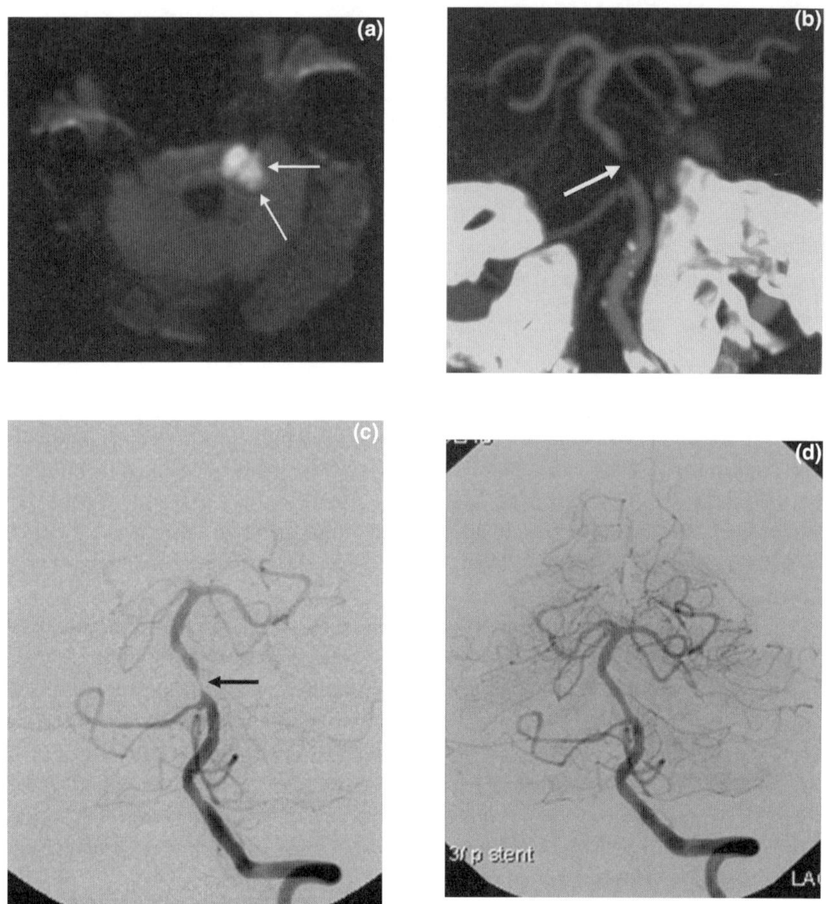

FIGURE 4.5 A 72-year-old man with medical history remarkable for hypertension and dyslipidemia presented with posterior circulation infarct (**a**). CTA and posterior circulation angiography (left vertebral artery injection) performed demonstrated severe mid-basilar artery stenosis (**b** and **c**). Left vertebral artery injection demonstrated near-complete reversal of the stenosis after a drug-eluting balloon expandable stent (Cypher, Cordis Johnson & Johnson) was deployed (**d**).

The *Possis AngioJet system* (Posis Medical Inc., Minneapolis, MN) is a rheolytic thrombectomy device that uses high-pressure saline jets to create a distal Venturi suction which gently agitates the clot face. The generated clot fragments are then sucked into the access catheter. At Massachusetts General Hospital, a 5 French Possis AngioJet catheter was used to successfully treat three patients who presented with acute stroke in the setting of ICA occlusion. Patency of the carotid artery was re-established in two patients. In the third patient, the device was able to create a channel through the column of thrombus, allowing intracranial access.[97] The NeuroJet (Posis Medical Inc.) is a smaller, single-channel device, specifically developed to be used in the intracranial circulation. Unfortunately, issues with vessel dissection and inability to navigate through the carotid siphon were noted in a pilot study for acute ischemic stroke, and the trial was discontinued.[77,98] Other vortex aspiration devices have been developed for the extracerebral circulation, using high-pressure streams to generate Venturi forces that physically fragment, draw in, and aspirate thrombi, including the Oasis (Boston Scientific), the Amplatz Thrombectomy Device (Microvena Corp.), and the Hydrolyzer (Cordis).[98]

The Penumbra stroke system (Penumbra Inc., San Leandro, CA) includes two different revascularization options: (1) thrombus debulking and aspiration may be achieved by a reperfusion catheter that aspirates the clot while a separator device fragments it, and (2) direct thrombus extraction may be performed by a ring retriever while a balloon guide catheter is used to temporarily arrest flow. This system has been tested in a pilot trial in Europe. Twenty patients (mean NIHSS 21) with a total of 21 vessel occlusions (7 ICA, 5 MCA, and 9 Basilar) were treated up to 8 hours after symptom onset. Recanalization prior to IA lysis was achieved in all cases (48% TIMI 2; 52% TIMI 3). Seven patients were also treated with IA UK or rt-PA. Good outcome at 30 days (defined as mRS ≤ 2 or NIHSS 4-point improvement) was demonstrated in 42%. The mortality rate was 45%, but there were no device-related deaths.[99] There was one asymptomatic SAH and three symptomatic ICHs. A prospective, single-arm, multicenter trial is being conducted in the United States and Europe currently.

Flow Augmentation

The NeuroFlo device (CoAxia Inc., Maple Grove, MN) is a dual balloon catheter uniquely designed for partial occlusion of the aorta above and below the origin of the renal arteries (Fig. 4.6). Through mechanisms that have yet to be elucidated, this device increases global cerebral perfusion within minutes of balloon inflation, with little or no increase in mean arterial blood pressure. The ongoing Safety and Efficacy of NeuroFlo Technology in Ischemic Stroke (SENTIS) trial is a prospective, controlled, randomized, multicenter trial of NeuroFlo treatment plus standard medical management versus standard medical management in stroke patients with NIHSS scores between 5 and 18, within 10 hours of symptom onset. A second pilot clinical trial, Flo24, will study the effect of perfusion augmentation in patients who present with an MRI PWI–DWI mismatch between 8 and 24 hours after last seen well.

CONCLUSION

The efficacy of IV thrombolysis in patients with moderate-to-severe strokes due to proximal arterial occlusions is restricted by several factors, including the relatively short therapeutic window, poor recanalization rates as the clot burden increases, restrictive eligibility criteria, and the risk of intracerebral hemorrhage. Endovascular techniques improve the rates of recanalization in this patient population, and appear to increase the likelihood of a good functional outcome. Intravenous thrombolysis

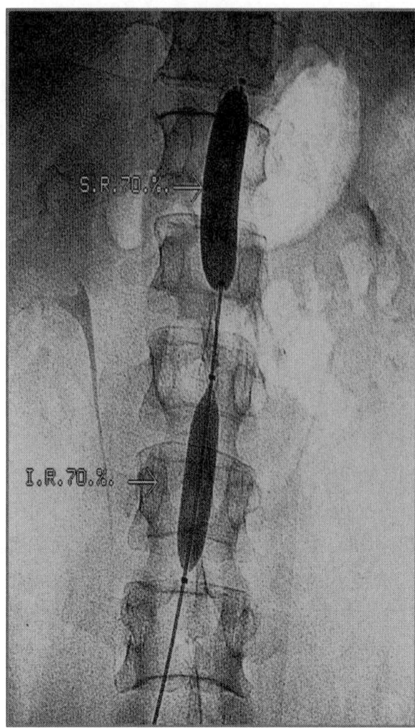

FIGURE 4.6 The NeuroFlo device with its dual balloon catheter uniquely designed for partial occlusion of the aorta above and below the origin of the renal arteries.

with rt-PA should be initiated in all eligible patients presenting within 3 hours of stroke onset, and considered as a "bridge" to IAT for appropriate patients with verified proximal vessel occlusions. Mechanical thrombolysis has become a powerful adjunct to IA infusion of chemical thrombolytics, and should be considered as primary therapy in patients who have contraindications to chemical thrombolysis or who present late (up to 8 hours in the anterior circulation). The time window for IAT in the posterior circulation has not been well established, and at this point a judicious decision should be made on a case-by-case basis. The emerging neuroimaging techniques that identify territory at risk, such as CT and MRI perfusion, are under active investigation to establish triage criteria for patient selection in IAT. These methods may eventually define a subgroup of patients who will benefit from late IV or IA thrombolysis.

REFERENCES

1. Recommendations on stroke prevention, diagnosis, and therapy. Report of the WHO Task Force on Stroke and other Cerebrovascular Disorders. *Stroke* 1989;20:1407–1431.
2. Tissue plasminogen activator for acute ischemic stroke. The National Institute of Neurological Disorders and Stroke rt-PA Stroke Study Group. *N Engl J Med* 1995; 333:1581–1587.

3. Practice advisory: thrombolytic therapy for acute ischemic stroke–summary statement. Report of the Quality Standards Subcommittee of the American Academy of Neurology. *Neurology* 1996;47:835–839.
4. Adams HP Jr, Brott TG, Furlan AJ, Gomez CR, Grotta J, Helgason CM, Kwiatkowski T, Lyden PD, Marler JR, Torner J, Feinberg W, Mayberg M, Thies W. Guidelines for thrombolytic therapy for acute stroke: a supplement to the guidelines for the management of patients with acute ischemic stroke. A statement for healthcare professionals from a Special Writing Group of the Stroke Council, American Heart Association. *Circulation* 1996; 94:1167–1174.
5. Wardlaw JM, Zoppo G, Yamaguchi T, Berge E. Thrombolysis for acute ischaemic stroke. *Cochrane Database Syst Rev* 2003;CD000213.
6. Hacke W, Donnan G, Fieschi C, Kaste M, von Kummer R, Broderick JP, Brott T, Frankel M, Grotta JC, Haley EC Jr, Kwiatkowski T, Levine SR, Lewandowski C, Lu M, Lyden P, Marler JR, Patel S, Tilley BC, Albers G, Bluhmki E, Wilhelm M, Hamilton S; ATLANTIS Trials Investigators; ECASS Trials Investigators; NINDS rt-PA Study Group Investigators. Association of outcome with early stroke treatment: pooled analysis of ATLANTIS, ECASS, and NINDS rt-PA stroke trials. *Lancet* 2004;363:768–774.
7. Hacke W. The results of the joint analysis of two phase II trials on desmoteplase in acute ischemic stroke with treatment 3 to 9 hours after stroke onset. 14th European Stroke Conference. Bologna, Italy, May 2005.
8. Wolpert SM, Bruckmann H, Greenlee R, Wechsler L, Pessin MS, del Zoppo GJ. Neuroradiologic evaluation of patients with acute stroke treated with recombinant tissue plasminogen activator. The rt-PA Acute Stroke Study Group. *Am J Neuroradiol* 1993;14:3–13.
9. Caplan LR, Mohr JP, Kistler JP, Koroshetz W. Should thrombolytic therapy be the first-line treatment for acute ischemic stroke? Thrombolysis—not a panacea for ischemic stroke. *N Engl J Med* 1997;337:1309–1310 [discussion 1313].
10. Haley Jr EC, Lewandowski C, Tilley BC. Myths regarding the NINDS rt-PA Stroke Trial: setting the record straight. *Ann Emerg Med* 1997;30:676–682.
11. Saver JL. Number needed to treat estimates incorporating effects over the entire range of clinical outcomes: novel derivation method and application to thrombolytic therapy for acute stroke. *Arch Neurol* 2004;61:1066–1070.
12. Barnwell SL, Clark WM, Nguyen TT, O'Neill OR, Wynn ML, Coull BM. Safety and efficacy of delayed intraarterial urokinase therapy with mechanical clot disruption for thromboembolic stroke. *Am J Neuroradiol* 1994;15:1817–1822.
13. Smith WS, Sung G, Starkman S, Saver JL, Kidwell CS, Gobin YP, Lutsep HL, Nesbit GM, Grobelny T, Rymer MM, Silverman IE, Higashida RT, Budzik RF, Marks MP; MERCI Trial Investigators. Safety and efficacy of mechanical embolectomy in acute ischemic stroke: results of the MERCI trial. *Stroke* 2005;36:1432–1438.
14. Mayer TE, Hamann GF, Brueckmann H. Mechanical extraction of a basilar-artery embolus with the use of flow reversal and a microbasket. *N Engl J Med* 2002;347: 769–770.
15. Yu W, Binder D, Foster-Barber A, Malek R, Smith WS, Higashida RT. Endovascular embolectomy of acute basilar artery occlusion. *Neurology* 2003;61:1421–1423.
16. Ueda T, Hatakeyama T, Kohno K, Kumon Y, Sakaki S. Endovascular treatment for acute thrombotic occlusion of the middle cerebral artery: local intra-arterial thrombolysis combined with percutaneous transluminal angioplasty. *Neuroradiology* 1997;39:99–104.
17. Qureshi Al, Siddiqui AM, Kim SH, Hanel RA, Xavier AR, Kirmani JF, Suri MF, Boulos AS, Hopkins LN. Reocclusion of recanalized arteries during intra-arterial thrombolysis for acute ischemic stroke. *AJNR Am J Neuroradiol* 2004; 25:322–328.

18. Sussman BJ, Fitch TS. Thrombolysis with fibrinolysin in cerebral arterial occlusion. *J Am Med Assoc* 1958;167:1705–1709.

19. Lisboa RC, Jovanovic BD, Alberts MJ. Analysis of the safety and efficacy of intra-arterial thrombolytic therapy in ischemic stroke. *Stroke* 2002;33:2866–2871.

20. Nedeltchev K, Fischer U, Arnold M, Ballinari P, Haefeli T, Kappeler L, Brekenfeld C, Remonda L, Schroth G, Mattle HP. Long-term effect of intra-arterial thrombolysis in stroke. *Stroke* 2006;37:3002-3007.

21. Brekenfeld C, Remonda L, Nedeltchev K, v Bredow F, Ozdoba C, Wiest R, Arnold M, Mattle HP, Schroth G. Endovascular neuroradiological treatment of acute ischemic stroke: techniques and results in 350 patients. *Neurol Res* 2005; 27 (Suppl. 1):S29–S35.

22. del Zoppo GJ, Higashida RT, Furlan AJ, Pessin MS, Rowley HA, Gent M. PROACT: a phase II randomized trial of recombinant pro-urokinase by direct arterial delivery in acute middle cerebral artery stroke. PROACT Investigators. Prolyse in Acute Cerebral Thromboembolism. *Stroke* 1998;29:4–11.

23. Furlan A, Higashida R, Wechsler L, Gent M, Rowley H, Kase C, Pessin M, Ahuja A, Callahan F, Clark WM, Silver F, Rivera F. Intra-arterial prourokinase for acute ischemic stroke. The PROACT II study: a randomized controlled trial. Prolyse in Acute Cerebral Thromboembolism. *JAMA* 1999;282:2003–2011.

24. Kase CS, Furlan AJ, Wechsler LR, Higashida RT, Rowley HA, Hart RG, Molinari GF, Frederick LS, Roberts HC, Gebel JM, Sila CA, Schulz GA, Roberts RS, Gent M. Cerebral hemorrhage after intra-arterial thrombolysis for ischemic stroke: the PROACT II trial. *Neurology* 2001; 57:1603–1610.

25. Hill MD, Kent DM, Hinchey J, Rowley H, Buchan AM, Wechsler LR, Higashida RT, Fischbein NJ, Dillon WP, Gent M, Firszt CM, Schulz GA, Furlan AJ; PROACT-2 Investigators. Sex-based differences in the effect of intra-arterial treatment of stroke: analysis of the PROACT-2 study. *Stroke* 2006;37:2322–2325.

26. Arnold M, Nedeltchev K, Mattle HP, Loher TJ, Stepper F, Schroth G, Brekenfeld C, Sturzenegger M, Remonda L. Intra-arterial thrombolysis in 24 consecutive patients with internal carotid artery T occlusions. *J Neurol Neurosurg Psychiatry* 2003; 74:739–742.

27. Zaidat OO, Suarez Jl, Santillan C, Sunshine JL, Tarr RW, Paras VH, Selman WR, Landis DM. Response to intra-arterial and combined intravenous and intra-arterial thrombolytic therapy in patients with distal internal carotid artery occlusion. *Stroke* 2002;33:1821–1826.

28. Zeumer H, Hacke W, Ringelstein EB. Local intraarterial thrombolysis in vertebrobasilar thromboembolic disease. *Am J Neuroradiol* 1983;4:401–404.

29. Furlan A, Higashida R. Intra-arterial thrombolysis in acute ischemic Stroke. In: Mohr JP, Choi DW, Grotta JC, et al., eds. *Stroke: Pathophysiology, Diagnosis, and Management.* 4th ed. Philadelphia, PA: Churchill Livingstone; 2004 p. 943–951.

30. Lindsberg PJ, Mattle HP. Therapy of basilar artery occlusion: a systematic analysis comparing intra-arterial and intravenous thrombolysis. *Stroke* 2006;37:922–928.

31. Lewandowski CA, Frankel M, Tomsick TA, Broderick J, Frey J, Clark W, Starkman S, Grotta J, Spilker J, Khoury J, Brott T. Combined intravenous and intra-arterial r-TPA versus intra-arterial therapy of acute ischemic stroke: Emergency Management of Stroke (EMS) Bridging Trial. *Stroke* 1999;30:2598–2605.

32. Ernst R, Pancioli A, Tomsick T, Kissela B, Woo D, Kanter D, Jauch E, Carrozzella J, Spilker J, Broderick J. Combined intravenous and intra-arterial recombinant tissue plasminogen activator in acute ischemic stroke. *Stroke* 2000;31:2552–2557.

33. Suarez Jl, Zaidat OO, Sunshine JL, Tarr R, Selman WR, Landis DM. Endovascular administration after intravenous infusion of thrombolytic agents for the treatment of patients with acute ischemic strokes. *Neurosurgery* 2002;50:251–259 [discussion 259–260].
34. Combined intravenous and intra-arterial recanalization for acute ischemic stroke: the Interventional Management of Stroke Study. *Stroke* 2004;35:904–911.
35. Keris V, Rudnicka S, Vorona V, Enina G, Tilgale B, Fricbergs J. Combined intraarterial/intravenous thrombolysis for acute ischemic stroke. *Am J Neuroradiol* 2001;22:352–358.
36. Hill MD, Barber PA, Demchuk AM, Newcommon NJ, Cole-Haskayne A, Ryckborst K, Sopher L, Button A, Hu W, Hudon ME, Morrish W, Frayne R, Sevick RJ, Buchan AM. Acute intravenous–intra-arterial revascularization therapy for severe ischemic stroke. *Stroke* 2002;33:279–282.
37. Investigators TII. Preliminary Results of IMS II Trial. *Stroke* 2006; 37:708.
38. Broderick J, Tomsick T. The IMS trials. *Endovasc Today* 2006:1–3.
39. Smith WS. Safety of mechanical thrombectomy and intravenous tissue plasminogen activator in acute ischemic stroke. Results of the multi Mechanical Embolus Removal in Cerebral Ischemia (MERCI) trial, part I. *Am J Neuroradiol* 2006; 27: 1177–1182.
40. Lev MH, Farkas J, Gemmete JJ, Hossain ST, Hunter GJ, Koroshetz WJ, Gonzalez RG. Acute stroke: improved nonenhanced CT detection—benefits of soft-copy interpretation by using variable window width and center level settings. *Radiology* 1999;213:150–155.
41. Hacke W, Kaste M, Fieschi C, Toni D, Lesaffre E, von Kummer R, Boysen G, Bluhmki E, Hoxter G, Mahagne MH. Intravenous thrombolysis with recombinant tissue plasminogen activator for acute hemispheric stroke. The European Cooperative Acute Stroke Study (ECASS). *JAMA.* 1995;274:1017–1025.
42. Hunter GJ, Silvennoinen HM, Hamberg LM, Koroshetz WJ, Buonanno FS, Schwamm LH, Rordorf GA, Gonzalez RG. Whole-brain CT perfusion measurement of perfused cerebral blood volume in acute ischemic stroke: probability curve for regional infarction. *Radiology* 2003;227:725–730.
43. Wintermark M, Reichhart M, Thiran JP, Maeder P, Chalaron M, Schnyder P, Bogousslavsky J, Meuli R. Prognostic accuracy of cerebral blood flow measurement by perfusion computed tomography, at the time of emergency room admission, in acute stroke patients. *Ann Neurol* 2002;51:417–432.
44. Selim M, Kumar S, Fink J, Schlaug G, Caplan LR, Linfante I. Seizure at stroke onset: should it be an absolute contraindication to thrombolysis? *Cerebrovasc Dis* 2002;14:54–57.
45. Ay H, Buonanno FS, Rordorf G, Schaefer PW, Schwamm LH, Wu O, Gonzalez RG, Yamada K, Sorensen GA, Koroshetz WJ. Normal diffusion-weighted MRI during stroke-like deficits. *Neurology* 1999;52:1784–1792.
46. Schaefer PW. Applications of DWI in clinical neurology. *J Neurol Sci* 2001;186 (Suppl. 1):S25–S35.
47. Schaefer PW, Hassankhani A, Putman C, Sorensen AG, Schwamm L, Koroshetz W, Gonzalez RG. Characterization and evolution of diffusion MR imaging abnormalities in stroke patients undergoing intra-arterial thrombolysis. *Am J Neuroradiol* 2004;25:951–957.
48. Kidwell CS, Alger JR, Saver JL. Beyond mismatch: evolving paradigms in imaging the ischemic penumbra with multimodal magnetic resonance imaging. *Stroke* 2003; 34:2729–2735.
49. Schellinger PD, Fiebach JB, Hacke W. Imaging-based decision making in thrombolytic therapy for ischemic stroke: present status. *Stroke* 2003;34:575–583.
50. Davis SM, Butcher KS, Parsons MW, Barbar PA, Gerraty R, Frayne J, Talman P, Bladin C, Levi C, Herkes G, Watson J, Hankey G, Chalk J, Schultz D, Kimber T, Fink J, Muir K.

Echoplanar Imaging Thrombolysis Evaluation Trial: Epithet. 28th International Stroke Conference, Phoenix, Arizona, USA; February 2003.

51. Khatri P, Broderick J, Khoury JC, Carrozzella J, Tomsick T, for the IMS-1 and 2 Investigators. Microcatheter contrast injections during intra-arterial thrombolysis increase intracranial hemorrhage risk. International Stroke Conference; Kissimmee, Florida; 2006.
52. Greer DM, Koroshetz WJ, Cullen S, Gonzalez RG, Lev MH. Magnetic resonance imaging improves detection of intracerebral hemorrhage over computed tomography after intra-arterial thrombolysis. *Stroke* 2004;35:491–495.
53. Zeumer H, Freitag HJ, Zanella F, Thie A, Arning C. Local intra-arterial fibrinolytic therapy in patients with stroke: urokinase versus recombinant tissue plasminogen activator (r-TPA). *Neuroradiology* 1993;35:159–162.
54. Qureshi Al, Siddiqui AM, Suri MF, Kim SH, Ali Z, Yahia AM, Lopes DK, Boulos AS, Ringer AJ, Saad M, Guterman LR, Hopkins LN. Aggressive mechanical clot disruption and low-dose intra-arterial third-generation thrombolytic agent for ischemic stroke: a prospective study. *Neurosurgery* 2002;51:1319–1327 [discussion 1327–1319].
55. Cornu C, Boutitie F, Candelise L, Boissel JP, Donnan GA, Hommel M, Jaillard A, Lees KR. Streptokinase in acute ischemic stroke: an individual patient data meta-analysis: The Thrombolysis in Acute Stroke Pooling Project. *Stroke* 2000;31:1555–1560.
56. Kaur J, Zhao Z, Klein GM, Lo EH, Buchan AM. The neurotoxicity of tissue plasminogen activator? *J Cereb Blood Flow Metab* 2004;24:945–963.
57. Haley Jr EC, Lyden PD, Johnston KC, Hemmen TM. A pilot dose-escalation safety study of tenecteplase in acute ischemic stroke. *Stroke* 2005;36:607–612.
58. Hoh BL, Nogueira RG, O'Donnell J, Pryor JC, Rabinov JD, Hirsch JA, Rordorf GA, Buonanno FS, Koroshetz WJ, Schwamm LH. Intra-arterial thrombolysis for acute stroke: com parison of era using urokinase versus era not using urokinase at a single center. Seventh Joint Meeting of the AANS/ CNS Section on Cerebrovascular Surgery and the American Society of Interventional and Therapeutic Neuroradiology; San Diego, CA, USA; February, 2004.
59. Eckert B, Kucinski T, Neumaier-Probst E, Fiehler J, Rother J, Zeumer H. Local intra-arterial fibrinolysis in acute hemispheric stroke: effect of occlusion type and fibrinolytic agent on recanalization success and neurological outcome. *Cerebrovasc Dis* 2003;15:258–263.
60. Deitcher SR, Toombs CF. Non-clinical and clinical characterization of a novel acting thrombolytic: alfimeprase. *Pathophysiol Haemost Thromb* 2005;34:215–220.
61. Lapchak PA, Araujo DM, Pakola S, Song D, Wei J, Zivin JA. Microplasmin: a novel thrombolytic that improves behavioral outcome after embolic strokes in rabbits. *Stroke* 2002;33:2279–2284.
62. Sherman DG, Atkinson RP, Chippendale T, Levin KA, Ng K, Futrell N, Hsu CY, Levy DE. Intravenous ancrod for treatment of acute ischemic stroke: the STAT study: a randomized controlled trial. Stroke Treatment with Ancrod Trial. *JAMA* 2000;283:2395–2403.
63. Alexandrov AV, Grotta JC. Arterial reocclusion in stroke patients treated with intravenous tissue plasminogen activator. *Neurology* 2002;59:862–867.
64. Abciximab in acute ischemic stroke: a randomized, double-blind, placebo-controlled, dose-escalation study. The Abciximab in Ischemic Stroke Investigators. *Stroke* 2000; 31:601–609.
65. Eckert B, Koch C, Thomalla G, Roether J, Zeumer H. Acute basilar artery occlusion treated with combined intravenous Abciximab and intra-arterial tissue plasminogen activator: report of 3 cases. *Stroke* 2002;33:1424–1427.

66. Lee DH, Jo KD, Kim HG, Choi SJ, Jung SM, Ryu DS, Park MS. Local intraarterial urokinase thrombolysis of acute ischemic stroke with or without intravenous abciximab: a pilot study. *J Vasc Interv Radiol* 2002;13:769–774.
67. Deshmukh VR, Fiorella DJ, Albuquerque FC, Frey J, Flaster M, Wallace RC, Spetzler RF, McDougall CG. Intra-arterial thrombolysis for acute ischemic stroke: preliminary experience with platelet glycoprotein IIb/IIIa inhibitors as adjunctive therapy. *Neurosurgery* 2005;56:46–54 [discussion 54–45].
68. Mangiafico S, Cellerini M, Nencini P, Gensini G, Inzitari D. Intravenous glycoprotein IIb/IIIa inhibitor (tirofiban) followed by intra-arterial urokinase and mechanical thrombolysis in stroke. *Am J Neuroradiol* 2005;26:2595–2601.
69. Qureshi Al, Harris-Lane P, Kirmani JF, Janjua N, Divani AA, Mohammad YM, Suarez Jl, Montgomery MO. Intra-arterial reteplase and intravenous abciximab in patients with acute ischemic stroke: an open-label, dose-ranging, phase I study. *Neurosurgery* 2006;59:789–796 [discussion 796–787].
70. Bergui M, Stura G, Daniele D, Cerrato P, Berardino M, Bradac GB. Mechanical thrombolysis in ischemic stroke attributable to basilar artery occlusion as first-line treatment. *Stroke* 2006;37:145–150.
71. Kerber CW, Barr JD, Berger RM, Chopko BW. Snare retrieval of intracranial thrombus in patients with acute stroke. *J Vasc Interv Radiol* 2002;13:1269–1274.
72. Ueda T, Sakaki S, Nochide I, Kumon Y, Kohno K, Ohta S. Angioplasty after intra-arterial thrombolysis for acute occlusion of intracranial arteries. *Stroke* 1998;29:2568–2574.
73. Nakano S, Iseda T, Yoneyama T, Kawano H, Wakisaka S. Direct percutaneous transluminal angioplasty for acute middle cerebral artery trunk occlusion: an alternative option to intra-arterial thrombolysis. *Stroke* 2002;33:2872–2876.
74. Abou-Chebl A, Bajzer CT, Krieger DW, Furlan AJ, Yadav JS. Multimodal therapy for the treatment of severe ischemic stroke combining GPIIb/IIIa antagonists and angioplasty after failure of thrombolysis. *Stroke* 2005;36:2286–2288.
75. Nogueira RG, Schwamm LH, Buonanno FS, Koroshetz WJ, Rabinov JD, Pryor JC, Hirsch JA. Angioplasty of acute occluded intracranial arteries with low-pressure silicone balloons. ASITN 3rd Annual Course and Workshops; San Juan, Puerto Rico; August 2006.
76. Berlis A, Lutsep H, Barnwell S, Norbash A, Wechsler L, Jungreis CA, Woolfenden A, Redekop G, Hartmann M, Schumacher M. Mechanical thrombolysis in acute ischemic stroke with endovascular photoacoustic recanalization. *Stroke* 2004;35:1112–1116.
77. Nesbit GM, Luh G, Tien R, Barnwell SL. New and future endovascular treatment strategies for acute ischemic stroke. *J Vasc Interv Radiol* 2004;15:S103–S110.
78. Lutsep H. Mechanical thrombolysis in acute stroke: emedicine; November 2, 2006.
79. Gralla J, Schroth G, Remonda L, Nedeltchev K, Slotboom J, Brekenfeld C. Mechanical thrombectomy for acute ischemic stroke: thrombus-device interaction, efficiency, and complications *in vivo*. *Stroke* 2006;37:3019–3024.
80. Chapot R. First experience with the Catch, a new device for cerebral thrombectomy. *Intervent Neuroradiol* 2005;11(Suppl. 2):58.
81. Hans Henkes JR, Lowens S, Miloslavski E, Roth C, Reith W, Kühne D. A device for fast mechanical clot retrieval from intracranial arteries (Phenox Clot Retriever). *Neurocrit Care* 2006;5:134–140.
82. Schumacher HC, Meyers PM, Yavagal DR, Harel NY, Elkind MS, Mohr JP, Pile-Spellman J. Endovascular mechanical thrombectomy of an occluded superior

division branch of the left MCA for acute cardioembolic stroke. *Cardiovasc Intervent Radiol* 2003;26:305–308.

83. Veznedaroglu E, Levy EI. Endovascular management of acute symptomatic intracranial arterial occlusion. *Neurosurgery* 2006;59:S242–S250.
84. Henkes H, Lowens S, Preiss H, Reinartz J, Miloslavski E, Kuhne D. A new device for endovascular coil retrieval from intracranial vessels: alligator retrieval device. *Am J Neuroradiol* 2006;27:327–329.
85. Mahon BR, Nesbit GM, Barnwell SL, Clark W, Marotta TR, Weill A, Teal PA, Qureshi AI. North American clinical experience with the EKOS MicroLysUS infusion catheter for the treatment of embolic stroke. *Am J Neuroradiol* 2003;24:534–538.
86. Groups TTeaftIIIS. ASITN/JSCVS Annual Meeting; Orlando, Florida; February 2006.
87. Alexandrov AV, Molina CA, Grotta JC, Garami Z, Ford SR, Alvarez-Sabin J, Montaner J, Saqqur M, Demchuk AM, Moye LA, Hill MD, Wojner AW; CLOTBUST Investigators. Ultrasound-enhanced systemic thrombolysis for acute ischemic stroke. *N Engl J Med* 2004;351:2170–2178.
88. Levy El, Ecker RD, Horowitz MB, Gupta R, Hanel RA, Sauvageau E, Jovin TG, Guterman LR, Hopkins LN. Stent-assisted intracranial recanalization for acute stroke: early results. *Neurosurgery* 2006;58:458–463 [discussion 458–463].
89. Levy El, Sauvageau E, Hanel RA, Parikh R, Hopkins LN. Self-expanding versus balloon-mounted stents for vessel recanalization following embolic occlusion in the canine model: technical feasibility study. *Am J Neuroradiol* 2006;27:2069–2072.
90. Jea B. ASITN/JSCVS Annual Meeting; *Orlando, Florida*; February 2006.
91. Fitzsimmons BF, Becske T, Nelson PK. Rapid stent-supported revascularization in acute ischemic stroke. *Am J Neuroradiol.* 2006;27:1132–1134.
92. Sauvageau E, Levy EI. Self-expanding stent-assisted middle cerebral artery recanalization: technical note. *Neuroradiology* 2006;48:405–408.
93. Henkes H, Miloslavski E, Lowens S, Reinartz J, Liebig T, Kuhne D. Treatment of intracranial atherosclerotic stenoses with balloon dilatation and self-expanding stent deployment (WingSpan). *Neuroradiology* 2005;47:222–228.
94. Jovin TG, Gupta R, Uchino K, Jungreis CA, Wechsler LR, Hammer MD, Tayal A, Horowitz MB. Emergent stenting of extracranial internal carotid artery occlusion in acute stroke has a high revascularization rate. *Stroke* 2005; 36:2426–2430.
95. Chapot R, Houdart E, Rogopoulos A, Mounayer C, Saint-Maurice JP, Merland JJ. Thromboaspiration in the basilar artery: report of two cases. *Am J Neuroradiol* 2002;23:282–284.
96. Lutsep HL, Clark WM, Nesbit GM, Kuether TA, Barnwell SL. Intraarterial suction thrombectomy in acute stroke. *Am J Neuroradiol* 2002;23:783–786.
97. Bellon RJ, Putman CM, Budzik RF, Pergolizzi RS, Reinking GF, Norbash AM. Rheolytic thrombectomy of the occluded internal carotid artery in the setting of acute ischemic stroke. *Am J Neuroradiol* 2001; 22:526–530.
98. Molina CA, Saver JL. Extending reperfusion therapy for acute ischemic stroke: emerging pharmacological, mechanical, and imaging strategies. *Stroke* 2005;36:2311–2320.
99. Bose A, Jansen O. Clinical safety and performance of the penumbra stroke system: a novel device for the treatment of acute stroke due to large vessel occlusive disease. European Stroke Conference; Brussels, Belgium; May 2006.

5

NONTHROMBOLYTIC ACUTE STROKE THERAPIES

Aneesh B. Singhal, Larami MacKenzie, and Joshua M. Levine

INTRODUCTION

The past few years have witnessed significant advances in the field of acute stroke therapy. As discussed in other chapters, the therapeutic efficacy of early thrombolysis using intravenous tissue plasminogen activator (IV rt-PA) has been confirmed in randomized multicenter trials and in the community hospital setting. The data regarding safety and efficacy of intra-arterial thrombolysis are being investigated. While early arterial recanalization is undoubtedly the most potent strategy to reduce brain injury after stroke, it needs to be accomplished rapidly (within 3 hours for IV rt-PA) to reduce the risk of potentially fatal complications such as brain hemorrhage. The narrow time window for administering IV rt-PA, and the high risk for complications, has curtailed its use to less than 4–5% of patients in the United States. While efforts to increase the time window and safety of rt-PA are ongoing, it is also important to develop alternative nonthrombolytic (neuroprotective) stroke treatments that may be more applicable to the majority of stroke patients in whom thrombolysis is not a viable option.

Theoretically, neuroprotection after stroke can be achieved using pharmaceutical or physiological therapies that inhibit biochemical, metabolic, or cellular pathways of ischemic cell death. The major mechanisms of ischemic cell death include excitotoxicity and acidotoxicity, oxidative and nitrosative stress, apoptosis, inflammation, and peri-infarct deplorarization.[1–3] These fundamental cell death mechanisms are complex and overlapping, affect gray matter and white matter in different ways, and evolve together over time to mediate injury in neurons, glial

Acute Ischemic Stroke: An Evidence-based Approach, Edited by David M. Greer.

cells, and vascular structures (Fig. 5.1). The individual contribution of each pathway toward the overall stroke-related injury varies[4] and is highly dependent on the duration and the severity of ischemia. Knowledge gained from over five decades of basic science research has revealed multiple molecular and biochemical targets within each of these fundamental cell death pathways. Neuroprotective drugs have been developed for many of these targets. While no agent has proved efficacious in phase III clinical trials, it is recognized that these trials had many shortcomings, such as small sample sizes or poor patient selection. The encouraging results of animal studies, combined with advances in clinical trial design, raise hope that successful neuroprotection will be achieved in the near future. In this chapter, we review the major nonthrombolytic or neuroprotective approaches to stroke management, including pharmaceutical drug trials and physiological approaches.

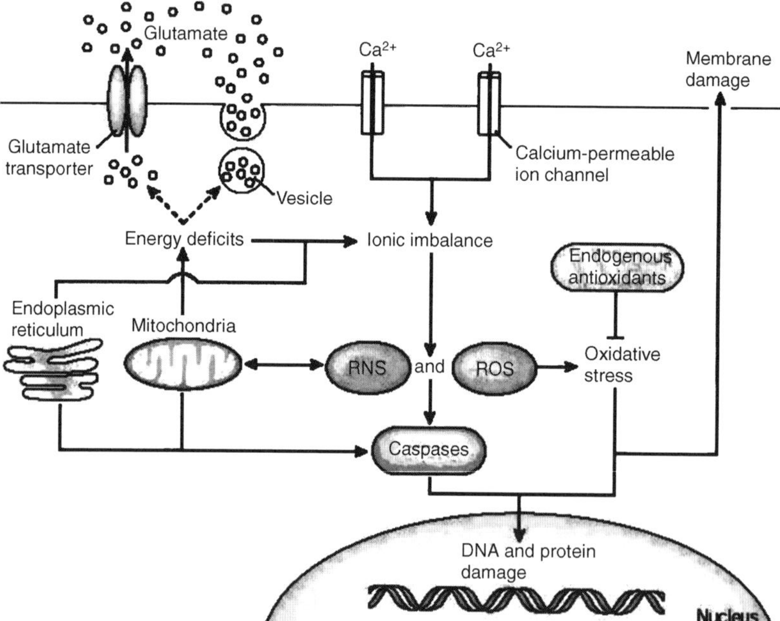

FIGURE 5.1 Major pathways implicated in ischemic cell death: excitotoxicity, ionic imbalance, oxidative and nitrosative stresses, and apoptotic-like mechanisms. There is extensive interaction and overlap between multiple mediators of cell injury and cell death. After ischemic onset, loss of energy substrates leads to mitochondrial dysfunction and generation of reactive oxygen species (ROS) and reactive nitrogen species (RNS). Additionally, energy deficits lead to ionic imbalance and excitotoxic glutamate efflux and build up of intracellular calcium. Downstream pathways ultimately include direct free radical damage to membrane lipids, cellular proteins, and DNA, as well as calcium-activated proteases, plus caspase cascades that dismantle a wide range of homeostatic, reparative, and cytoskeletal proteins. (Reprinted with permission from reference 1.)

PREVIOUS STROKE NEUROPROTECTIVE TRIALS

Over the past 15 years, over 85 phase II and phase III drug trials have been conducted to investigate the clinical efficacy of stroke neuroprotective drugs that target one or more pathways of cell death.[5] These drugs were developed based on the promising results of over a thousand experimental studies in animal stroke models.[6] Unfortunately, no drug has survived the challenge of clinical testing. The most notable failure is the SAINT-II trial of NXY-059, a free radical scavenger. Rodent and primate studies had shown remarkable efficacy with this drug, and the initial SAINT-I trial in Australasia and Europe showed that NXY-059 improved functional outcome after acute stroke and reduced the risk of thrombolytic-associated hemorrhage.[7] The field of stroke neuroprotection was optimistic that SAINT-II, the largest ever acute stroke trial, would yield positive results. However, like numerous other trials of nonthrombolytic drugs, SAINT-II proved to be a negative trial and the company (Astra-Zeneca) terminated plans to further investigate the potential of this drug to treat stroke. Previous drugs that failed clinical trials include the lipid peroxidation inhibitor tirilazad mesylate,[8] the ICAM-1 antibody enlimomab,[9] the recombinant basic fibroblast growth factor Trafermin,[10] the sodium channel blocker fosphenytoin, the calcium channel blocker nimodipine,[11] the GABA agonist clomethiazole,[12,13] the glutamate antagonist and sodium channel blocker lubeluzole,[14] the competitive NMDA antagonist selfotel,[15] and several noncompetitive NMDA antagonists (dextrorphan, gavestinel, aptiganel, and eliprodil).

The failure of these predominantly industry-sponsored clinical trials has been devastating for the field of stroke neuroprotection. Some of these failures may indeed be attributable to the lack of efficacy of the drug being tested. However, these past failures have also exposed the shortcomings of clinical trial designs, such as inadequate sample sizes, poor patient selection, and suboptimal choice of outcome measures. Efforts are underway to understand and address the reasons behind the failure of previous trials. The results of a recent meta-analysis[6] indicate that the process of preclinical testing and drug selection for clinical trials was inadequate, and more stringent guidelines have been proposed.[6,16,17] Neuroimaging is being advocated as a means to optimize patient selection, and attention is being paid to developing clinical outcome measures that are more sensitive and better suited for the drug being tested.[18] The focus is shifting toward the use of drugs and physiological strategies as adjunctive therapies that expand the therapeutic time window for thrombolysis, and the development of combination therapies that target multiple rather than a single pathway of cell death. These and other advances provide reason to remain optimistic about the future of stroke neuroprotection. While a detailed review of past failures is beyond the scope of this chapter, the following sections provide a summary of a few highly promising drugs that failed clinical testing and a review of ongoing phase II and phase III clinical trials.

PHARMACEUTICAL DRUG TRIALS

Antioxidants/Free Radical Scavengers

A trial of Ebselen PZ51, a selenoorganic compound with glutathione peroxidase-like action, is currently in phase III of clinical trial. A small, randomized, double-blind, placebo-controlled trial of Ebselen initiated within 48 hours after stroke suggested protective efficacy as measured by the Glascow Outcome Scale (GOS) and Barthel Index (BI) at 1 month ($p = 0.023$), but not at 3 months ($p = 0.056$). Better clinical outcomes were observed if Ebselen administration was initiated less than 24 hours after symptom onset, but not greater than 24 hours.[19] The Edaravone Acute Infarction Study (EAIS), a double-blind, randomized, placebo-controlled study looking at the effect of Edaravone (MCI-186) administered within 72 hours after ischemic stroke onset, yielded promising results (modified Rankin Scale [mRS] score significantly improved; $p = 0.0382$).[20] The agent has been clinically available in Japan since 2001; however, it has not been followed up with either further study or clinical usage in the United States. A recent Japanese study of Edaravone in cardioembolic stroke suggested it may only be useful in patients with mild stroke (National Institutes of Health Stroke Scale (NIHSS) score < 8); however, the trend toward long-term function seemed not to favor Edaravone.[21]

Metal cations play a key role in free radical propagation and endothelial and lipid injury. Deferoxamine, an iron chelator, is under phase I investigation as a neuroprotectant after acute stroke. Because iron is the catalyst of the Fenton cycle, deferoxamine–iron binding could act as an indirect free-radical scavenger. Additionally, deferoxamine is thought to stabilize hypoxia-inducible factor-1 (HIF-1), one of the transcription factors that increases the expression of erythropoietin and vascular endothelial growth factor. In a rat model of middle cerebral artery (MCA) stroke, deferoxamine administration as late as 24 hours after stroke onset has been shown to reduce infarct volume by as much as 28% and to improve functional recovery.[22] DP-b99 is a lipophilic membrane-activated metal cation chelator. It has been shown to be safe in humans and has entered a phase IIb trial, looking at neuroprotective effects when administered within 9 hours of stroke.[23]

GABA Agonism

The Early GABAergic Activation in Stroke Trial (EGASIS) looked at the use of diazepam administration within 12 hours after both ischemic and hemorrhagic stroke onset. The rationale for diazepam use includes both its inhibitory effect on harmful neuronal nitric oxide synthase activity and on neuronal hyperpolarization by increased GABA-A-mediated chloride conductance. Although the treatment seemed to worsen hemorrhagic stroke outcome due to an increase in pneumonia and death, in the subgroup of ischemic stroke there was a trend toward statistical significance for the primary endpoint of functional independence at 3 months. Importantly, in the ischemic stroke subgroup, diazepam treatment did show significance for the secondary endpoint of "complete recovery." For unclear reasons, cardioembolic strokes had a better response to treatment.[24] At this stage it is difficult to interpret this favorable *post hoc* analysis, particularly when determination of cardioembolic stroke etiology is difficult in the hyperacute setting. The utility of acute GABA agonism using diazepam cannot be settled without further study, which might be limited by the lack of patent protection.

Serotonin Agonists

Repinotan or BAYx3702 is a potent 5HT-1a receptor agonist that binds to pre- and postsynaptic serotonin receptors. It is believed to exert neuroprotection directly via G protein-coupled inwardly rectifying potassium channels which hyperpolarize neurons, block glutamate release, and reduce neuronal firing rates.[25] In experimental stroke models, it reduces infarct volume when administered up to 5 hours after stroke onset. A phase II trial demonstrated safety, and there was a trend toward beneficial effect on functional outcome at 3 months when started within 6 hours of stroke onset and continued for 72 hours.[26] Repinotan is currently being evaluated in several phase III trials including the Repinotan Stroke Study, the Repinotan in Acute Ischemic Stroke trial, and the Repinotan-Randomized Exposure Controlled Trial (RECT). Piclozotan, or SUN N4057, another selective 5HT-1a receptor agonist, has been shown to be neuroprotective in a rat model of transient MCA occlusion.[27] Patients are currently being recruited for a phase IIb trial looking at both 6-hour and 6–9 hour windows in patients with a demonstrable ischemic penumbra on perfusion–diffusion imaging.

Statins

3-Hydroxy-3-methylglutaryl–coenzyme A (HMG-CoA) reductase inhibitors (statins) have been shown to improve vascular outcomes due to their cholesterol-lowering effects as well as multiple pleiotropic effects.[28] In high-risk populations, statin therapy is known to reduce the risk of vascular events such as myocardial infarction and stroke. A meta-analysis of 10 trials involving 79,494 subjects[29] showed that statin therapy reduced the incidence of stroke by 18%, major coronary events by 27%, and all-cause mortality by 15%. The SPARCL trial recently showed that high-dose HMG-CoA reductase inhibitors prevent recurrent stroke and transient ischemic attacks.[30]

In rodent stroke models, statin pretreatment has been shown to reduce infarct volumes and improve outcomes.[31,32] Similarly, several clinical studies have shown that prior statin use reduced the severity of acute ischemic stroke and myocardial infarction.[33–36] Recent studies indicate that benefit can be achieved even when treatment is initiated after the onset of symptoms. In rodents, atorvastatin and simvastatin have been shown to reduce the growth of ischemic lesions, enhance functional outcome, and induce brain plasticity when administered after stroke onset.[37,38] A retrospective analysis of the population-based Northern Manhattan Stroke Study (NOMASS)[39] showed that patients using lipid-lowering agents at the time of ischemic stroke have a lower incidence of in-hospital stroke progression and reduced 90-day mortality rates. Retrospective analysis of data of the phase III citicoline trial showed that poststroke statin use (123 patients) predicted good functional outcome (measured by mRS and NIHSS scores) at 3 months.[40] Clinical trials have also provided some evidence of improved poststroke outcomes with statin use. A small pilot study from Spain showed significant improvement in the 3-day and 90-day NIHSS scores in patients treated with simvastatin 3–12 hours after stroke onset, as compared to placebo-treated patients.[41] Adding to these data, several groups have reported that statins reduce the incidence and severity of vasospasm after subarachnoid hemorrhage.[42,43] Furthermore, recent animal and human studies of subarachnoid hemorrhage and ischemic stroke indicate that statin withdrawal may have deleterious effects.[44,45] Based on these preliminary data, clinical trials of statin therapy in acute stroke have been initiated. The FASTER Trial, looking at combination antiplatelet/statin therapy started within 24 hours after minor stroke/TIA, may better address the effect of statin use in the acute setting, although the trial is designed to look at stroke recurrence.

Platelet Inhibition

The GP IIb–IIIa complex inhibitor Tirofiban has been used as an adjunct to thrombolysis in a number of small case series reports.[46] A small transcranial Doppler (TCD) study suggests that it reduces microembolization from unstable carotid plaque.[47] In an open pilot study, Tirofiban administered within 9 hours after stroke onset blocked the conversion of ischemic penumbra to mature infarction.[48] A phase III study (SETIS) has started recruiting patients to investigate its efficacy versus aspirin within the 6-hour window.

Anti-Inflammatory Agents

"Anakinra/Kineret," an IL-1 receptor antagonist approved for use in rheumatoid arthritis, was recently evaluated in a small phase II trial. When initiated within 6 hours after stroke onset, Anakinra treatment yielded promising preliminary results: it was deemed safe with demonstrable biologic activity and likely favorable clinical outcome.[49]

Erythropoietin (EPO)

EPO is considered one of the most promising stroke therapeutic agents. The mechanistic pathways by which EPO provides its neuroprotective effects remain to be fully elucidated; however, it is hypothesized that they involve an EPO receptor distinct from that activated in erythropoiesis. EPO has pleiotropic effects: it has been shown to cross the blood–brain barrier, protect against ischemia–reperfusion injury by inhibiting apoptosis and hypoxia, and enhance angiogenesis. When directly administered into the brain, EPO reduces neurologic dysfunction in rodent models of stroke, and reduces infarct volumes by 75% when administered systemically up to 3 hours after arterial occlusion. In a small ($n = 40$), randomized, double-blind, placebo-controlled trial of EPO administered intravenously between 2 hours and 40 minutes and 7 hours and 55 minutes after stroke symptom onset, the agent was found to be safe, and treatment correlated with a reduction in NIHSS score between baseline and day 30 after stroke.[50] Furthermore, there was a strong trend toward functional improvement as measured by mRS and BI (Fig. 5.2) and infarct reduction on brain MRI, as well as a significant reduction in the neuronal injury marker S100beta in the EPO arm 30 days after infarct.

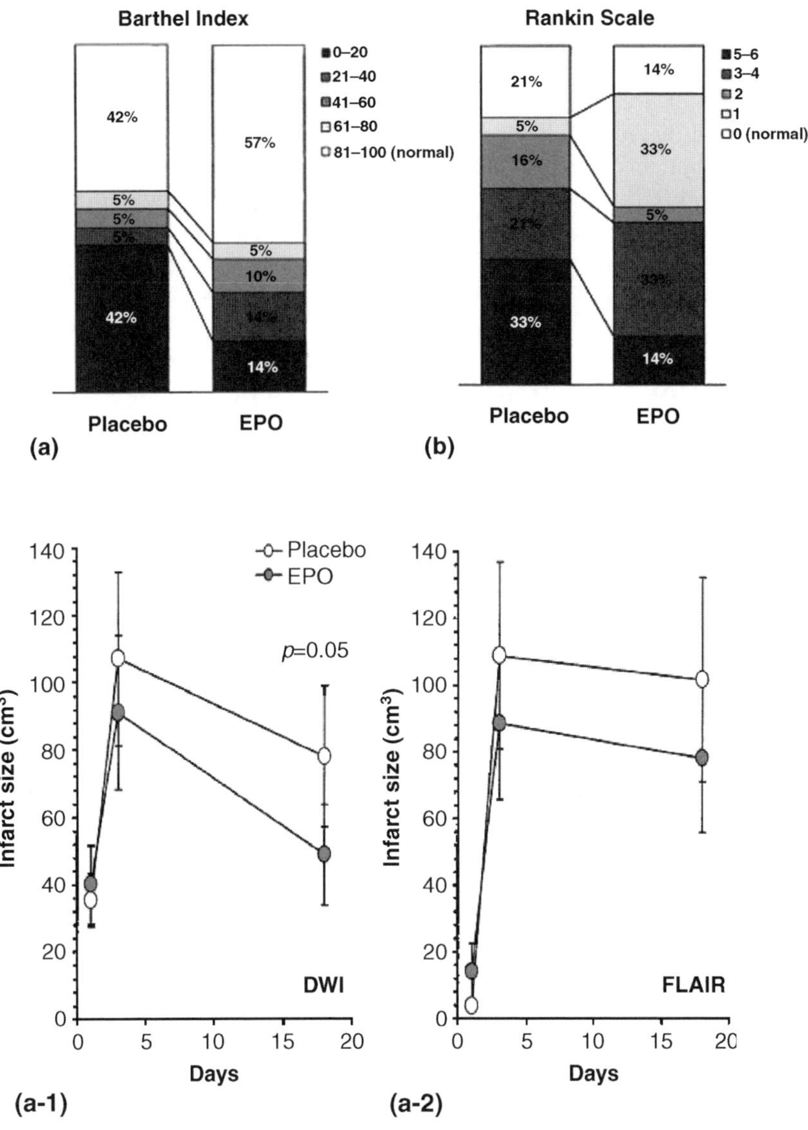

FIGURE 5.2 Clinical outcome of patients in the double-blind, proof-of-concept trial evaluating EPO in acute stroke. (**a**) Barthel Index (rhEPO vs. placebo, $p < 0.05$). (**b**) Modified Rankin Scale (rhEPO vs. placebo, $p < 0.07$) on day 30. Dead patients received the worst possible score. Evolution of lesion size of patients in the efficacy trial of Albumin in acute stroke. ((a-1) and DWI and (a-2) FLAIR.) (Reprinted with permission from reference 50.)

Citicoline

Citicoline (cytidine-5′-diphosphocholine or CDP-choline) is an intermediate in the biosynthesis of phosphatidylcholine and is a neuronal membrane stabilizer. Citicoline showed immense promise in animal studies and in several phase II clinical trials. However, a phase III efficacy trial failed to show benefit. Despite this negative result, many believe that citicoline still holds promise as a stroke therapy. This is because in a *post hoc* analysis, citicoline was found to reduce ischemic lesion growth on diffusion-weighted MRI (DWI) when administered orally within 24 hours of ischemic stroke[52], and a meta-analysis of four citicoline trials showed that a good outcome at 3 months was achieved in 25.2% of citicoline-treated patients versus 20.2% of controls (odds ratio [OR] 1.33; 95% confidence interval [CI] 1.10–1.62; $p = 0.0034$).[53] The International Citicoline Trial on Acute Stroke (ICTUS) is an ongoing study designed to examine the neuroprotective effects of citicoline on clinical outcome after stroke when administered intravenously within 24 hours after stroke, followed by oral dosing.

NONPHARMACEUTICAL APPROACHES

Albumin

Ginsberg's pioneering animal research has shown that albumin infusions enhance red cell perfusion and suppress thrombosis and leukocyte adhesion in the microcirculation, particularly during the early reperfusion phase.[54] Albumin also improves microcirculatory flow, plasma viscosity, red cell deformability, and oxygen transport capacity. In addition, albumin has potent antioxidant and antiapoptotic effects. In experimental stroke, albumin has been shown to reduce infarct size, improve neurofunction scores, and reduce brain edema.[55] In the Albumin in Acute Stroke (ALIAS) phase II trial, an open-labeled, dose-escalation, nonrandomized pilot clinical trial conducted at two centers in North America, albumin was found to be safe and effective in reducing stroke-related brain injury.[56,57] Eighty-two subjects with an NIHSS>6 received 25% albumin within 16 hours of stroke onset in two doses, 0.34–1.03 and 1.37–2.05 g/kg. Nearly half of the patients (42) also received rt-PA. The probability of a good clinical outcome at 3 months was greater in the high-dose cohort than in the low-dose cohort (relative risk [RR] 1.81; 95% CI 1.11–2.94), and compared to the NINDS rt-PA Stroke Study cohort (RR 1.95; 95% CI 1.47–2.57). The high-dose albumin cohort members who received concomitant rt-PA were three times more likely to achieve a good outcome than those subjects receiving both lower dose albumin and rt-PA, suggesting a synergistic effect between albumin and rt-PA. Over the course of 3 months after treatment, the NIHSS scores progressively improved in the high-dose albumin group, but did not improve in the low-dose cohort (Fig. 5.3a), achieving statistically significant improvement in the high-dose albumin/rt-PA cohort. Both with and without rt-PA, the distribution of functional outcome scores (mRS scores) in the high- and low-dose albumin groups favored the high-dose albumin cohort (Fig. 5.3b), where 68.2% of patients in the

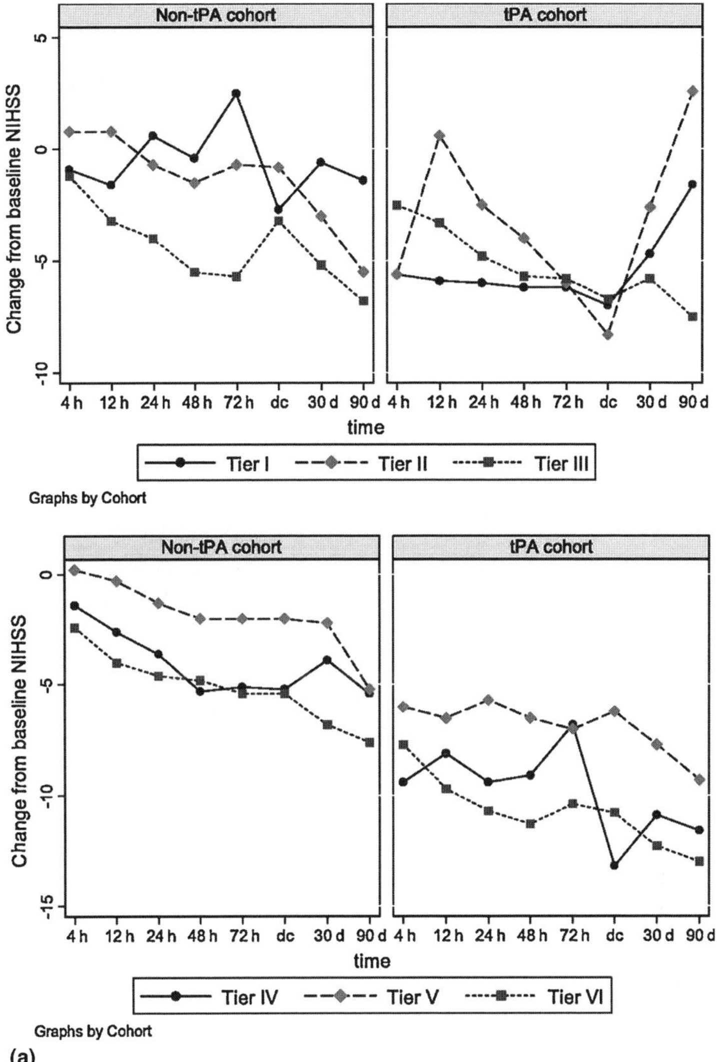

FIGURE 5.3 The Albumin in Acute Stroke (ALIAS) Phase II Trial. Data represent mean ± SEM. p-Value according to multiple regression analysis. Dead patients have been censored. (a) Mean change in NIH Stroke Scale score over time since treatment in rt-PA and non-rt-PA cohorts receiving the three lowest doses (Tiers I, 0.34 mg/kg; II, 0.68 mg/kg; III, 1.03 mg/kg) and three highest doses of albumin (Tiers IV, 1.37 mg/kg; V, 1.71 mg/kg; VI, 2.03 mg/kg).

high-dose albumin/rt-PA group had a good outcome at 3 months (mRS 0–1). In 13% of the patients who received high-dose albumin, the major side effect was pulmonary edema, which was responsive to diuresis. Based on these encouraging results, the phase III multicenter ALIAS trial has been initiated.

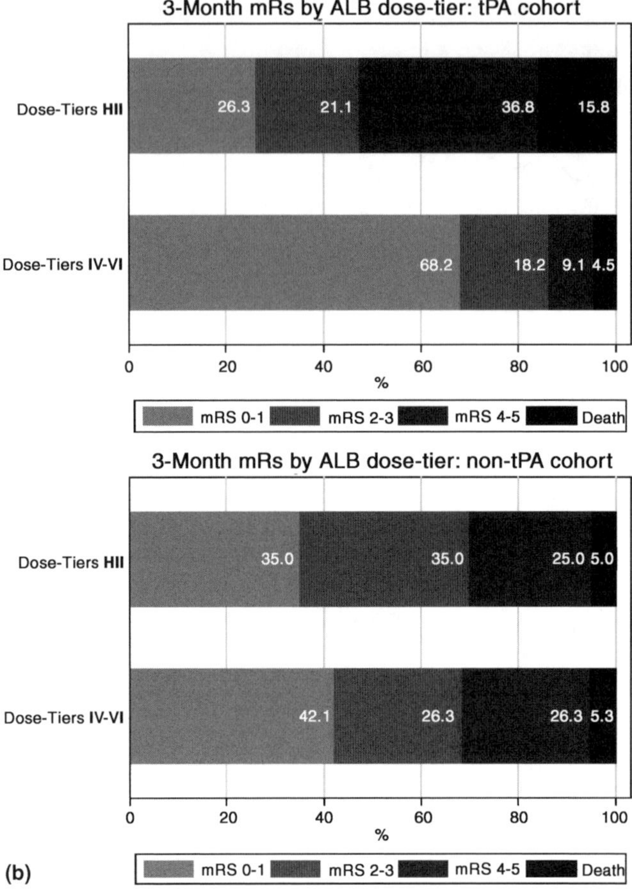

FIGURE 5.3 (*Continued*) (b) Distribution of modified Rankin Scale (mRS) scores at 3 months in the lower (I–III) and higher (IV–VI) albumin dose tiers for the rt-PA and non-rt-PA cohorts. (Reprinted with permission from reference 57.)

Magnesium

Magnesium has many neuroprotective properties. It inhibits presynaptic glutamate release,[58] blocks NMDA receptors,[59] antagonizes calcium channels, and maintains cerebral blood flow.[60] In animal models, intravenous magnesium administered as late as 6 hours after stroke onset reduced infarct volumes.[61,62] In pilot clinical studies, magnesium was found to reduce death and disability from stroke, raising expectations that magnesium could be a safe and inexpensive treatment.[63] *Intravenous MAGnesium Efficacy in Stroke* (IMAGES) was a large multicenter trial involving 2589 patients treated with IV magnesium or normal saline (placebo) within 12 hours after acute stroke. The primary clinical outcome, death or disability at 3 months, was not improved by magnesium, although some benefit was observed in subcortical (lacunar) strokes.[64] *MR-IMAGES* is an ongoing substudy designed to assess whether magnesium reduces the frequency of infarct growth on serial MRI studies. *Field Administration of Stroke Therapy–Magnesium* (FAST-MAG) is an ongoing phase III trial designed to determine whether ultra-early initiation of intravenous magnesium sulfate supplementation by paramedics is neuroprotective.[65]

Transcranial Doppler Ultrasound

The therapeutic principal of TCD is based on using ultrasound energy to disrupt clot by increasing clot surface area and consequent exposure to thrombolytic agents. Initial attempts at using ultrasound were mired by safety issues. The TRUMB study (Transcranial Low-Frequency Ultrasound Mediated Thrombolysis in Brain Ischemia Study) utilized 300 kHz ultrasound with concurrent rt-PA. The phase II trial was abandoned after 93% of patients developed brain hemorrhage. However, subsequent efforts using a different range of ultrasound energy focused at the site of arterial obstruction have shown positive results. The Combined Lysis of Thrombus in Brain Ischemia Using Transcranial Ultrasound and Systemic t-PA (CLOTBUST) phase II study demonstrated complete arterial recanalization within 2 hours in 49% of patients treated with TCD and rt-PA compared to 30% recanalization in the group that received rt-PA alone.[66] There was a nonsignificant trend toward clinical recovery within 2 hours in 29% of patients receiving the combination, compared to 21% in those receiving rt-PA alone. In addition, a 3-month mRS score of 0–1 was found in 42% of the patients with combined therapy compared to 29% who received rt-PA alone (Fig. 5.4). In another phase II trial of TCD-assisted thrombolysis, the addition of multiple boluses of microbubbles to the 2-hours middle cerebral artery TCD insonation facilitated and accelerated recanalization.[67] Two additional trials of microbubbles with TCD (MUST and NANOART) are ongoing.

Decompressive Craniectomy

Malignant or life-threatening MCA territory infarction occurs in up to 10% of strokes and is associated with an 80% mortality rate. Stroke progression and

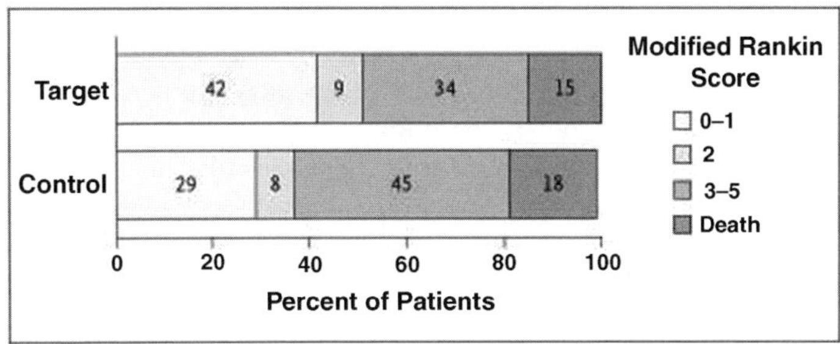

FIGURE 5.4 Outcomes at 3 months in the CLOTBUST trial. Favorable outcomes were defined as a score of 0–1 on the modified Rankin Scale, indicating little or no disability. A total of 42% of patients in the target group who were eligible for follow-up and 29% of those in the control group met these criteria. Other outcomes included a modified Rankin Score of 2 (9% in the target group vs. 8% in the control group); a score of 3–5 (34% in the target group vs. 45% in the control group); and death (15% in the target group vs. 18% in the control group). (Reprinted with permission from reference 66.)

extension into the anterior and posterior cerebral artery territories results in massive brain edema and elevated intracerebral pressures, ultimately causing brain herniation. Theoretically, patients with impending malignant edema may benefit from decompressive craniectomy to reduce intracranial pressure and prevent herniation. Predicting malignant MCA edema is therefore important and multiple investigators have attempted to predict the development of malignant brain edema using techniques such as CT, magnetic resonance imaging (MRI), positron emission tomography (PET), and microdialysis. Multiple case series have identified predictors, such as presence of a third nerve palsy, depth of coma, presence of posturing, and the age of the patient to identify which patients will fare well with surgery. As with thrombolysis, it seems intuitive that the earlier the intervention, the greater the likelihood of preserving the penumbra and promoting a good outcome. Nonrandomized studies have shown that decompressive hemicraniectomy improves survival rates. A pooled analysis of 93 patients with malignant MCA infarction undergoing surgery within 48 hours from three ongoing randomized controlled trials in Europe (DECIMAL, DESTINY, HAMLET) was recently published.[68] An mRS score of 4 or lower was achieved in 75% operated patients versus 24% of controls (pooled absolute risk reduction or ARR 51%; 95% CI 34–69); an mRS of 3 or lower in 43% versus 21% (ARR 23%; 95% CI 5–41), and survival in 78% versus 29% (ARR 50%; 95% CI 33–67).

COMBINATION THERAPY FOR STROKE

Targeting a single cell death pathway has so far proved unsuccessful. Efforts are now being directed toward combining drugs that target distinct pathways in order to enhance the degree of neuroprotection. Various neuroprotective combinations have been used with some success in animal models, including the co-administration of an NMDA receptor antagonist with GABA receptor agonists,[69] citicholine,[70] free radical scavengers,[71] cyclohexamide,[72] caspase inhibitors,[73] or growth factors such as fibroblast growth factor (bFGF).[74] Synergy is also observed with two different antioxidants,[75] and with citicoline plus basic bFGF.[76] Caspase inhibitors delivered with bFGF or an NMDA receptor antagonist have been shown to potentially extend the therapeutic window for thrombolysis with lower effective doses.[77]

Another rationale for combination drug therapy is that agents that decrease reperfusion injury, reduce postischemic hemorrhage, and inhibit downstream targets in cell death cascades may prove useful in increasing the efficacy and safety of thrombolytic drugs such as rt-PA. Synergistic or additive effects have been reported with the combination of thrombolytics with free radical scavengers,[78] AMPA receptor antagonists,[79] NMDA blockers,[80] MMP inhibitors,[81] citicoline,[82] topiramate,[83] antileukocytic adhesion antibodies,[84] and antithrombotics.[85] Two recent clinical trials have reported the feasibility and safety of intravenous rt-PA combined with neuroprotectants, albumin, clomethiazole,[86] and lubeluzole.[87] However, in the SAINT trial[7] the combination of NXY-059 and rt-PA did not yield any clinical benefit over rt-PA treatment alone.

PHYSIOLOGICAL STRATEGIES

Hypothermia

As with all molecular and biochemical pathways, the major mechanisms of cell death are temperature-dependent. Hypothermia can protect against multiple deleterious processes, including oxidative stress, inflammation, lipid peroxidation, and activation of cysteine or serine proteases.[88–94] Each degree of temperature decline reduces the rate of cellular respiration, oxygen demand, carbon dioxide production by 10%.[95] Preclinical and clinical results have been encouraging, making hypothermia an attractive physiological therapy that targets multiple injury mechanisms. However, the therapeutic time window for hypothermia is narrow.[96] In one study, hypothermia proved beneficial if initiated 30 minutes before stroke onset, but not 10 minutes after stroke onset.[97]

While moderate hypothermia (28–32°C) is technically difficult and fraught with complications, recent experimental studies have shown that small decreases in the core temperature (from normothermia to 33–36°C) are safe and sufficient to reduce neuronal death. In humans, improved functional recovery and reduced mortality were achieved in two randomized clinical trials of mild hypothermia in survivors of out-of-hospital cardiac arrest.[98,99] With prolonged cooling (12–48 hours), substantial neuroprotection can be achieved in focal as well as global cerebral ischemia.[100,101] In a nonrandomized pilot study of 25 patients with acute, large, complete MCA infarction, mild hypothermia significantly reduced intracranial pressure from 20.9 to 13.4 mm Hg, leading to an increase in cerebral perfusion pressure from 68 to 78 mm Hg. Mortality was reduced to 44% versus approximately 80% in historical controls.[102] Radiologically, moderate hypothermia attenuates infarct volumes on MRI in rats[103] and causes regression of ischemic injury in humans with MCA stroke.[104]

Based on these results, additional controlled trials are now underway to test the therapeutic impact of hypothermia combined with thrombolysis. The results of a recent trial (Cooling for Acute Ischemic Brain Damage [COOL-AID])[105] suggest that the combination of intra-arterial thrombolysis plus mild hypothermia via external cooling is safe, although mean time to achieve the target temperature was 3.5 ± 1.5 hours. Use of an intravascular inferior vena cava heat exchange catheter is also safe, and cooling may be achieved more quickly (77 ± 44 minutes).[106] The two COOL-AID trials (external cooling vs. inferior vena cava cooling) were not designed to determine efficacy. Use of a cooling helmet has also been found to be safe, and can achieve brain temperature reduction of 1.84°C/hours of cooling, requiring a mean of 3.4 hours to achieve temperatures below 34°C.[107] Several single- and multi-center randomized trials are underway in patients with ischemic and hemorrhagic stroke: Intravascular Cooling for the Treatment of Stroke-Longer window (ICTuS-L), Nordic Cooling Stroke Study (NOCSS), Controlled Hypothermia in Large Infarction (CHILI), and the Combined Cytoprotection rt-PA Stroke Trial investigating the efficacy of caffeine, ethanol, and cooling via a femoral catheter for 24 hours with or without rt-PA.

Hyperoxia

Reduced blood supply after ischemic stroke severely decreases the cellular levels of oxygen and consequently disrupts the function of numerous energy-dependent processes that are required to preserve cellular integrity. Increasing brain tissue oxygenation is therefore considered a rational stroke treatment strategy. Oxygen has distinct advantages over pharmaceutical agents: it easily diffuses across the blood–brain barrier, acts on multiple cell death pathways, and high doses are well tolerated without major safety concerns, at least when administered for short durations. Brain oxygenation can be increased either by delivering oxygen at high atmospheric pressures using specialized chambers (hyperbaric oxygen therapy or HBO), inhaling high concentrations of oxygen (normobaric oxygen therapy or NBO), and by injecting perfluorocarbons, synthetic hemoglobins, and aqueous oxygen solutions. HBO has been extensively studied and showed remarkable efficacy in animal studies[108–116]; however, it failed to show clinical efficacy in three small human trials.[117–119] These trials had several shortcomings, including limited sample size, the use of excessive chamber pressures, delayed time to therapy, poor patient selection, and questionable choice of outcome measures. Most investigators believe that HBO can be effective in mitigating stroke-related injury; however, the failure of these trials as well as practical limitations of HBO have reduced the enthusiasm for using it in the acute stroke setting. Recent studies have shown that significant neuroprotection can be achieved even with NBO, or the simple delivery of high concentrations of oxygen via a face mask.[120–127] NBO has several advantages: it is widely available, simple to administer, noninvasive, well tolerated, inexpensive, and can be started promptly after stroke onset by paramedics in the field. Unlike many other drugs or physiological strategies, NBO may be used in patients undergoing thrombolysis. Animal data suggest that it can be used to extend the narrow time window for administering thrombolytic agents (Fig. 5.5). A pilot human clinical trial showed encouraging results, with NBO-treated patients showing reversal of diffusion-weighted MRI abnormalities, reduction in infarct volumes, and improvement in neurofunction scores during the period of oxygen administration (Fig. 5.6).[126] Based on these encouraging results, a multicenter, randomized, double-blind, placebo-controlled trial has been initiated.

Induced Hypertension

The phenomenon of cerebral autoregulation in the healthy brain maintains constant cerebral blood flow the face of wide fluctuations in arterial blood pressure. However, the ischemic brain loses its capacity to autoregulate and becomes sensitive to blood pressure manipulation. This is most relevant in the ischemic penumbra, where raising mean arterial pressure has been shown to improve cerebral perfusion, with a concomitant return of electrical activity. In animal models of focal cerebral ischemia, induced hypertension therapy augmented cerebral blood flow, attenuated brain injury, and improved neurological function.[128,129] In humans, spontaneous hypertension is commonly observed in the setting of critical carotid artery stenosis, and lowering blood pressure can result in infarct extension and neurological deterioration.[130] Induced hypertension is commonly used to improve perfusion in

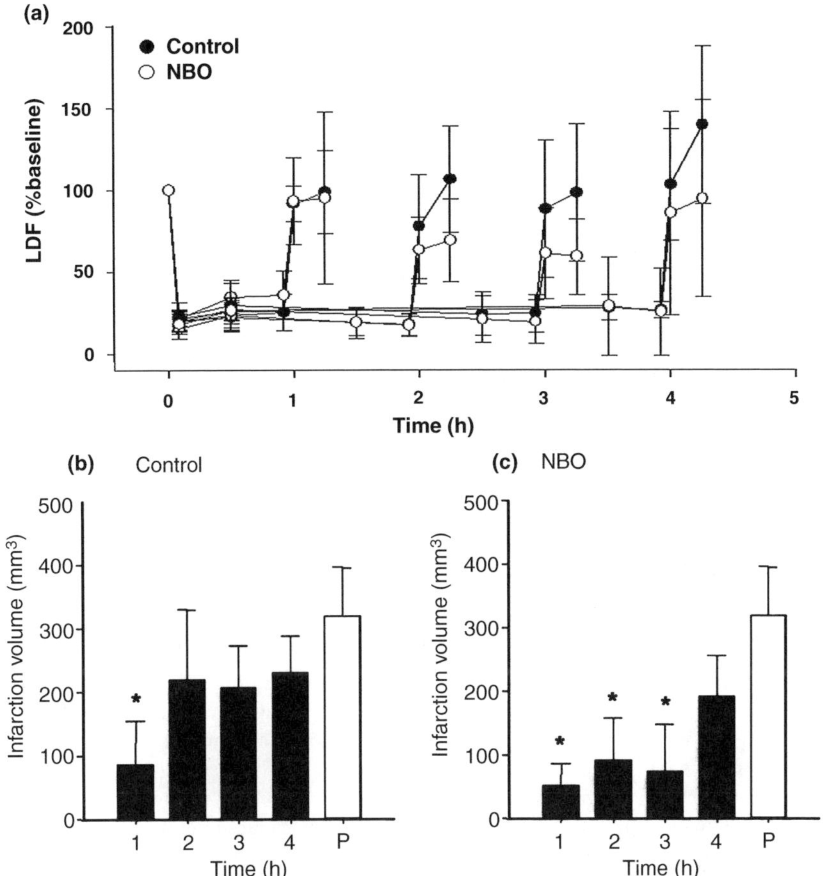

FIGURE 5.5 (**a**) Comparison of ischemia–reperfusion profiles in various control and NBO groups. LDF cerebral perfusion data are calculated as a percentage of pre-ischemic baselines (mean ± S.D.). NBO did not lead to any statistically significant differences in ischemia or reperfusion. (**b**) Forty-eight-hour infarct volumes (mean + SD) in control transient ischemia rats compared with untreated permanent focal cerebral ischemia. In this model, the reperfusion window is about 1–2 hours. $*p < 0.05$ vs. permanent ischemia. (**c**) Forty-eight-hour infarct volumes (mean + S.D.) in NBO-treated transient ischemia rats compared with untreated permanent focal cerebral ischemia. NBO increased the reperfusion window to about 3–4 hours. $*p < 0.05$ vs. permanent ischemia. (Reprinted with permission from reference 124.)

the ischemic distal arterial territory in patients with vasospasm after aneurysmal subarachnoid hemorrhage.[131]

Based upon this rationale, the effect of pharmacologically induced hypertension on clinical and imaging outcomes is being investigated in patients with acute stroke.[132–134] In one study, patients with significant diffusion–perfusion "mismatch" on MRI, large vessel occlusive disease, and fluctuating neurological deficits were found to be more likely to respond. Induced hypertension correlated with improved cortical cerebral

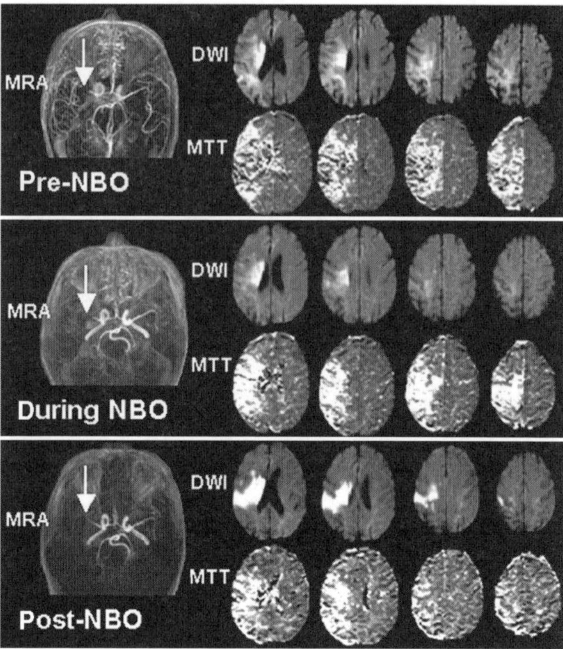

FIGURE 5.6 Serial MRI findings in a patient with cardio embolic right MCA stroke treated with NBO for 8 hours. *Top:* Baseline (pre-NBO) MRI, 13.1 hours postsymptom onset, shows a large DWI lesion, a larger MTT lesion, and MCA occlusion (arrow) on head MRA. *Middle:* A second MRI after 3.75 hours (during-NBO) shows 36% reduction in the DWI lesion, stable MTT deficit, and persistent MCA occlusion. *Bottom:* A third MRI after 24 hours (post-NBO) shows reappearance of DWI abnormality in some areas of previous reversal; MTT image shows partial reperfusion (39% MTT volume reduction, mainly in the ACA territory); MRA shows partial MCA recanalization. (Reprinted with permission from reference 126.)

perfusion and improvement in clinical tests of cortical function.[135,136] A two-center safety trial of pharmacologically induced hypertension enrolled 11 subjects. Raising mean arterial blood pressure to 30% above baseline resulted in an improvement of mean NIHSS from 10 to 8.4. Two patients developed asymptomatic postischemic brain hemorrhage and one patient showed evidence of myocardial infarction. Although these complications were not attributed to treatment in this trial, induced hypertension therapy has theoretical risks, including postischemic brain hemorrhage, myocardial ischemia, cardiac arrhythmias, and peripheral ischemia from vasopressor-induced vasoconstriction. A major limitation of induced hypertension as an acute stroke treatment is that it cannot be used as an adjunct to patients receiving thrombolysis because of the risk of precipitating intracerebral hemorrhage.

Glucose Management

Between 20% and 50% of acute stroke patients are hyperglycemic at presentation.[137] The degree of hyperglycemia correlates with both mortality and functional outcome,[138] even despite successful recanalization after thrombolysis.[139] In experimental models of cerebral ischemia, hyperglycemia is shown to exacerbate ischemic neuronal injury through a variety of mechanisms. Hyperglycemia amplifies extracellular glutamate accumulation, especially in the cortex,[140] impairs lipid metabolism,[141] reduces perfusion to the penumbra, promotes calcium influx through NMDA receptors, cytotoxic edema, oxidative stress, and free-radical production, and increases inflammation including expression of metalloproteinases (MMPs).[142] The Glucose Insulin in Stroke Trial suggests that administration of glucose, insulin, and potassium during the first 24 hours after stroke onset is safe; this pilot study was underpowered to determine efficacy.[143] Three studies addressing aggressive insulin therapy for euglycemia, the Glucose Regulation in Acute Stroke Patients Trial (GRASP), Glucose Insulin in Stroke Trial-UK (GIST-UK), and Treatment of Hyperglycemia in Ischemic Stroke (THIS), are ongoing.

SUMMARY

Although the efficacy of intravenous rt-PA in ischemic stroke has been established through several studies, the vast minority of stroke patients remain ineligible for thrombolysis. Efforts are underway to find a safe and effective neuroprotective therapy that can be applied to the broader stroke population. Basic science research has elucidated several fundamental pathways of cell death, each providing an array of molecular and biochemical targets for pharmaceutical intervention. Over 85 stroke neuroprotective drug trials have been conducted; however, not a single trial has yielded positive results, and consequently the field of stroke neuroprotection is viewed with pessimism. It is important to understand that these clinical trials had several shortcomings, and their failure may not reflect the nonefficacy of neuroprotective drugs. Much knowledge has been gained from prior efforts. The importance of factors such as thorough preclinical testing, proper patient selection, the choice of outcome measures, and the use of advanced CT- and MRI-based neuroimaging tools is now widely recognized. Contemporary efforts are focusing on the development of combination therapies that target the entire neurovascular unit, and adjunctive therapies that can be used to enhance the safety and efficacy of thrombolysis. A broad range of pharmaceutical agents and physiological strategies are currently being investigated. Some of these studies have already yielded encouraging results that are being confirmed in phase III trials. The exciting advances in neuroprotection research, combined with the efforts to increase stroke awareness, increase the application of thrombolytics, and improve general stroke care through the creation of specialized stroke units, raise hope that we will soon be successful in reducing the enormous global burden of stroke-related death and disability.

REFERENCES

1. Lo EH, Dalkara T, Moskowitz MA. Mechanisms, challenges and opportunities in stroke. *Nat Rev Neurosci* 2003;4:399–415.

2. Syntichaki P, Tavernarakis N. The biochemistry of neuronal necrosis: rogue biology? *Nat Rev Neurosci* 2003;4:672–684.
3. Singhal AB, Lo EH, Dalkara T, Moskowitz MA. Advances in stroke neuroprotection: hyperoxia and beyond. *Neuroimaging Clin N Am* 2005;15:697–720, xii–xiii.
4. Dirnagl U, Iadecola C, Moskowitz MA. Pathobiology of ischaemic stroke: an integrated view. *Trends Neurosci* 1999;22:391–397.
5. Kidwell CS, Liebeskind DS, Starkman S, Saver JL. Trends in acute ischemic stroke trials through the 20th century. *Stroke* 2001;32:1349–1359.
6. O'Collins VE, Macleod MR, Donnan GA, Horky LL, van der Worp BH, Howells DW. 1,026 experimental treatments in acute stroke. *Ann Neurol* 2006;59:467–477.
7. Lees KR, Zivin JA, Ashwood T, Davalos A, Davis SM, Diener HC, Grotta J, Lyden P, Shuaib A, Hardemark HG, Wasiewski WW. Nxy-059 for acute ischemic stroke. *N Engl J Med* 2006;354:588–600.
8. The RANTTAS Investigators. A randomized trial of tirilazad mesylate in patients with acute stroke (RANTTAS). *Stroke* 1996;27:447–453.
9. Enlimomab Acute Stroke Trial Investigators. Use of anti-icam-1 therapy in ischemic stroke: results of the enlimomab acute stroke trial. *Neurology* 2001;57:1428–1434.
10. Bogousslavsky J, Victor SJ, Salinas EO, Pallay A, Donnan GA, Fieschi C, Kaste M, Orgogozo JM, Chamorro A, Desmet A. Fiblast (trafermin) in acute stroke: results of the European-Australian phase ii/iii safety and efficacy trial. *Cerebrovasc Dis* 2002;14:239–251.
11. The American Nimodipine Study Group. Clinical trial of nimodipine in acute ischemic stroke. *Stroke* 1992;23:3–8.
12. Wahlgren NG, Ranasinha KW, Rosolacci T, Franke CL, van Erven PM, Ashwood T, Claesson L. Clomethiazole acute stroke study (class): results of a randomized, controlled trial of clomethiazole versus placebo in 1360 acute stroke patients. *Stroke* 1999;30:21–28.
13. Lyden P, Shuaib A, Ng K, Levin K, Atkinson RP, Rajput A, Wechsler L, Ashwood T, Claesson L, Odergren T, Salazar-Grueso E. Clomethiazole acute stroke study in ischemic stroke (class-i): final results. *Stroke* 2002;33:122–128.
14. Diener HC, Cortens M, Ford G, Grotta J, Hacke W, Kaste M, Koudstaal PJ. Lubeluzole in acute ischemic stroke treatment: a double-blind study with an 8-hour inclusion window comparing a 10-mg daily dose of lubeluzole with placebo. *Stroke* 2000;31:2543–2551.
15. Davis SM, Lees KR, Albers GW, Diener HC, Markabi S, Karlsson G, Norris J. Selfotel in acute ischemic stroke: possible neurotoxic effects of an NMDA antagonist. *Stroke* 2000;31:347–354.
16. Fisher M, Albers GW, Donnan GA, Furlan AJ, Grotta JC, Kidwell CS, Sacco RL, Wechsler LR. Enhancing the development and approval of acute stroke therapies: stroke therapy academic industry roundtable. *Stroke* 2005;36:1808–1813.
17. Fisher M, Hanley DF, Howard G, Jauch EC, Warach S. Recommendations from the stair v meeting on acute stroke trials, technology and outcomes. *Stroke* 2007;38:245–248.
18. Cramer SC, Koroshetz WJ, Finklestein SP. The case for modality-specific outcome measures in clinical trials of stroke recovery-promoting agents. *Stroke* 2007;38:1393–1395.
19. Yamaguchi T, Sano K, Takakura K, Saito I, Shinohara Y, Asano T, Yasuhara H. Ebselen in acute ischemic stroke: a placebo-controlled, double-blind clinical trial. Ebselen study group. *Stroke* 1998;29:12–17.

20. Edavarone acute infarction study group. Effect of a novel free radical scavenger, edaravone (mci-186), on acute brain infarction. Randomized, placebo-controlled, double-blind study at multicenters. *Cerebrovasc Dis* 2003;15:222–229.

21. Inatomi Y, Takita T, Yonehara T, Fujioka S, Hashimoto Y, Hirano T, Uchino M. Efficacy of edaravone in cardioembolic stroke. *Intern Med* 2006;45:253–257.

22. Freret T, Valable S, Chazalviel L, Saulnier R, Mackenzie ET, Petit E, Bernaudin M, Boulouard M, Schumann-Bard P. Delayed administration of deferoxamine reduces brain damage and promotes functional recovery after transient focal cerebral ischemia in the rat. *Eur J Neurosci* 2006;23:1757–1765.

23. Rosenberg G, Angel I, Kozak A. Clinical pharmacology of dp-b99 in healthy volunteers: first administration to humans. *Br J Clin Pharmacol* 2005;60:7–16.

24. Lodder J, van Raak L, Hilton A, Hardy E, Kessels A. Diazepam to improve acute stroke outcome: results of the early gaba-ergic activation study in stroke trial. A randomized double-blind placebo-controlled trial. *Cerebrovasc Dis* 2006;21: 120–127.

25. Mauler F, Fahrig T, Horvath E, Jork R. Inhibition of evoked glutamate release by the neuroprotective 5-ht(1a) receptor agonist bay x 3702 *in vitro* and *in vivo*. *Brain Res* 2001;888:150–157.

26. Teal P, Silver FL, Simard D. The brains study: safety, tolerability, and dose-finding of repinotan in acute stroke. *Can J Neurol Sci* 2005;32:61–67.

27. Kamei K, Maeda N, Nomura K, Shibata M, Katsuragi-Ogino R, Koyama M, Nakajima M, Inoue T, Ohno T, Tatsuoka T. Synthesis, sar studies, and evaluation of 1,4-benzoxazepine derivatives as selective 5-ht1a receptor agonists with neuroprotective effect: discovery of piclozotan. *Bioorg Med Chem* 2006;14:1978–1992.

28. Liao JK, Laufs U. Pleiotropic effects of statins. *Annu Rev Pharmacol Toxicol* 2005;45: 89–118.

29. Cheung BM, Lauder IJ, Lau CP, Kumana CR. Meta-analysis of large randomized controlled trials to evaluate the impact of statins on cardiovascular outcomes. *Br J Clin Pharmacol* 2004;57:640–651.

30. Amarenco P, Bogousslavsky J, Callahan 3rd A, Goldstein LB, Hennerici M, Rudolph AE, Sillesen H, Simunovic L, Szarek M, Welch KM, Zivin JA. High-dose atorvastatin after stroke or transient ischemic attack. *N Engl J Med* 2006;355:549–559.

31. Amin-Hanjani S, Stagliano NE, Yamada M, Huang PL, Liao JK, Moskowitz MA. Mevastatin, an HMG-CoA reductase inhibitor, reduces stroke damage and upregulates endothelial nitric oxide synthase in mice. *Stroke* 2001;32:980–986.

32. Laufs U, Gertz K, Huang P, Nickenig G, Bohm M, Dirnagl U, Endres M. Atorvastatin upregulates type III nitric oxide synthase in thrombocytes, decreases platelet activation, and protects from cerebral ischemia in normocholesterolemic mice. *Stroke* 2000;31:2442–2449.

33. Jonsson N, Asplund K. Does pretreatment with statins improve clinical outcome after stroke? A pilot case-referent study. *Stroke* 2001;32:1112–1115.

34. Greisenegger S, Mullner M, Tentschert S, Lang W, Lalouschek W. Effect of pretreatment with statins on the severity of acute ischemic cerebrovascular events. *J Neurol Sci* 2004;221:5–10.

35. Marti-Fabregas J, Gomis M, Arboix A, Aleu A, Pagonabarraga J, Belvis R, Cocho D, Roquer J, Rodriguez A, Garcia MD, Molina-Porcel L, Diaz-Manera J, Marti-Vilalta JL.

Favorable outcome of ischemic stroke in patients pretreated with statins. *Stroke* 2004;35:1117–1121.

36. Yoon SS, Dambrosia J, Chalela J, Ezzeddine M, Warach S, Haymore J, Davis L, Baird AE. Rising statin use and effect on ischemic stroke outcome. *BMC Med* 2004;2:4.
37. Chen J, Zhang ZG, Li Y, Wang Y, Wang L, Jiang H, Zhang C, Lu M, Katakowski M, Feldkamp CS, Chopp M. Statins induce angiogenesis, neurogenesis, and synaptogenesis after stroke. *Ann Neurol* 2003;53:743–751.
38. Sironi L, Cimino M, Guerrini U, Calvio AM, Lodetti B, Asdente M, Balduini W, Paoletti R, Tremoli E. Treatment with statins after induction of focal ischemia in rats reduces the extent of brain damage. *Arterioscler Thromb Vasc Biol* 2003;23:322–327.
39. Elkind MS, Flint AC, Sciacca RR, Sacco RL. Lipid-lowering agent use at ischemic stroke onset is associated with decreased mortality. *Neurology* 2005;65:253–258.
40. Moonis M, Kane K, Schwiderski U, Sandage BW, Fisher M. HMG-CoA reductase inhibitors improve acute ischemic stroke outcome. *Stroke* 2005;36:1298–1300.
41. Montaner J, Chacon P, Krupinski J, et al. Safety and efficacy of statins in the acute phase of ischemic stroke: the mistics trial. *Stroke* 2004;35:293.
42. Parra A, Kreiter KT, Williams S, Sciacca R, Mack WJ, Naidech AM, Commichau CS, Fitzsimmons BF, Janjua N, Mayer SA, Connolly Jr. ES, Effect of prior statin use on functional outcome and delayed vasospasm after acute aneurysmal subarachnoid hemorrhage: a matched controlled cohort study. *Neurosurgery* 2005;56:476–484 [discussion 476–484].
43. Tseng MY, Czosnyka M, Richards H, Pickard JD, Kirkpatrick PJ. Effects of acute treatment with pravastatin on cerebral vasospasm, autoregulation, and delayed ischemic deficits after aneurysmal subarachnoid hemorrhage: a phase II randomized placebo-controlled trial. *Stroke* 2005;36:1627–1632.
44. Gertz K, Laufs U, Lindauer U, Nickenig G, Bohm M, Dirnagl U, Endres M. Withdrawal of statin treatment abrogates stroke protection in mice. *Stroke* 2003;34:551–557.
45. Singhal AB, Topcuoglu MA, Dorer DJ, Ogilvy CS, Carter BS, Koroshetz WJ. Ssri and statin use increases the risk for vasospasm after subarachnoid hemorrhage. *Neurology* 2005;64:1008–1013.
46. Junghans U, Seitz RJ, Wittsack HJ, Aulich A, Siebler M. Treatment of acute basilar artery thrombosis with a combination of systemic alteplase and tirofiban, a nonpeptide platelet glycoprotein IIb/IIIa inhibitor: report of four cases. *Radiology* 2001;221: 795–801.
47. Junghans U, Siebler M. Cerebral microembolism is blocked by tirofiban, a selective nonpeptide platelet glycoprotein IIb/IIIa receptor antagonist. *Circulation* 2003;107:2717–2721.
48. Junghans U, Seitz RJ, Ritzl A, Wittsack HJ, Fink GR, Freund HJ, Siebler M. Ischemic brain tissue salvaged from infarction by the GP IIb/IIIa platelet antagonist tirofiban. *Neurology* 2002;58:474–476.
49. Emsley HC, Smith CJ, Georgiou RF, Vail A, Hopkins SJ, Rothwell NJ, Tyrrell PJ. A randomised phase II study of interleukin-1 receptor antagonist in acute stroke patients. *J Neurol Neurosurg Psychiatry* 2005;76:1366–1372.
50. Ehrenreich H, Hasselblatt M, Dembowski C, Cepek L, Lewczuk P, Stiefel M, Rustenbeck HH, Breiter N, Jacob S, Knerlich F, Bohn M, Poser W, Ruther E, Kochen M, Gefeller O, Gleiter C, Wessel TC, De Ryck M, Itri L, Prange H, Cerami A, Brines M, Siren

AL. Erythropoietin therapy for acute stroke is both safe and beneficial. *Mol Med* 2002;8:495–505.

51. Clark WM, Wechsler LR, Sabounjian LA, Schwiderski UE. A phase III randomized efficacy trial of 2000 mg citicoline in acute ischemic stroke patients. *Neurology* 2001;57:1595–1602.
52. Warach S, Pettigrew LC, Dashe JF, Pullicino P, Lefkowitz DM, Sabounjian L, Harnett K, Schwiderski U, Gammans R. Effect of citicoline on ischemic lesions as measured by diffusion-weighted magnetic resonance imaging. Citicoline 010 investigators. *Ann Neurol* 2000;48:713–722.
53. Davalos A, Castillo J, Alvarez-Sabin J, Secades JJ, Mercadal J, Lopez S, Cobo E, Warach S, Sherman D, Clark WM, Lozano R. Oral citicoline in acute ischemic stroke: an individual patient data pooling analysis of clinical trials. *Stroke* 2002;33:2850–2857.
54. Belayev L, Pinard E, Nallet H, Seylaz J, Liu Y, Riyamongkol P, Zhao W, Busto R, Ginsberg MD. Albumin therapy of transient focal cerebral ischemia: *in vivo* analysis of dynamic microvascular responses. *Stroke* 2002;33:1077–1084.
55. Belayev L, Liu Y, Zhao W, Busto R, Ginsberg MD. Human albumin therapy of acute ischemic stroke: marked neuroprotective efficacy at moderate doses and with a broad therapeutic window. *Stroke* 2001;32:553–560.
56. Ginsberg MD, Hill MD, Palesch YY, Ryckborst KJ, Tamariz D. The alias pilot trial: a dose-escalation and safety study of albumin therapy for acute ischemic stroke—I: physiological responses and safety results. *Stroke* 2006;37:2100–2106.
57. Palesch YY, Hill MD, Ryckborst KJ, Tamariz D, Ginsberg MD. The alias pilot trial: a dose-escalation and safety study of albumin therapy for acute ischemic stroke—II: neurologic outcome and efficacy analysis. *Stroke* 2006;37:2107–2114.
58. Lin JY, Chung SY, Lin MC, Cheng FC. Effects of magnesium sulfate on energy metabolites and glutamate in the cortex during focal cerebral ischemia and reperfusion in the gerbil monitored by a dual-probe microdialysis technique. *Life Sci* 2002;71:803–811.
59. Nowak L, Bregestovski P, Ascher P, Herbet A, Prochiantz A. Magnesium gates glutamate-activated channels in mouse central neurones. *Nature* 1984;307:462–465.
60. Chi OZ, Pollak P, Weiss HR. Effects of magnesium sulfate and nifedipine on regional cerebral blood flow during middle cerebral artery ligation in the rat. *Arch Int Pharmacodyn Ther* 1990;304:196–205.
61. Izumi Y, Roussel S, Pinard E, Seylaz J. Reduction of infarct volume by magnesium after middle cerebral artery occlusion in rats. *J Cereb Blood Flow Metab* 1991;11:1025–1030.
62. Marinov MB, Harbaugh KS, Hoopes PJ, Pikus HJ, Harbaugh RE. Neuroprotective effects of preischemia intraarterial magnesium sulfate in reversible focal cerebral ischemia. *J Neurosurg* 1996;85:117–124.
63. Muir KW, Lees KR. A randomized, double-blind, placebo-controlled pilot trial of intravenous magnesium sulfate in acute stroke. *Stroke* 1995;26:1183–1188.
64. Muir KW, Lees KR, Ford I, Davis S. Magnesium for acute stroke (intravenous magnesium efficacy in stroke trial): randomised controlled trial. *Lancet* 2004;363:439–445.
65. Saver JL, Kidwell C, Eckstein M, Starkman S. Prehospital neuroprotective therapy for acute stroke: results of the field administration of stroke therapy-magnesium (fast-mag) pilot trial. *Stroke* 2004;35:e106–e108.

66. Alexandrov AV, Molina CA, Grotta JC, Garami Z, Ford SR, Alvarez-Sabin J, Montaner J, Saqqur M, Demchuk AM, Moye LA, Hill MD, Wojner AW. Ultrasound-enhanced systemic thrombolysis for acute ischemic stroke. *N Engl J Med* 2004;351:2170–2178.
67. Molina CA, Ribo M, Rubiera M, Montaner J, Santamarina E, Delgado-Mederos R, Arenillas JF, Huertas R, Purroy F, Delgado P, Alvarez-Sabin J. Microbubble administration accelerates clot lysis during continuous 2-MHz ultrasound monitoring in stroke patients treated with intravenous tissue plasminogen activator. *Stroke* 2006;37:425–429.
68. Vahedi K, Hofmeijer J, Juettler E, Vicaut E, George B, Algra A, Amelink GJ, Schmiedeck P, Schwab S, Rothwell PM, Bousser MG, van der Worp HB, Hacke. Early decompressive surgery in malignant infarction of the middle cerebral artery: a pooled analysis of three randomised controlled trials. *Lancet Neurol* 2007;6:215–222.
69. Lyden PD, Jackson-Friedman C, Shin C, Hassid S. Synergistic combinatorial stroke therapy: a quantal bioassay of a gaba agonist and a glutamate antagonist. *Exp Neurol* 2000;163:477–489.
70. Onal MZ, Li F, Tatlisumak T, Locke KW, Sandage Jr, BW, Fisher M. Synergistic effects of citicoline and mk-801 in temporary experimental focal ischemia in rats. *Stroke* 1997;28:1060–1065.
71. Barth A, Barth L, Newell DW. Combination therapy with mk-801 and alpha-phenyl-tert-butyl-nitrone enhances protection against ischemic neuronal damage in organotypic hippocampal slice cultures. *Exp Neurol* 1996;141:330–336.
72. Du C, Hu R, Csernansky CA, Liu XZ, Hsu CY, Choi DW. Additive neuroprotective effects of dextrorphan and cycloheximide in rats subjected to transient focal cerebral ischemia. *Brain Res* 1996;718:233–236.
73. Ma J, Endres M, Moskowitz MA. Synergistic effects of caspase inhibitors and mk-801 in brain injury after transient focal cerebral ischaemia in mice. *Br J Pharmacol* 1998;124:756–762.
74. Barth A, Barth L, Morrison RS, Newell DW. Bfgf enhances the protective effects of mk-801 against ischemic neuronal injury *in vitro*. *Neuroreport* 1996;7:1461–1464.
75. Schmid-Elsaesser R, Hungerhuber E, Zausinger S, Baethmann A, Reulen HJ. Neuroprotective efficacy of combination therapy with two different antioxidants in rats subjected to transient focal ischemia. *Brain Res* 1999;816:471–479.
76. Schabitz WR, Li F, Irie K, Sandage Jr, BW, Locke KW, Fisher M. Synergistic effects of a combination of low-dose basic fibroblast growth factor and citicoline after temporary experimental focal ischemia. *Stroke* 1999;30:427–431 [discussion 431–422].
77. Ma J, Qiu J, Hirt L, Dalkara T, Moskowitz MA. Synergistic protective effect of caspase inhibitors and bfgf against brain injury induced by transient focal ischaemia. *Br J Pharmacol* 2001;133:345–350.
78. Asahi M, Asahi K, Wang X, Lo EH. Reduction of tissue plasminogen activator-induced hemorrhage and brain injury by free radical spin trapping after embolic focal cerebral ischemia in rats. *J Cereb Blood Flow Metab* 2000;20:452–457.
79. Meden P, Overgaard K, Sereghy T, Boysen G. Enhancing the efficacy of thrombolysis by ampa receptor blockade with nbqx in a rat embolic stroke model. *J Neurol Sci* 1993;119:209–216.
80. Zivin JA, Mazzarella V. Tissue plasminogen activator plus glutamate antagonist improves outcome after embolic stroke. *Arch Neurol* 1991;48:1235–1238.

81. Sumii T, Lo EH. Involvement of matrix metalloproteinase in thrombolysis-associated hemorrhagic transformation after embolic focal ischemia in rats. *Stroke* 2002;33:831–836.
82. Andersen M, Overgaard K, Meden P, Boysen G, Choi SC. Effects of citicoline combined with thrombolytic therapy in a rat embolic stroke model. *Stroke* 1999;30:1464–1471.
83. Yang Y, Li Q, Shuaib A. Enhanced neuroprotection and reduced hemorrhagic incidence in focal cerebral ischemia of rat by low dose combination therapy of urokinase and topiramate. *Neuropharmacology* 2000;39:881–888.
84. Bowes MP, Rothlein R, Fagan SC, Zivin JA. Monoclonal antibodies preventing leukocyte activation reduce experimental neurologic injury and enhance efficacy of thrombolytic therapy. *Neurology* 1995;45:815–819.
85. Shuaib A, Yang Y, Nakada MT, Li Q, Yang T. Glycoprotein IIb/IIIa antagonist, murine 7e3 f(ab′) 2, and tissue plasminogen activator in focal ischemia: evaluation of efficacy and risk of hemorrhage with combination therapy. *J Cereb Blood Flow Metab* 2002;22:215–222.
86. Lyden P, Jacoby M, Schim J, Albers G, Mazzeo P, Ashwood T, Nordlund A, Odergren T. The clomethiazole acute stroke study in tissue-type plasminogen activator-treated stroke (class-t): final results. *Neurology* 2001;57:1199–1205.
87. Grotta J. Combination therapy stroke trial: recombinant tissue-type plasminogen activator with/without lubeluzole. *Cerebrovasc Dis* 2001;12:258–263.
88. Astrup J, Siesjo BK, Symon L. Thresholds in cerebral ischemia–the ischemic penumbra. *Stroke* 1981;12:723–725.
89. Cardell M, Boris-Moller F, Wieloch T. Hypothermia prevents the ischemia-induced translocation and inhibition of protein kinase c in the rat striatum. *J Neurochem* 1991;57:1814–1817.
90. Globus MY, Busto R, Lin B, Schnippering H, Ginsberg MD. Detection of free radical activity during transient global ischemia and recirculation: effects of intraischemic brain temperature modulation. *J Neurochem* 1995;65:1250–1256.
91. Krieger DW, Yenari MA. Therapeutic hypothermia for acute ischemic stroke: what do laboratory studies teach us? *Stroke* 2004;35:1482–1489.
92. Han HS, Karabiyikoglu M, Kelly S, Sobel RA, Yenari MA. Mild hypothermia inhibits nuclear factor-kappab translocation in experimental stroke. *J Cereb Blood Flow Metab* 2003;23:589–598.
93. Wang GJ, Deng HY, Maier CM, Sun GH, Yenari MA. Mild hypothermia reduces ICAM-1 expression, neutrophil infiltration and microglia/monocyte accumulation following experimental stroke. *Neuroscience* 2002;114:1081–1090.
94. Han HS, Qiao Y, Karabiyikoglu M, Giffard RG, Yenari MA. Influence of mild hypothermia on inducible nitric oxide synthase expression and reactive nitrogen production in experimental stroke and inflammation. *J Neurosci* 2002;22: 3921–3928.
95. Prosser CL. Temperature. In: Prosser CL, editor *Comparative animal physiology.* Philadelphia: WB Saunders; 1973. p 362–428.
96. Markarian GZ, Lee JH, Stein DJ, Hong SC. Mild hypothermia: therapeutic window after experimental cerebral ischemia. *Neurosurgery* 1996;38:542–550 [discussion 551].
97. Welsh FA, Harris VA. Postischemic hypothermia fails to reduce ischemic injury in gerbil hippocampus. *J Cereb Blood Flow Metab* 1991;11:617–620.

98. The Hypothermia After Cardiac Arrest Study Group. Mild therapeutic hypothermia to improve the neurologic outcome after cardiac arrest. *N Engl J Med* 2002;346:549–556.

99. Bernard SA, Gray TW, Buist MD, Jones BM, Silvester W, Gutteridge G, Smith K. Treatment of comatose survivors of out-of-hospital cardiac arrest with induced hypothermia. *N Engl J Med* 2002;346:557–563.

100. Ginsberg MD. Hypothermic neuroprotection in cerebral ischemia. In: Welch KMA, Caplan LR, Reis DJ, Siesjo BK, Weir B, editors *Primer on cerebrovascular diseases*. San Diego: Academic Press; 1997. p 272–275.

101. Corbett D, Hamilton M, Colbourne F. Persistent neuroprotection with prolonged postischemic hypothermia in adult rats subjected to transient middle cerebral artery occlusion. *Exp Neurol* 2000;163:200–206.

102. Schwab S, Schwarz S, Spranger M, Keller E, Bertram M, Hacke W. Moderate hypothermia in the treatment of patients with severe middle cerebral artery infarction. *Stroke* 1998;29:2461–2466.

103. Kollmar R, Henninger N, Bardutzky J, Schellinger PD, Schabitz WR, Schwab S. Combination therapy of moderate hypothermia and thrombolysis in experimental thromboembolic stroke—an MRI study. *Exp Neurol* 2004;190:204–212.

104. Berger C, Schramm P, Schwab S. Reduction of diffusion-weighted MRI lesion volume after early moderate hypothermia in ischemic stroke. *Stroke* 2005;36:e56–e58.

105. Krieger DW, De Georgia MA, Abou-Chebl A, Andrefsky JC, Sila CA, Katzan IL, Mayberg MR, Furlan AJ. Cooling for acute ischemic brain damage (cool aid): an open pilot study of induced hypothermia in acute ischemic stroke. *Stroke* 2001;32:1847–1854.

106. De Georgia MA, Krieger DW, Abou-Chebl A, Devlin TG, Jauss M, Davis SM, Koroshetz WJ, Rordorf G, Warach S. Cooling for acute ischemic brain damage (cool aid): a feasibility trial of endovascular cooling. *Neurology* 2004;63:312–317.

107. Wang H, Olivero W, Lanzino G, Elkins W, Rose J, Honings D, Rodde M, Burnham J, Wang D. Rapid and selective cerebral hypothermia achieved using a cooling helmet. *J Neurosurg* 2004;100:272–277.

108. Badr AE, Yin W, Mychaskiw G, Zhang JH. Dual effect of hbo on cerebral infarction in mcao rats. *Am J Physiol Regul Integr Comp Physiol* 2001;280:R766–R770.

109. Burt JT, Kapp JP, Smith RR. Hyperbaric oxygen and cerebral infarction in the gerbil. *Surg Neurol* 1987;28:265–268.

110. Lou M, Eschenfelder CC, Herdegen T, Brecht S, Deuschl G. Therapeutic window for use of hyperbaric oxygenation in focal transient ischemia in rats. *Stroke* 2004;35:578–583.

111. Veltkamp R, Warner DS, Domoki F, Brinkhous AD, Toole JF, Busija DW. Hyperbaric oxygen decreases infarct size and behavioral deficit after transient focal cerebral ischemia in rats. *Brain Res* 2000;853:68–73.

112. Sunami K, Takeda Y, Hashimoto M, Hirakawa M. Hyperbaric oxygen reduces infarct volume in rats by increasing oxygen supply to the ischemic periphery. *Crit Care Med* 2000;28:2831–2836.

113. Schabitz WR, Schade H, Heiland S, Kollmar R, Bardutzky J, Henninger N, Muller H, Carl U, Toyokuni S, Sommer C, Schwab S. Neuroprotection by hyperbaric oxygenation after experimental focal cerebral ischemia monitored by mr-imaging. *Stroke* 2004;35:1175–1179.

114. Roos JA, Jackson-Friedman C, Lyden P. Effects of hyperbaric oxygen on neurologic outcome for cerebral ischemia in rats. *Acad Emerg Med* 1998;5:18–24.

115. Kawamura S, Yasui N, Shirasawa M, Fukasawa H. Therapeutic effects of hyperbaric oxygenation on acute focal cerebral ischemia in rats. *Surg Neurol* 1990;34:101–106.

116. Weinstein PR, Anderson GG, Telles DA. Results of hyperbaric oxygen therapy during temporary middle cerebral artery occlusion in unanesthetized cats. *Neurosurgery* 1987;20:518–524.

117. Anderson DC, Bottini AG, Jagiella WM, Westphal B, Ford S, Rockswold GL, Loewenson RB. A pilot study of hyperbaric oxygen in the treatment of human stroke. *Stroke* 1991;22:1137–1142.

118. Nighoghossian N, Trouillas P, Adeleine P, Salord F. Hyperbaric oxygen in the treatment of acute ischemic stroke. A double-blind pilot study. *Stroke* 1995;26:1369–1372.

119. Rusyniak DE, Kirk MA, May JD, Kao LW, Brizendine EJ, Welch JL, Cordell WH, Alonso RJ. Hyperbaric oxygen therapy in acute ischemic stroke: results of the hyperbaric oxygen in acute ischemic stroke trial pilot study. *Stroke* 2003;34:571–574.

120. Flynn EP, Auer RN. Eubaric hyperoxemia and experimental cerebral infarction. *Ann Neurol* 2002;52:566–572.

121. Singhal AB, Dijkhuizen RM, Rosen BR, Lo EH. Normobaric hyperoxia reduces mri diffusion abnormalities and infarct size in experimental stroke. *Neurology* 2002;58: 945–952.

122. Singhal AB, Wang X, Sumii T, Mori T, Lo EH. Effects of normobaric hyperoxia in a rat model of focal cerebral ischemia–reperfusion. *J Cereb Blood Flow Metab* 2002;22: 861–868.

123. Liu S, Shi H, Liu W, Furuichi T, Timmins GS, Liu KJ. Interstitial po2 in ischemic penumbra and core are differentially affected following transient focal cerebral ischemia in rats. *J Cereb Blood Flow Metab* 2004;24:343–349.

124. Kim HY, Singhal AB, Lo EH. Normobaric hyperoxia extends the reperfusion window in focal cerebral ischemia. *Ann Neurol* 2005;57:571–575.

125. Ratai EM, Benner T, Sorensen AG, Vangel M, Koroshetz WJ, Schaefer PW, Lo EH, Gonzalez RG, Singhal AB. Therapeutic effects of normobaric hyperoxia in acute stroke: multivoxel MR-spectroscopy and adc correlations on serial imaging. *13th Scientific Meeting of the International Society of Magnetic Resonance in Medicine*; 2005.

126. Singhal AB, Benner T, Roccatagliata L, Koroshetz WJ, Schaefer PW, Lo EH, Buonanno FS, Gonzalez RG, Sorensen AG. A pilot study of normobaric oxygen therapy in acute ischemic stroke. *Stroke* 2005;36:797–802.

127. Henninger N, Bouley J, Nelligan JM, Sicard KM, Fisher M. Normobaric hyperoxia delays perfusion/diffusion mismatch evolution, reduces infarct volume, and differentially affects neuronal cell death pathways after suture middle cerebral artery occlusion in rats. *J Cereb Blood Flow Metab* 2007; Epub Feb 21.

128. Hayashi S, Nehls DG, Kieck CF, Vielma J, DeGirolami U, Crowell RM. Beneficial effects of induced hypertension on experimental stroke in awake monkeys. *J Neurosurg* 1984;60:151–157.

129. Cole DJ, Matsumura JS, Drummond JC, Schell RM. Focal cerebral ischemia in rats: effects of induced hypertension, during reperfusion, on cbf. *J Cereb Blood Flow Metab* 1992;12:64–69.

130. Fischberg GM, Lozano E, Rajamani K, Ameriso S, Fisher MJ. Stroke precipitated by moderate blood pressure reduction. *J Emerg Med* 2000;19:339–346.

131. Kassell NF, Peerless SJ, Durward QJ, Beck DW, Drake CG, Adams HP. Treatment of ischemic deficits from vasospasm with intravascular volume expansion and induced arterial hypertension. *Neurosurgery* 1982;11:337–343.

132. Rordorf G, Cramer SC, Efird JT, Schwamm LH, Buonanno F, Koroshetz WJ. Pharmacological elevation of blood pressure in acute stroke. Clinical effects and safety. *Stroke* 1997;28:2133–2138.

133. Rordorf G, Koroshetz WJ, Ezzeddine MA, Segal AZ, Buonanno FS. A pilot study of drug-induced hypertension for treatment of acute stroke. *Neurology* 2001;56:1210–1213.

134. Hillis AE, Ulatowski JA, Barker PB, Torbey M, Ziai W, Beauchamp NJ, Oh S, Wityk RJ. A pilot randomized trial of induced blood pressure elevation: effects on function and focal perfusion in acute and subacute stroke. *Cerebrovasc Dis* 2003;16:236–246.

135. Hillis AE, Wityk RJ, Beauchamp NJ, Ulatowski JA, Jacobs MA, Barker PB. Perfusion-weighted MRI as a marker of response to treatment in acute and subacute stroke. *Neuroradiology* 2004;46:31–39.

136. Hillis AE, Barker PB, Beauchamp NJ, Winters BD, Mirski M, Wityk RJ. Restoring blood pressure reperfused wernicke's area and improved language. *Neurology* 2001;56:670–672.

137. Woo J, Lam CW, Kay R, Wong AH, Teoh R, Nicholls MG. The influence of hyperglycemia and diabetes mellitus on immediate and 3-month morbidity and mortality after acute stroke. *Arch Neurol* 1990;47:1174–1177.

138. Gray CS, Taylor R, French JM, Alberti KG, Venables GS, James OF, Shaw DA, Cartlidge NE, Bates D. The prognostic value of stress hyperglycaemia and previously unrecognized diabetes in acute stroke. *Diabet Med* 1987;4:237–240.

139. Leigh R, Zaidat OO, Suri MF, Lynch G, Sundararajan S, Sunshine JL, Tarr R, Selman W, Landis DM, Suarez JI. Predictors of hyperacute clinical worsening in ischemic stroke patients receiving thrombolytic therapy. *Stroke* 2004;35:1903–1907.

140. Li PA, Shuaib A, Miyashita H, He QP, Siesjo BK, Warner DS. Hyperglycemia enhances extracellular glutamate accumulation in rats subjected to forebrain ischemia. *Stroke* 2000;31:183–192.

141. Katsura K, Rodriguez de Turco EB, Siesjo BK, Bazan NG. Effects of hyperglycemia and hypercapnia on lipid metabolism during complete brain ischemia. *Brain Res* 2004;1030:133–140.

142. Garg R, Chaudhuri A, Munschauer F, Dandona P. Hyperglycemia, insulin, and acute ischemic stroke: a mechanistic justification for a trial of insulin infusion therapy. *Stroke* 2006;37:267–273.

143. Scott JF, Robinson GM, French JM, O'Connell JE, Alberti KG, Gray CS. Glucose potassium insulin infusions in the treatment of acute stroke patients with mild to moderate hyperglycemia: the glucose insulin in stroke trial (GIST). *Stroke* 1999; 30:793–799.

6

SURGICAL MANAGEMENT OF ACUTE STROKE PATIENTS

Alim P. Mitha, Carlos E. Sanchez, and Christopher S. Ogilvy

INTRODUCTION

Acute stroke patients may benefit from a number of surgical procedures designed to either reperfuse tissue at risk of infarction (the so-called "ischemic penumbra") or prevent the damaging effects of secondary processes on adjacent functional tissue. The decision of which surgical procedure to employ is largely based on the site of the culprit lesion and the size and territory of infracted brain tissue. Whether a role exists for surgical intervention in any given acute stroke case is often the most difficult question to answer, and depends on the patient's clinical status, time since symptom onset, imaging findings, and a variety of other patient- and surgeon-specific factors. For these reasons, the team managing the patient, including the neurosurgeon, must be familiar with the indications and outcomes of current medical and surgical treatment strategies for acute ischemic stroke. This chapter will focus on patient selection, timing, and outcomes after surgical therapy for acute ischemic stroke patients, including early carotid endarterectomy (CEA), extracranial–intracranial (EC-IC) arterial bypass, decompressive hemicraniectomy, posterior fossa decompression, and intracranial embolectomy.

EARLY CAROTID ENDARTERECTOMY

CEA involves exposure of the carotid bifurcation in the neck to a point along the internal carotid artery (ICA) beyond which the atherosclerotic plaque terminates.

Acute Ischemic Stroke: An Evidence-based Approach, Edited by David M. Greer.

Arteriotomy, removal of the plaque, and careful closure of the arteriotomy are carried out using a microvascular technique, ensuring minimal residual stenosis or flow disturbance. The operation can be performed under local or general anesthesia, and several variations of the procedure exist, including eversion endarterectomy.[1] Maintaining cerebral perfusion during the procedure by shunting can be done on a routine or selective basis. Intraoperative decision-making can also be assisted by various methods of monitoring, including electroencephalography, carotid stump pressure, somatosensory-evoked potentials, transcranial Doppler, and cerebral oximetry. Finally, the arteriotomy closure can be done primarily or, in the case of smaller vessels, by using a patch to increase lumen size.

Patient Selection

CEA is a proven and effective therapy for preventing stroke in patients with symptomatic, severe carotid artery stenosis causing transient ischemic attacks (TIAs), or nondisabling strokes.[2,3] In the setting of an acute stroke, indications for early CEA include a high-grade carotid stenosis, nondisabling symptoms, and a patent intracranial ICA. Early CEA is usually not performed in patients with depressed levels of consciousness or severely disabling strokes due to generally poor outcomes.[4] While an abnormal computed tomography (CT) scan in patients with minor stroke does not correlate well with perioperative morbidity, a large radiographic infarct (roughly greater than one third of the middle cerebral artery (MCA) territory) is a contraindication to early CEA since these patients are at highest risk of poor outcome related to reperfusion injury and hemorrhagic complications.[5–7] Importantly, early CEA is not absolutely contraindicated after recent administration of intravenous tissue plasminogen activator, and can be safely performed in appropriate patients.[7] In the setting of an acute stroke, early CEA should also be considered for contralateral ICA stenosis, even though it may be asymptomatic, in order to prevent further restriction of cerebral perfusion after symptomatic ipsilateral ICA occlusion.[4] Improvements in imaging techniques are also allowing for better patient selection for early CEA. Mismatches between magnetic resonance (MR) diffusion-weighted imaging (DWI) and perfusion-weighted imaging (PWI) demonstrating a large ischemic penumbra may identify those patients who will most benefit from early reperfusion.[4,8]

Timing

The timing of CEA after ischemic stroke has been a controversial issue. In 1969, the Joint Study of Extracranial Arterial Occlusion reported 42% mortality after CEA in patients with neurological deficits of less than 2 weeks duration, compared with 5% mortality in patients with more than 2 weeks of symptoms.[2,7] Early evidence also demonstrated an increased risk of intracerebral hemorrhage after early CEA in patients with acute stroke.[9–11] This led to the conclusion that most complications occurred with early surgical intervention, and resulted in a traditional 4–6 week delay for CEA after an acute stroke. In retrospect, however, there were major problems with patient selection in these earlier reports. Many of the patients suffered from profound neurological deficits or had complete arterial occlusions.[9,10,12] Furthermore, the extent of cerebral damage was not recognized in many of the reports originating prior to the advent of CT imaging.[6]

More recent reports conclude that early CEA after a nondisabling ischemic stroke can be performed with perioperative mortality and stroke rates comparable to those of delayed CEA. In a subgroup analysis by the North American Symptomatic Carotid Endarterectomy Trial (NASCET) investigators, 42 patients who underwent early CEA (<30 days after stroke) were compared with 58 patients who underwent delayed CEA (>30 days), and no overall difference was demonstrated in the perioperative stroke rate (4.8% vs. 5.2%).[7,13] Another recent prospective randomized study of 86 patients showed no difference in either perioperative stroke (2% in both groups) or survival rates (mean 23 months follow-up) between patients randomized to early or delayed CEA.[6]

In patients with recurrent hemispheric symptoms due to severe and/or irregular carotid stenosis, urgent CEA should be considered because of the significant risk of a major disabling stroke.[14] While the period of highest risk has yet to be clearly defined and much of the current evidence suggests similar perioperative morbidity and mortality rates between early and delayed CEA, most clinicians now advocate early CEA for patients with a high-grade stenosis and an acute nondisabling stroke. Patients with a symptomatic severe carotid stenosis have a 7.5% per month risk of disabling stroke following an initial acute stroke.[15] Furthermore, the risk at 30 days is highest for large artery atherosclerotic disease compared with cardioembolic and small vessel ischemic disease.[16] Complications of interval anticoagulation therapy (which may give rise to hemorrhagic conversion), interruption of physical therapy programs, and stress endured by some patients in the waiting period have also been cited as reasons for early CEA.[6] The risk of major disabling stroke in patients presenting with recurrent hemispheric symptoms within the initial days of acute stroke, especially those presenting in a crescendo fashion with severe and/or irregular carotid stenosis, makes early CEA an important consideration.[17]

While early CEA is considered to be relatively safe, it may not always be necessary. For instance, early surgery can be deferred in patients who are medically unstable or for those whose cardiac or respiratory status requires optimization. In the NASCET study, the rate of ipsilateral stroke at 1 month for medically treated patients with high-grade stenoses was only 3.3% and was even lower (1.7%) in patients with near-occlusions.[2,7] Even in patients with free-floating intraluminal thrombus, anticoagulant therapy is a well tolerated and reasonable first step, given that these patients are at particularly high risk for perioperative stroke.[14,18,19] Hence, there is little evidence for a true emergency CEA, even in the setting of acute stroke.

EXTRACRANIAL/INTRACRANIAL ARTERIAL BYPASS

EC-IC arterial bypass involves the use of general anesthesia, open craniotomy, and end-to-side anastomosis of the superficial temporal artery to a branch of the middle cerebral artery (MCA) (Fig. 6.1). Currently, this technique is being used primarily in the setting of intracranial aneurysm therapy, moyamoya disease, and

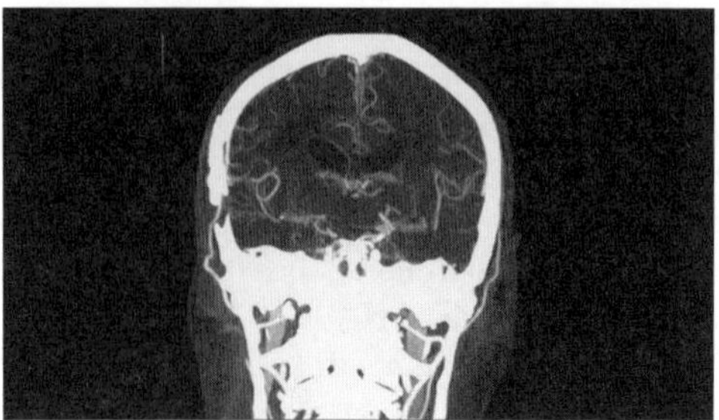

FIGURE 6.1 CT angiography of an EC–IC bypass, showing the new intracranial course of the right superficial temporal artery, anastamosed to the middle cerebral artery M2 segment.

preservation of vascular flow during tumor removal.[20] EC-IC arterial bypass was previously advocated in patients with ICA stenosis or occlusion, carotid siphon stenosis, MCA occlusion, and peripheral branch MCA occlusion. Moreover, early reports and clinical studies supported its use in patients with TIAs, prolonged reversible ischemic neurological deficits, and completed infarcts.[21] However, in 1985 an international randomized study of 1377 patients by the EC-IC Bypass Study Group subsequently demonstrated a lack of benefit in patients with atherosclerotic disease of the carotid and middle cerebral arteries.[22]

Failure of the trial to demonstrate a benefit for EC-IC bypass was unexpected, since many who performed the procedure had already concluded it to be useful and effective.[23] The study itself was well designed, involved a large number of patients, had a perfect follow-up record, and a high bypass patency rate. No distinction was made, however, between the hemodynamic or embolic origin of cerebral and retinal ischemic events. More importantly, physiological imaging was not used in the selection of patients for the procedure. Given that the study was not specifically designed to measure a benefit in neurologic function, which may occur if blood flow to the ischemic penumbra was restored, patients selected using physiological parameters could still demonstrate a clinical benefit from EC-IC bypass.

In a study by Powers et al.[24] on 29 EC–IC bypass patients compared to 23 nonsurgical patients, selection criteria on the basis of reduced cerebral perfusion pressure by positron emission tomography (PET) failed to prove beneficial. However, this was a nonrandomized trial, and compared with the nonsurgical group, surgical patients had more TIAs, multiple TIAs, fewer ICA occlusions without recurrent symptoms, and symptoms within 30 days prior to entry into the study. Stronger evidence seems to support the use of physiological methods of imaging to select patients for EC-IC bypass. For instance, the St. Louis Carotid Occlusion Study demonstrated that increased oxygen extraction fraction (OEF) measured by PET predicts subsequent ipsilateral stroke in patients with symptomatic carotid occlusion.[25] In other studies, postoperative improvement in regional cerebral blood flow detected by PET correlated with clinical improvement.[26,27]

The potential benefit of EC-IC bypass, therefore, has not been well studied in acute stroke patients carefully selected using newer physiological methods, including PET, xenon CT, single-photon emission computed tomography (SPECT), or CT or MR perfusion.[5] Ongoing trials such as the Carotid Occlusion Surgery Study (COSS), the entry criteria of which include recent symptomatic occlusion of the ICA and increased OEF measured by PET, may help to clarify the benefit of emergency EC-IC bypass for selected patients (Figure 6.2). The Japanese EC-IC Bypass Trial (JET) is another ongoing randomized trial of EC-IC bypass in patients with severe hemodynamic failure measured by SPECT. Although final results are pending, JET preliminarily demonstrates a reduced incidence of major stroke or death in the 2-year period after surgery.[28,29]

With respect to timing of surgery, there is little evidence to either support or challenge the use of emergent EC-IC bypass in the setting of acute cerebral ischemia. The EC-IC Bypass Study results do not apply to acute atherosclerotic stroke patients, since patients within 8 weeks of an acute cerebral ischemic event were excluded.[30] In a study by Engel et al.,[21] patients presenting with progressive strokes who were surgically treated within 3–4 weeks following symptom onset had the least benefit. Other studies have not convincingly shown improved outcome with the use of emergency EC-IC bypass.[31,32]

In the emergency situation, we believe this technique can be successfully employed in selected patients with symptomatic ischemia due to dissection or atherosclerotic disease despite being on maximal medical therapy. We have also seen patients with carotid occlusion and an isolated cerebral hemisphere (poor collateral flow) benefit from EC-IC bypass. Any potential benefit, however, must

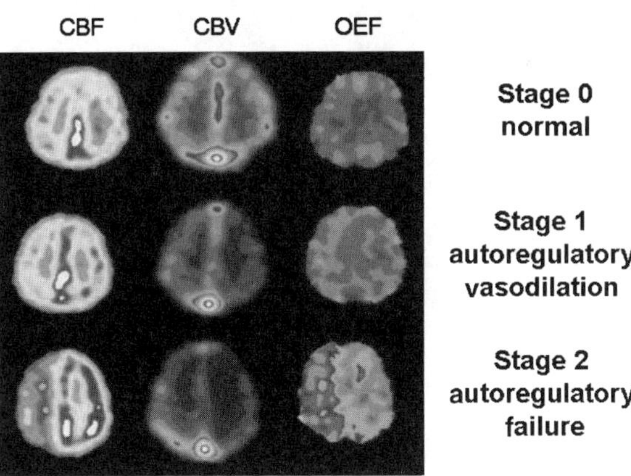

FIGURE 6.2 Oxygen extraction fraction (OEF) positron emission tomography (PET) study, showing increased fraction of oxygen use in the right hemisphere of this patient with an ipsilateral flow-limiting lesion. In the initial stage of decreasing cerebral blood flow (CBF), compensatory vasodilation occurs so that the cerebral blood volume (CBV) remains relatively stable. However, as this mchanism begins to fail with progressively decreased CBF, the OEF increases, giving an indication of how tenuous the situation may be over the long term. (Courtesy of Dr. William Powers, with permission.)

be balanced with the risk of surgery and the possibility of hemorrhage from reperfusion of the ischemic territory.

DECOMPRESSIVE HEMICRANIECTOMY

Decompressive hemicraniectomy is primarily intended to treat the high intracranial pressure associated with massive MCA infarction and subsequent swelling (Fig. 6.3). Focal areas of ischemia may result when intracranial pressure is greater than 20 mm Hg, and global ischemia can occur when intracranial pressure exceeds 50 mm Hg.[33] Therefore, removal of a large part of the calvarium, theoretically reducing intracranial hypertension, ongoing ischemia, and preventing swollen tissue from displacing healthier neighboring tissue, may benefit some patients following large territory MCA infarction.

The procedure typically involves a wide bone removal of the cranial vault, measuring roughly 13 cm in antero-posterior dimensions and from the floor of the middle cranial fossa to at least 9 cm superiorly. After opening of the dura, an anterior temporal lobectomy is usually performed, with or without resection of any necrotic avascular tissue.[34] This is followed by loose closure of the dura with allograft or pericranium. The bone flap can be either stored in the preperitoneal fat, or refrigerated in antibiotic solution and replaced after the edema has subsided. Decompressive hemicraniectomy is usually done with the patient being treated in the ICU setting and in conjunction with other aggressive medical therapies. Success of the procedure

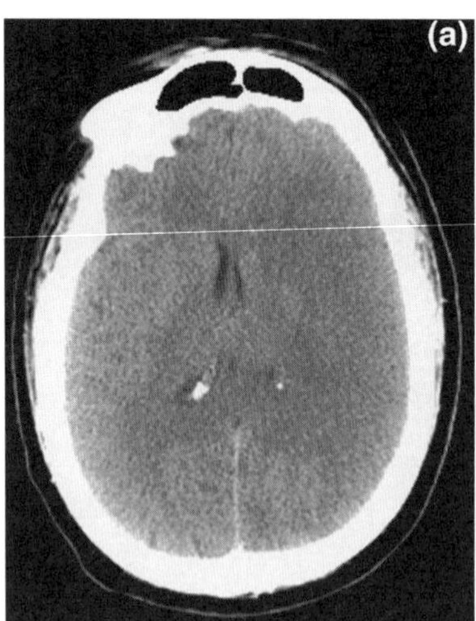

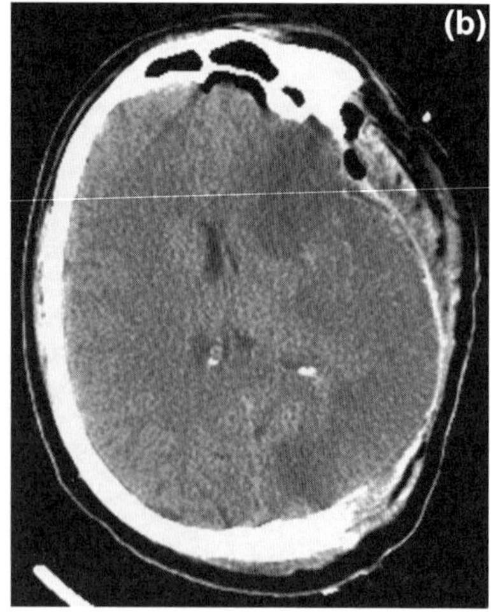

FIGURE 6.3 (**a**) Thirty-eight-year-old male presenting with new onset headache, hand numbness, and visual changes, deteriorating to aphasia and right hemiparesis over 3 hours. This CT demonstrates a large left MCA infarct with hypoattenuation in the MCA territory, loss of normal gray–white matter differentiation, partial effacement of the frontal horn of the left lateral ventricle, and sulcal effacement within the left frontal and parietal lobes. (**b**) Postoperative CT after decompressive hemicraniectomy and left anterior temporal lobectomy.

depends on the degree of decompression achieved, and a repeat operation may be necessary for clinical and/or radiographic evidence of persistent herniation.

Patient Selection

Decompressive hemicraniectomy has been shown to reduce mortality and improve outcome in patients with malignant MCA infarction.[34–36] It is usually reserved for patients with large territory supratentorial infarction who subsequently develop severe symptomatic brain swelling, and should be limited to those patients who experience a clinically progressive course. Signs of uncal herniation, including pupillary abnormalities or a deterioration in level of consciousness, should prompt the physician to consider this surgical option, since these patients tend to be refractory to conventional medical management of ICP. Furthermore, ventriculostomy is not a good option by itself because it can exacerbate focal brain shifts due to mass effect from the swelling.

Not all patients with MCA infarction, however, will develop severe brain swelling and herniation. Significant edema occurs in only 10–13% of all proximal MCA infarctions, but results in a mortality rate higher than 80%.[33–36] The risk of developing severe brain swelling is greatest in the first 24–48 hours and is associated with younger age, nausea and vomiting in the first 24 hours, early hypodensity on CT, increased amount of MCA territory involved (>50%), National Institutes of Health Stroke Scale (NIHSS) score of $\geq$15 for right hemispheric MCA infarction and $\geq$20 for left hemisphere infarct, and a midline shift of more than 10 mm at the level of the septum pellucidum.[33,35]

Younger age at presentation has consistently correlated with a better outcome after decompressive hemicraniectomy.[33,34,37,38] In one study of 42 patients (mean age of 50 years, range 15–73), Rabinstein et al.[39] showed an odds ratio for poor outcome of 2.9 per 10-year increase in age. Another study showed that 70% of patients 40 years or younger had Glasgow Outcome Scale (GOS) scores of 4 or 5, a level achieved in only 20% of patients older than 55 years. Furthermore, while decompressive hemicraniectomy is generally indicated for nondominant hemispheric infarction, younger patients with dominant hemisphere infarction may also benefit. In those with dominant hemisphere infarctions and preserved language function who subsequently deteriorate, decompressive hemicraniectomy can also be considered; however, patients initially presenting with global aphasia are generally not good candidates.

Timing

Interestingly, studies have not conclusively demonstrated a benefit of hemicraniectomy for patients who are surgically treated before developing signs and symptoms of herniation.[34,36] Schwab et al.[36] studied 63 patients who underwent hemicraniectomy for acute MCA infarction. Although the mortality rate for patients undergoing early surgery (<24 hours after stroke symptom onset) was lower than for patients who underwent surgery after the first signs of herniation (16% vs. 34%, respectively), there was no significant difference in outcome between early surgery and late surgery with mean Barthel Index scores of 70 and 63, respectively. Early decompression, however, also led to a significant reduction in length of stay in the intensive care unit (7.4 days vs. 13.3 days).

The concern with early surgery is that not all patients with large territory infarction will develop malignant cerebral edema and signs of herniation. Furthermore, some patients with raised ICP from infarct-related cerebral edema will improve with medical treatment alone. Hence, many patients chosen to undergo early hemicraniectomy might do so unnecessarily. On the contrary, waiting for signs of herniation, such as pupillary dilatation, may cause an unnecessary delay in management. Robertson et al.[35] suggest that patients who are at higher risk of developing malignant cerebral edema should undergo early hemicraniectomy and duraplasty, while those patients with signs of herniation should also undergo anterior temporal lobectomy and resection of nonviable tissue.

Although the questions of how early to perform the procedure and which patients will most benefit from decompressive hemicraniectomy are currently addressed by retrospective studies or case series, several prospective randomized trials, such as Hemicraniectomy and Durotomy upon Deterioration from Infarction Related Swelling Trial (HEADDFIRST) and Hemicraniectomy after Middle Cerebral Artery Infarction with Life-threatening Edema Trial (HAMLET), are ongoing. Results of these studies will hopefully aid clinicians in making better decisions regarding a patient's candidacy for, and outcome after, the aggressive procedure.[40] Until better eligibility criteria are defined, all patients with either dominant or nondominant large territory MCA infarction should be evaluated for potential decompressive hemicraniectomy on a case-by-case basis and by a team comprised of neurosurgeons, stroke neurologists, and intensive care specialists. Furthermore, it is important to have early discussions with the patient and their family regarding options for management in any case that could potentially be treated by decompressive hemicraniectomy. These discussions should take place prior to potential deterioration in the patient's condition, since surgical decompression should be undertaken emergently once signs of herniation develop.

POSTERIOR FOSSA DECOMPRESSION

Decompression of the posterior fossa is the infratentorial equivalent of a decompressive hemicraniectomy. It is primarily intended for cerebellar infarction, usually in the distribution of the posterior inferior cerebellar artery (PICA), and typically involves the removal of bone overlying the infarcted tissue (Fig. 6.4).[41] Opening of the dura and evacuation of necrotic tissue is frequently done, but it depends on the timing of surgery and the clinical scenario. A frontal horn ventriculostomy is also typically placed at the time of surgery; however, its use alone in the management of cerebellar infarction may result in upward herniation of tissue and is generally not recommended.

Although surgery can improve outcome in patients with imminent infratentorial herniation, the selection of patients, timing of surgery, and the type of surgery is widely disputed and treated differently across institutions.[10,42–44] Following

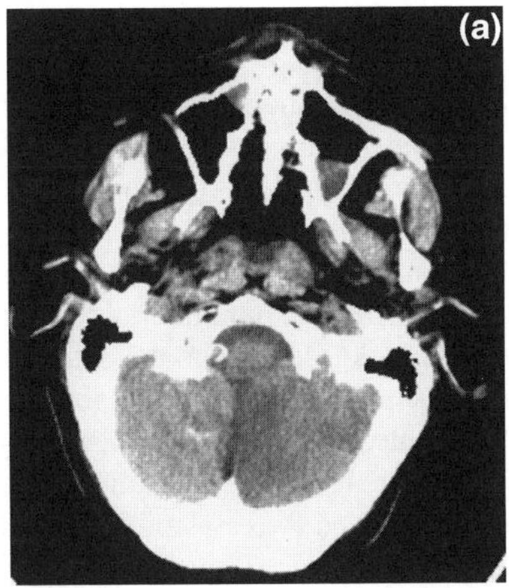

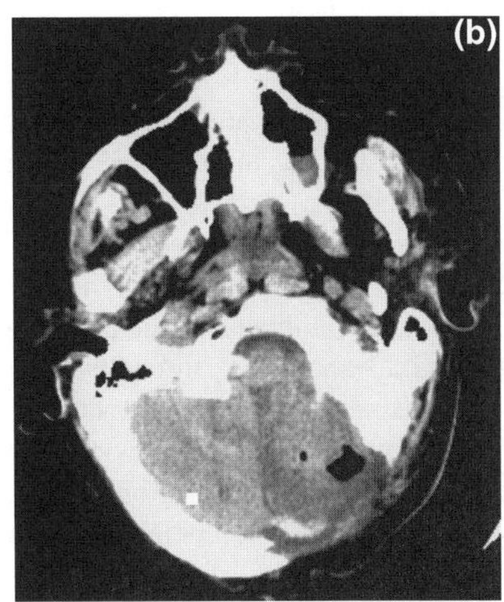

FIGURE 6.4 (**a**) Seventy-eight-year-old woman presenting with new onset vertigo and gait unsteadiness. Hypoattenuation of the left cerebellar hemisphere consistent with infarction. (**b**) Postoperative CT after suboccipital craniectomy and partial resection of the left cerebellar hemisphere.

cerebellar stroke, patients should be monitored closely in a neurological intensive care unit or specialized neurological ward for clinical signs of worsening. After the first 72–96 hours, further deterioration is unlikely.[45] If signs of deterioration develop, they can be managed initially with osmotic agents, such as hypertonic saline or mannitol. Within the confines of the posterior fossa, however, the development of significant edema following acute infarction is unpredictable and may be catastrophic, resulting in deterioration due to direct mass effect on the brainstem, obstructive hydrocephalus by fourth ventricle compression, or occlusion of the cerebral aqueduct secondary to upward herniation of the vermis.[46]

Emergent surgery should be strongly considered for patients who present with signs of brainstem compression, increased intracranial pressure, or hydrocephalus.[47] In patients who are initially neurologically stable then subsequently decline, only a brief trial of medical therapy should precede emergent surgical intervention since irreversible brainstem injury can occur rapidly. In addition, clinical judgment taking into account the size of infarcted territory and time since ictus should be exercised in order to expedite decompression in patients prior to significant deterioration and permanent tissue damage. For example, in an obtunded patient with massive cerebellar infarction, posterior fossa decompression is essential.

Specific predictive factors for outcome after surgical intervention have not been well defined in the literature. In one prospective, multicenter observational study of 95 patients, the state of consciousness was the only predictive factor retained in a logistic regression analysis.[42] In this study, there was a 2.8-fold increased risk for poor outcome for each increase on a three-step scale (awake/drowsy, somnolent/stuporous, and comatose), and good outcomes (modified Rankin Scale score ≤ 2) were achieved in 86%, 76%, and 47% of patients within each group, respectively.

INTRACRANIAL EMBOLECTOMY

Intracranial embolectomy involves the use of general anesthesia, open craniotomy, and arteriotomy for the retrieval of embolic material. In the past, it has been used most frequently to remove solid embolus from the proximal MCA, although reports of successful embolectomy of other intracranial vessels also exist.[5,30,48–50] Its use has decreased in recent years, primarily due to the increased and more effective use of intravenous recombinant tissue plasminogen activator (rt-PA), intra-arterial thrombolysis, and advancements in endovascular mechanical clot disruption and extraction. The Mechanical Embolus Removal in Cerebral Ischemia (MERCI) device, for example, is a new endovascular device being used for mechanical embolus removal in patients who either are ineligible or have failed intravenous thrombolytic therapy.[51,52]

Currently, surgical embolectomy is a technique reserved for cases of failed endovascular intervention. These situations may arise if catheters cannot be navigated through the intracranial vasculature to the embolus, if they are unable to cross the occluded segment, or in cases of an embolized interventional device. The success of an open surgical procedure, however, also depends on the nature and severity of symptoms, interval since symptom onset, probable source of the embolus, location of occlusion, extent of collateral circulation, and general medical condition of the patient. This procedure is best reserved for patients in good medical condition who have failed attempts at endovascular embolectomy, and who present soon after the onset of symptoms with a proximally located solid embolus and good collateral circulation.[5]

In a report by Meyer et al.,[49] blood flow was successfully restored in 75% of patients undergoing urgent surgical MCA embolectomy. Although all patients had moderate-to-severe neurological deficits preoperatively, 10% subsequently had no neurologic deficit, 25% had minimal deficits, 35% were independent but had substantial deficits, 20% had a poor outcome, and 10% died.[5] In another report by Touho et al.,[50] best results were obtained when open embolectomy was performed within 6 hours after onset of symptoms.

CONCLUSION

Optimal stroke care requires a proactive, evidence-based, multidisciplinary team approach using a combination of medical, interventional and, in selected patients, neurosurgical care. The speed and uncertainty of evolving acute stroke are best addressed with vigilant preparedness, as well as family communication, education, and counseling. Although prospective, controlled data remain sparse for some neurosurgical procedures, there is a clear role for surgery in acute ischemic stroke. Continued evidence-based practice will further refine management and improve outcomes for these patients.

Financial Relationships and Grant Information

The authors have not received any financial support in conjunction with the generation of this submission and there are no grants pertinent to this paper. In addition, the authors have no personal or institutional financial interest in drugs, materials, or devices described in this submission.

REFERENCES

1. Connolly JE. The evolution of extracranial carotid artery surgery as seen by one surgeon over the past 40 years. *Surgeon* 2003;1:249–258.
2. Beneficial effect of carotid endarterectomy in symptomatic patients with high-grade carotid stenosis. North American Symptomatic Carotid Endarterectomy Trial Collaborators. *N Engl J Med* 1991;325:445–453.
3. Mrc European carotid surgery trial: interim results for symptomatic patients with severe (70–99%) or with mild (0–29%) carotid stenosis. European Carotid Surgery Trialists' Collaborative Group. *Lancet* 1991;337:1235–1243.
4. Aleksic M, Rueger MA, Lehnhardt FG, Sobesky J, Matoussevitch V, Neveling M, Heiss WD, Brunkwall J, Jacobs AH. Primary stroke unit treatment followed by very early carotid endarterectomy for carotid artery stenosis after acute stroke. *Cerebrovasc Dis* 2006;22:276–281.
5. Pikus HJ, Heros RC. Stroke: indications for emergent surgical intervention. *Clin Neurosurg* 1999;45:113–127.
6. Ballotta E, Da Giau G, Baracchini C, Abbruzzese E, Saladini M, Meneghetti G. Early versus delayed carotid endarterectomy after a nondisabling ischemic stroke: a prospective randomized study. *Surgery* 2002;131:287–293.
7. McPherson CM, Woo D, Cohen PL, Pancioli AM, Kissela BM, Carrozzella JA, Tomsick TA, Zuccarello M. Early carotid endarterectomy for critical carotid artery stenosis after thrombolysis therapy in acute ischemic stroke in the middle cerebral artery. *Stroke* 2001;32:2075–2080.
8. Krishnamurthy S, Tong D, McNamara KP, Steinberg GK, Cockroft KM. Early carotid endarterectomy after ischemic stroke improves diffusion/perfusion mismatch on magnetic resonance imaging: report of two cases. *Neurosurgery* 2003;52:238–241 [discussion 242].
9. Blaisdell WF, Clauss RH, Galbraith JG, Imparato AM, Wylie EJ. Joint study of extracranial arterial occlusion. IV. A review of surgical considerations. *JAMA* 1969;209:1889–1895.
10. Caplan LR, Skillman J, Ojemann R, Fields WS. Intracerebral hemorrhage following carotid endarterectomy: a hypertensive complication? *Stroke* 1978;9:457–460.
11. Giordano JM, Trout 3rd, HH, Kozloff L, DePalma RG. Timing of carotid artery endarterectomy after stroke. *J Vasc Surg* 1985;2:250–255.
12. Wylie EJ, Hein MF, Adams JE. Intracranial hemorrhage following surgical revascularization for treatment of acute strokes. *J Neurosurg* 1964;21:212–215.
13. Gasecki AP, Ferguson GG, Eliasziw M, Clagett GP, Fox AJ, Hachinski V, Barnett HJ. Early endarterectomy for severe carotid artery stenosis after a nondisabling stroke: Results from the North American symptomatic carotid endarterectomy trial. *J Vasc Surg* 1994;20:288–295.
14. Barnett HJ, Meldrum HE, Eliasziw M. The appropriate use of carotid endarterectomy. *CMAJ* 2002;166:1169–1179.

15. Blaser T, Hofmann K, Buerger T, Effenberger O, Wallesch CW, Goertler M. Risk of stroke, transient ischemic attack, and vessel occlusion before endarterectomy in patients with symptomatic severe carotid stenosis. *Stroke* 2002;33:1057–1062.

16. Lovett JK, Coull AJ, Rothwell PM. Early risk of recurrence by subtype of ischemic stroke in population-based incidence studies. *Neurology* 2004;62:569–573.

17. Findlay JM, Marchak BE, Pelz DM, Feasby TE. Carotid endarterectomy: a review. *Can J Neurol Sci* 2004;31:22–36.

18. Heros RC. Carotid endarterectomy in patients with intraluminal thrombus. *Stroke* 1988;19:667–668.

19. Buchan A, Gates P, Pelz D, Barnett HJ. Intraluminal thrombus in the cerebral circulation. Implications for surgical management. *Stroke* 1988;19:681–687.

20. Kawaguchi S, Okuno S, Sakaki T. Effect of direct arterial bypass on the prevention of future stroke in patients with the hemorrhagic variety of moyamoya disease. *J Neurosurg* 2000;93:397–401.

21. Engel S, Ferraz H. Indications and results of extra-intracranial arterial bypasses. *Int Surg* 1983;68:197–200.

22. Failure of extracranial–intracranial arterial bypass to reduce the risk of ischemic stroke. Results of an international randomized trial. The EC/IC Bypass Study Group. *N Engl J Med* 1985;313:1191–1200.

23. McDowell F, Flamm ES. EC/IC bypass study. *Stroke* 1986;17:1–2.

24. Powers WJ, Grubb Jr, RL, Raichle ME. Clinical results of extracranial–intracranial bypass surgery in patients with hemodynamic cerebrovascular disease. *J Neurosurg* 1989;70:61–67.

25. Grubb Jr, RL, Derdeyn CP, Fritsch SM, Carpenter DA, Yundt KD, Videen TO, Spitznagel EL, Powers WJ. Importance of hemodynamic factors in the prognosis of symptomatic carotid occlusion. *JAMA* 1998;280:1055–1060.

26. Nagata S, Fujii K, Matsushima T, Fukui M, Sadoshima S, Kuwabara Y, Abe H. Evaluation of EC–IC bypass for patients with atherosclerotic occlusive cerebrovascular disease: clinical and positron emission tomographic studies. *Neurol Res* 1991;13: 209–216.

27. Sasoh M, Ogasawara K, Kuroda K, Okuguchi T, Terasaki K, Yamadate K, Ogawa A. Effects of EC–IC bypass surgery on cognitive impairment in patients with hemodynamic cerebral ischemia. *Surg Neurol* 2003;59:455–460 [discussion 460–453].

28. Mizumura S, Nakagawara J, Takahashi M, Kumita S, Cho K, Nakajo H, Toba M, Kumazaki T. Three-dimensional display in staging hemodynamic brain ischemia for jet study: objective evaluation using see analysis and 3d-ssp display. *Ann Nucl Med* 2004;18:13–21.

29. Jinnouchi J, Toyoda K, Inoue T, Fujimoto S, Gotoh S, Yasumori K, Ibayashi S, Iida M, Okada Y. Changes in brain volume 2 years after extracranial–intracranial bypass surgery: a preliminary subanalysis of the japanese EC–IC trial. *Cerebrovasc Dis* 2006;22: 177–182.

30. Meyer FB, Piepgras DG, Sundt TM, Yanagihara T. Emergency embolectomy for acute embolic occlusion of the middle cerebral artery. *Clin Neurosurg* 1985;32:155–173.

31. Diaz FG, Ausman JI, Mehta B, Dujovny M, de los Reyes RA, Pearce J, Patel S. Acute cerebral revascularization. *J Neurosurg* 1985;63:200–209.

32. Crowell RM, Olsson Y. Effect of extracranial–intracranial vascular bypass graft on experimental acute stroke in dogs. *J Neurosurg* 1973;38:26–31.
33. Subramaniam S, Hill MD. Massive cerebral infarction. *Neurologist* 2005;11:150–160.
34. Curry Jr, WT, Sethi MK, Ogilvy CS, Carter BS. Factors associated with outcome after hemicraniectomy for large middle cerebral artery territory infarction. *Neurosurgery* 2005;56:681–692 [discussion 681–692].
35. Robertson SC, Lennarson P, Hasan DM, Traynelis VC. Clinical course and surgical management of massive cerebral infarction. *Neurosurgery* 2004;55:55–61 [discussion 61–52].
36. Schwab S, Steiner T, Aschoff A, Schwarz S, Steiner HH, Jansen O, Hacke W. Early hemicraniectomy in patients with complete middle cerebral artery infarction. *Stroke* 1998;29:1888–1893.
37. Leonhardt G, Wilhelm H, Doerfler A, Ehrenfeld CE, Schoch B, Rauhut F, Hufnagel A, Diener HC. Clinical outcome and neuropsychological deficits after right decompressive hemicraniectomy in mca infarction. *J Neurol* 2002;249:1433–1440.
38. Wijdicks EF, Diringer MN. Middle cerebral artery territory infarction and early brain swelling: progression and effect of age on outcome. *Mayo Clin Proc* 1998;73: 829–836.
39. Rabinstein AA, Mueller-Kronast N, Maramattom BV, Zazulia AR, Bamlet WR, Diringer MN, Wijdicks EF. Factors predicting prognosis after decompressive hemicraniectomy for hemispheric infarction. *Neurology* 2006;67:891–893.
40. Hofmeijer J, Amelink GJ, Algra A, van Gijn J, Macleod MR, Kappelle LJ, van der Worp HB. Hemicraniectomy after middle cerebral artery infarction with life-threatening edema trial (hamlet). Protocol for a randomised controlled trial of decompressive surgery in space-occupying hemispheric infarction. *Trials* 2006;7:29.
41. Laun A, Busse O, Calatayud V, Klug N. Cerebellar infarcts in the area of the supply of the pica and their surgical treatment. *Acta Neurochir (Wien)* 1984;71:295–306.
42. Jauss M, Krieger D, Hornig C, Schramm J, Busse O. Surgical and medical management of patients with massive cerebellar infarctions: results of the German-Austrian cerebellar infarction study. *J Neurol* 1999;246:257–264.
43. Ho SU, Kim KS, Berenberg RA, Ho HT. Cerebellar infarction: a clinical and ct study. *Surg Neurol* 1981;16:350–352.
44. Scotti G, Spinnler H, Sterzi R, Vallar G. Cerebellar softening. *Ann Neurol* 1980;8: 133–140.
45. Jensen MB, St. Louis EK. Management of acute cerebellar stroke. *Arch Neurol* 2005;62:537–544.
46. Tohgi H, Takahashi S, Chiba K, Hirata Y. Cerebellar infarction. Clinical and neuroimaging analysis in 293 patients. The Tohoku Cerebellar Infarction Study Group. *Stroke* 1993;24:1697–1701.
47. Tulyapronchote R, Malkoff MD, Selhorst JB, Gomez CR. Treatment of cerebellar infarction by decompression suboccipital craniectomy. *Stroke* 1993;24:478–480.
48. Findlay JM, Ashforth R, Dean N. "Malignant" carotid artery dissection. *Can J Neurol Sci* 2002;29:378–385.
49. Meyer FB, Piepgras DG, Sundt Jr, TM, Yanagihara T. Emergency embolectomy for acute occlusion of the middle cerebral artery. *J Neurosurg* 1985;62:639–647.

50. Touho H, Morisako T, Hashimoto Y, Karasawa J. Embolectomy for acute embolic occlusion of the internal carotid artery bifurcation. *Surg Neurol* 1999;51:313–320.

51. Smith WS. Safety of mechanical thrombectomy and intravenous tissue plasminogen activator in acute ischemic stroke. Results of the multi mechanical embolus removal in cerebral ischemia (MERCI) trial, part I. *Am J Neuroradiol* 2006;27:1177–1182.

52. Smith WS, Sung G, Starkman S, Saver JL, Kidwell CS, Gobin YP, Lutsep HL, Nesbit GM, Grobelny T, Rymer MM, Silverman IE, Higashida RT, Budzik RF, Marks MP. Safety and efficacy of mechanical embolectomy in acute ischemic stroke: results of the merci trial. *Stroke* 2005;36:1432–1438.

7

ANTITHROMBOTIC THERAPY FOR ACUTE STROKE

Orla Sheehan and Peter Kelly

HEPARIN AND HEPARINOIDS

Unfractionated Heparin

Heparin was discovered in 1916 by a medical student at Johns Hopkins University. While attempting to extract thromboplastic substances from various tissues he discovered a substance with powerful anticoagulant activity. This was named "heparin" because it was first extracted from the liver.

Unfractionated heparin (UFH) is a mixture of sulfated glycosaminoglycans with a range of molecular weights up to 40,000 Da. UFH inhibits the coagulation cascade nonspecifically at several sites by inhibiting factors IIa, IXa, Xa, XIa, XIIa.[1] It also inhibits platelet function by binding to von Willebrand Factor (vWF) and interfering with its platelet hemostatic properties.[2,3] It acts on both the intrinsic and the extrinsic pathways of the coagulation cascade by inhibiting thrombin-mediated conversion of fibrinogen to fibrin, thus potentiating the actions of antithrombin III, inhibiting activation of factor IX, and by activating factor X inhibitor (Fig. 7.1).

Heparin must be given parenterally as it is not absorbed by the gut due to the large size and charge of its constituent molecules. Because of its short half-life (approximately 1 hour) UFH must be given frequently or as a continuous infusion.

Hemorrhage is the main complication that can arise from heparin therapy. Other side effects include Heparin-Induced Thrombocytopenia Syndrome (HITS), local irritation, hypersensitivity reactions and with long-term use, alopecia, hypoaldosteronism, and osteoporosis.

Acute Ischemic Stroke: An Evidence-based Approach, Edited by David M. Greer.

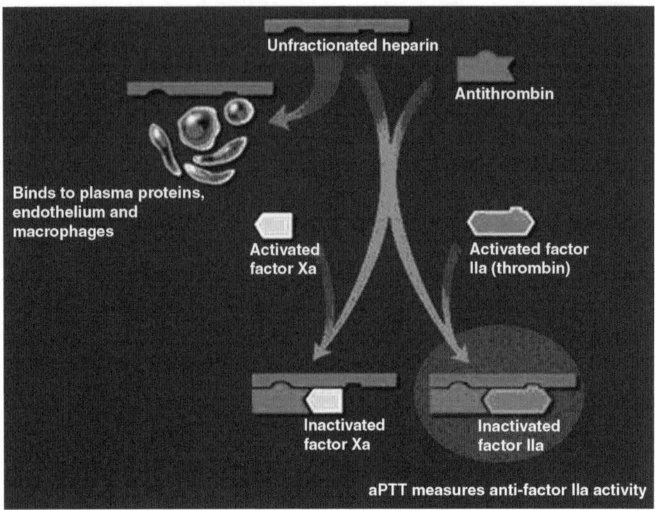

FIGURE 7.1 Effect of UFH and LMWH on factors IIa and Xa. Both types of heparin inactivate factor Xa by interacting with antithrombin. Longer chain UFH is able to inactivate factor IIa through formation of a tertiary complex, unlike LMWH. Compared with LMWH, UFH binds more to plasma proteins, endothelium, and macrophages, resulting in reduced bioavailability and greater variability to a given dose. UFH inactivates factors IIa and Xa and affects the PTT, a measure of anti-factor IIa activity. (Reprinted from the American Family Physician published by the American Academy of Family Physicians, February 15th, 1999, in an article entitled "Low-molecular-weight heparin in outpatient treatment of DVT.")

Low-Molecular-Weight Heparins and Heparinoids

The multiple effects of UFH on the coagulation cascade may increase its potential to cause hemorrhage.[4] Anticoagulants with more specific sites of action may confer a better safety profile. Two such anticoagulants are low-molecular-weight heparin (LMWH) and heparinoids.

Natural UFH consists of molecular chains of molecular weights varying from 5000 to more than 40,000 Da. In practice, its anticoagulant effect may be difficult to predict, requiring regular monitoring of the prothrombin time (PTT) and dose adjustment. In contrast, LMWHs consist of only short chains of polysaccharide having an average molecular weight of less than 8000 Da.

LMWHs are formed by various methods of fractionation or depolymerization of polymeric heparin (Table 7.1). Although they are enzymatically derived from UFH, they have a different site of action and can be administered subcutaneously. LMWHs exert their anticoagulant effect by inhibiting factor Xa and augmenting tissue-factor-pathway inhibitor, but minimally affect thrombin or factor IIa (Figs. 7.1 and 7.2).[4–6] Thus, the PTT, a measure of antithrombin (anti-factor IIa) activity, is not used to measure the activity of LMWHs.

Heparinoid is a term used to describe naturally occurring and synthetic glycosoaminoglycans of structure similar to heparin. Heparinoids have specific

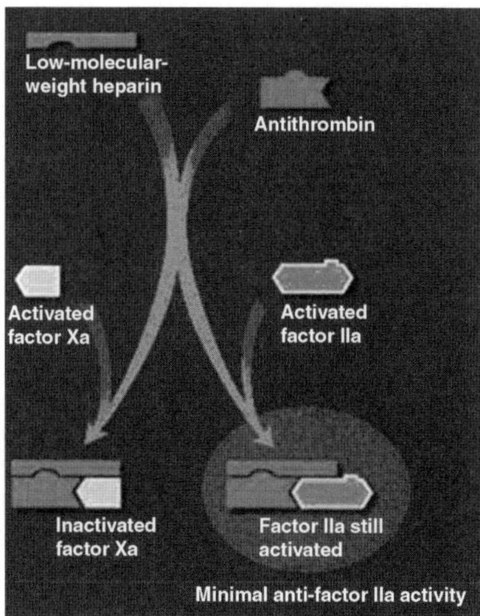

FIGURE 7.2 LMWH inhibits factor Xa and minimally affects factor IIa; thus, activated partial thromboplastin time is not used to measure its anticoagulant activity. (Reprinted from the American Family Physician published by the American Academy of Family Physicians, February 15th, 1999, in an article entitled "Low-molecular-weight heparin in outpatient treatment of DVT.")

antithrombin activity.[4,7] They are often used as an alternative to heparin in patients with HITS (Table 7.2).

Trials of Heparin in Acute Ischemic Stroke

Placebo-Controlled Trials of UFH, LMWH, and Heparinoids The International Stroke Trial (IST)[8] was a randomized, placebo-controlled trial of UFH (5000 or 12,500 IU twice daily) and aspirin (300 mg) in 19,435 unselected patients with acute stroke within 48 hours of symptom onset. Because of limited availability of neuroimaging, 33% of participants were enrolled with suspected but not proven ischemic stroke, some of whom may have suffered primary intracerebral hemorrhage (ICH).

TABLE 7.1 Commonly used LMWHs and Heparinoids.

Main LMWHs	Method of Preparation
Enoxaparin sodium	Benzylation followed by alkaline depolymerization
Dalteparin sodium	Nitrous acid depolymerization
Tinzaparin	Enzymatic depolymerization with heparinase
Nadroparin sodium	Nitrous acid depolymerization
Ardepatrin	Peroxidative depolymerization
Main heparinoid	Method of preparation
Danaparoid sodium	Prepared from animal gut mucosa; contains heparin sulfate (84%), dermatan sulfate (12%), and chondroitin sulfate (4%)

TABLE 7.2 Comparison of UFH and LMWH.

	UFH	LMWH
Administration	Intravenous	Subcutaneous
Bioavailabilty	Low, inconsistent	High, consistent
Elimination	Hepatic	Renal
Rate of HIT	More common	Rare
Monitoring of levels	Compulsory	Not required

In the heparin group, there were fewer recurrent ischemic strokes at 14 days (2.9% vs. 3.8%, $2p = 0.005$). This was offset by an increase in hemorrhagic strokes (1.2% vs. 0.4%, $2p < 0.00001$), resulting in a nonsignificant difference in death or nonfatal recurrent stroke at 14 days. The 12,500 IU dose of UFH was associated with more bleeding, more hemorrhagic strokes, and more deaths at 14 days. At 6 months the percentage dead or dependent was identical in both groups (62.9%).

Conflicting data were obtained from a randomized, placebo-controlled trial of 418 patients in which UFH was started within 3 hours of onset of symptoms as treatment for acute nonlacunar hemispheric cerebral infarction.[9] Patients were randomized to receive intravenous UFH or saline. In the heparin group, there were more independent patients as judged by a modified Rankin Scale (mRS) score of 0–2 (38.9% vs. 28.6%, $p = 0.025$). The incidence of symptomatic ICH (sICH) was greater in the heparin group (6.2% vs. 1.4%, $p = 0.008$) but no difference was found in rates of mortality or systemic hemorrhage between groups. This suggested a net benefit from UFH in this context, even after accounting for the increased frequency of sICH.

The Trial of Org 10172 in Acute Stroke Treatment (TOAST) was a randomized, double-blind, placebo-controlled trial of danaparoid in 1281 patients within 24 hours of onset of acute ischemic stroke.[10] A three-stage dosage regime was used to achieve plasma anti-factor Xa activity of 0.8 unit/mL. Favorable outcome was defined as the combination of a Glasgow Outcome Scale (GOS) score of 1 or 2 and a modified Barthel Index (BI) score of 12 or greater (on a scale of 0–20) at 3 months or 7 days. Very favorable outcome required the combination of a GOS score of 1 and a Barthel Index (BI) score of 19 or 20 at 3 months or 7 days.

The primary analysis showed no significant difference in the rate of favorable outcome at 3 months between the groups. Secondary analysis of 7-day outcomes found 59.2% of the heparinoid group compared to 54.3% of the placebo group with favorable outcome ($p = 0.07$) and 33.9% compared to 27.8% having a very favorable outcome ($p = 0.01$). Strokes due to large artery atherosclerosis (LAA) had significantly higher rates of favorable and very favorable outcome at 3 months among subjects who received the heparinoid ($p = 0.04$). No treatment effect was noted in other stroke subtypes. Although rates of neurological deterioration within the first 7 days were similar in both groups, more major bleeding events occurred within 10 days in the danaparoid group (33 events vs. 11 events, $p < 0.005$).

One meta-analysis examined the safety and efficacy of LMWH and heparinoids in 11 randomized trials of 3048 patients with acute ischemic stroke.[11] It reported a reduction in the incidence of deep venous thrombosis (DVT) (odds ratio (OR) 0.27,

95% CI 0.08–0.96) and symptomatic pulmonary embolism (PE) (OR 0.34, 95% CI 0.17–0.69), but an increase in major extracranial hemorrhage when compared to placebo (OR 2.17, 95% CI 1.10–4.28). Nonsignificant reductions in combined death and disability, as well as increases in case fatality and sICH were also observed. The authors concluded that insufficient evidence existed to support the routine use of LMWH in the management of patients with ischemic stroke.

The Cochrane Collaborators also reviewed acute anticoagulant therapy in 22 trials involving 23,547 patients.[12] Selection criteria were randomized trials comparing early anticoagulant therapy (started within 2 weeks of stroke onset) with control in patients with acute presumed or confirmed ischemic stroke. The anticoagulants included were UFH, LMWH, heparinoids, oral anticoagulants, and thrombin inhibitors. They found that, although anticoagulant therapy was associated with about 9 fewer recurrent ischemic strokes per 1000 patients treated, it was also associated with a similar sized 9 per 1000 patients increase in sICH. Similarly, anticoagulants prevented about 4 PEs per 1000, but this benefit was offset by an extra 9 major extracranial hemorrhages. They concluded that immediate anticoagulant therapy in patients with acute ischemic stroke is not associated with a net short- or long-term benefit.

Trials Comparing Heparin to Aspirin in Acute Stroke

The Heparin in Acute Embolic Stroke Trial (HAEST) was a multicenter, randomized trial of the effect of LMWH (dalteparin 100 IU/kg sc twice daily) or aspirin (160 mg once daily) for the acute treatment of 449 patients with ischemic stroke and atrial fibrillation (AF).[13] The primary outcome was the rate of recurrent stroke within 14 days. No difference in rates of early recurrence (8.5% dalteparin treated vs. 7.5% aspirin treated) or good 3-month functional outcome was found. The frequency of early sICH was 2.7% on dalteparin versus 1.8% on aspirin.

Tinzaparin in Acute Ischemic Stroke Trial (TAIST) was a randomized, double-blind trial that compared high-dose tinzaparin (175 IU/kg/day), medium-dose tinzaparin (100 IU/kg/day), or aspirin (300 mg/day) started within 48 hours of acute ischemic stroke, given for up to 10 days.[14] The proportion of patients independent at 6 months was similar in all the three groups (41.5% high-dose tinzaparin, 42.5% medium-dose tinzaparin, 42.5% aspirin). Rates of disability, case fatality, and neurological deterioration were also similar. No patients in the high-dose tinzaparin group developed a symptomatic DVT, but nine occurred in the aspirin group. A dose-dependent incidence of sICH was observed (seven with high-dose tinzaparin, three in the medium-dose tinzaparin group, and one in the aspirin group). Neither subtype-specific benefit of tinzaparin, nor a benefit on analysis of subgroups defined by age, gender, severity, or time to treatment onset was observed.

Trials of Unfractionated Heparin Compared to LMWH and Heparinoids

Relatively few data exist concerning the relative benefits of UFH, LMWH, and heparinoids in acute stroke treatment. In 2005, the Cochrane Collaboration reviewed trials comparing LMWHs or heparinoids with UFH in acute ischemic stroke.[15] Six trials involving 740 subjects were included. Four trials compared a heparinoid (danaparoid), one trial compared a LMWH (enoxaparin), and one trial compared an unspecified LMWH. In all cases, the control was UFH. Only trials in which treatment was started within 14 days of stroke onset were included.

Groups assigned to a LMWH or heparinoid had a significant reduction in the odds of DVT (OR 0.52, 95% CI 0.56–0.79). However, there were too few major events (PE, death, intracranial or extracranial hemorrhage) to provide a reliable estimate of other benefits or risks.

The PROTECT trial looked at certoparin, a LMWH, and compared it to UFH for the prevention of thromboembolic complications in patients with acute ischemic stroke.[16] It was a double-blinded trial of 545 patients randomized within 24 hours of stroke onset. Certoparin 3000 U anti-Xa once daily was compared to UFH 5000 IU sc three times daily, both given for 12–16 days. The rates of major thromboembolic events were 6.6% in the certoparin group compared with 8.8% in the UFH group, indicating noninferiority of certoparin ($p = 0.008$). There was no difference in major bleeding rates between groups (1.1% in certoparin vs. 1.8% in UFH group). It was concluded that certoparin was at least as effective and safe as UFH for the prevention of thromboembolic complications in this trial.

Combination Anticoagulant and Antiplatelet Therapy in Acute Stroke

The Cochrane group examined (a) whether the addition of UFH or LMWH to antiplatelet agents offers any net advantage over antiplatelet monotherapy for acute stroke, and (b) the effectiveness of anticoagulants compared to antiplatelets in acute ischemic stroke.[17] They included 4 trials of 16,558 patients, each of which specified aspirin (160–333 mg daily) as the control, and all of which randomized patients within 14 days of stroke onset. The anticoagulants tested were UFH and LMWH. Almost 98% of the patients were followed up for 6 months.

Compared with aspirin monotherapy, anticoagulant treatment was associated with a small but significant increase in the number of deaths at the end of follow-up (OR 1.10, 95% CI 1.01–1.29), equivalent to 20 more deaths per 1000 patients treated with anticoagulants. Subgroup analysis showed that the combination of low-dose UFH and aspirin was associated with a marginally significant reduced risk of any recurrent stroke (OR 0.75, 95% CI 0.56–1.03) and a marginally significant reduced risk of death at 14 days (OR 0.84, 95% CI 0.69–1.01), with no clear adverse effect on death at the end of follow-up.

As in previous reviews they also found an increased risk of sICH (OR 2.27, 95% CI 1.49–3.46), equivalent to 10 more (95% CI 0–10 more) sICHs per 1000 patients treated. An interaction by anticoagulant dose on sICH was observed ($p = 0.01$), with a greater risk in trials using high-dose anticoagulants (OR 3.24, 95% CI 2.09–5.04) as opposed to low-dose anticoagulants (OR 1.29, 95% CI 0.72–2.32). A similar dose–response relationship was observed when comparing UFH plus aspirin with aspirin monotherapy in the IST trial. Compared directly with aspirin, anticoagulants were associated with a nonsignificant increase in the risk of recurrent stroke (OR 1.20, 95% CI 0.99–1.46), equivalent to 10 more recurrent strokes per 1000 patients treated.

This was largely influenced by the high-dose UFH group in IST (OR 1.38, 95% CI 1.05–1.82). An interaction by UFH dose ($p = 0.01$) on recurrent stroke risk with combination UFH–aspirin therapy compared to aspirin monotherapy was observed, with a trend toward increased risk of recurrent stroke with high-dose UFH + aspirin (OR 1.22, 95% CI 0.92–1.62) and a trend toward reduced risk with low-dose UFH + aspirin (OR 0.75, 95% CI 0.56–1.03), equivalent to 10 fewer (95% CI 0–20 fewer) recurrent strokes per 1000 patients treated. They found a small, but significant benefit of LMWH over aspirin in the prevention of symptomatic DVT, equivalent to 10 (95% CI 0–30) fewer DVTs per 1000 patients treated. Compared with aspirin, anticoagulants were associated with nonsignificantly fewer symptomatic PEs (OR 0.85, 95% CI 0.55–1.32). There were fewer PEs with the combination of UFH and aspirin (OR 0.58, 95% CI 0.34–1.00), equivalent to 5 fewer (CI 0–10) PEs per 1000 patients treated. However, the overall incidence of symptomatic DVT and PE was low (1.1% and 0.7%).

Overall no evidence was found to support the claim that anticoagulants offer a net advantage over aspirin in patients with acute ischemic stroke. There was evidence, however, to suggest that combination anticoagulant and aspirin therapy was associated with a small increase in the number of deaths at the end of follow-up, equivalent to 20 more deaths per 1000 patients treated. This adverse effect can probably be attributed partly to the 10 extra sICHs, and the 5 extra major extracranial hemorrhages per 1000 patients treated with combination anticoagulant/aspirin therapy.

ASPIRIN

Mechanism

Aspirin exerts its antithrombotic effect by permanently inactivating the cyclooxygenase (COX) activity of prostaglandin H (PGH) synthase 1 and 2 (also referred to as COX-1 and COX-2). This irreversibly inhibits platelet TXA2 synthesis, requiring new platelet generation to restore previous levels. Vascular endothelial prostacyclin synthesis is also inhibited by aspirin, but not irreversibly as occurs in platelets. As higher doses of aspirin are needed to inhibit cyclooxygenase in vascular endothelium than in platelets, low-dose aspirin decreases TXA2 synthesis without a major reduction in prostacyclin synthesis.

Clinical Trials of Aspirin in Acute Ischemic Stroke

Three large randomized trials have examined the efficacy of aspirin treatment within 48 hours of stroke onset. IST compared 300 mg aspirin to no aspirin and also compared two doses of UFH to no heparin in a 3X2 factorial design.[18] IST found no significant difference in death and dependency at 6 months in patients treated with aspirin, heparin, or neither of these drugs. There was, however, a nonsignificant trend at 6 months toward a smaller percentage of the aspirin group being dead or dependent (62.2% vs. 63.5%, $2p = 0.07$). Secondary analysis revealed fewer recurrent ischemic strokes at 2 weeks among the aspirin-treated group (2.8% vs. 3.9%, $2p < 0.001$), which was not offset by any significant excess of hemorrhagic strokes (0.9% vs. 0.8%).

The Chinese Acute Stroke Trial (CAST) compared 160 mg aspirin to placebo given for 4 weeks to 21,106 patients with acute ischemic stroke[19] treated within 48 hours. Eighty-seven percent of patients had a brain computed tomography (CT) scan. The mortality rate after 1 month in the aspirin group was lower than in the placebo group (3.3% vs. 3.9%, $2p = 0.04$) with a reduction in the rate of recurrent ischemic stroke at 1 month (1.6% vs. 2.1%, $p = 0.01$). A small (nonsignificant) increase in hemorrhagic stroke in the aspirin-treated group was observed (0.21%, $p > 0.1$).

The reasons for the observed differences in mortality between aspirin-treated patients in IST and CAST are unclear. The findings may relate to baseline differences between the treated groups. CAST had a younger age profile (72% under 70 compared to 38% in IST), excluded some patients with severe stroke, and likely included more subjects with lacunar stroke, an etiology associated with lower mortality and less disability.

In the Multicenter Acute Stroke Trial Italy (MAST-I) study, 622 patients were randomized in a 2 × 2 factorial design to receive either a 1-hour infusion of 1.5 IU streptokinase or 300 mg aspirin or both, or neither.[20] Streptokinase (alone or with aspirin) was associated with a greater number of fatalities at 10 days (OR 2.7, 95% CI 1.7–4.3). In MAST-I, neither aspirin monotherapy nor combination therapy reduced the primary outcome of combined 6-month fatality and severe disability.

When the CAST collaborative group performed a meta-analysis of IST, CAST, and MAST-I, the trend seen in CAST and IST toward a beneficial effect of aspirin on the rate of death or dependency reached the threshold for statistical significance. Early aspirin therapy (160–300 mg/day) conferred an absolute reduction in the rate of recurrent ischemic stroke by 0.7% (7 per 1000 patients treated) ($p < 0.001$) and reduced the rate of death or dependency by 1.3% (13 per 1000 patients treated) ($2p = 0.007$). Aspirin caused about 2 hemorrhagic strokes among every 1000 patients treated, but prevented about 11 other strokes or deaths in hospital.

In addition, the approximately 1–2% risk of peristroke myocardial infarction was slightly reduced,[21] which increased the net clinical benefit of 9 per 1000 to about 10 favorable outcomes per 1000 treated.

Despite the low overall risk of the CAST population, the trial was large and included substantial numbers of patients at high risk of early death (e.g., 2600 of patients were drowsy or comotase at entry, of whom 16.2% randomized to aspirin died or suffered nonfatal recurrent stroke compared to 18.5% of placebo). It is reasonable to conclude that the results of CAST and IST can therefore be applied to both low- and high-risk patients following acute stroke.

In IST and CAST not all patients underwent brain imaging with CT before randomization. It was estimated that about 800 of the 40,000 included subjects in fact had ICH on subsequent imaging. The investigators found no indication in either trial that aspirin treatment led to a deterioration in clinical condition, leading the CAST group to suggest that the hazard of aspirin use in these patients cannot be large (Fig. 7.3).

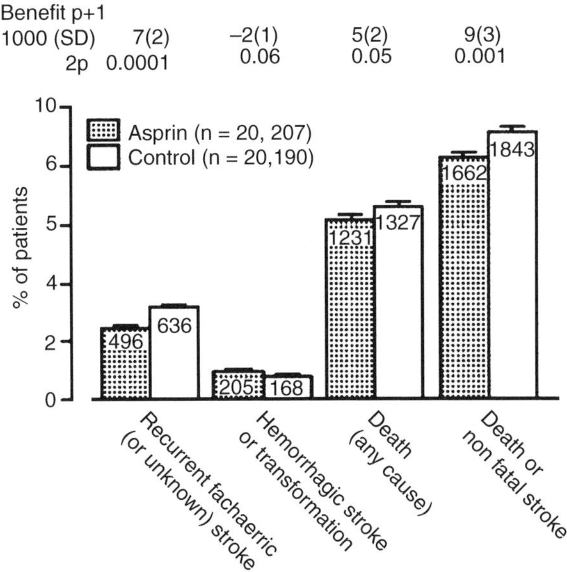

FIGURE 7.3 CAST, IST and MAST—overview of overall effects of early aspirin treatment in acute ischemic stroke on clinical events during scheduled treatment periods. (From reference 19, with permission.)

GLYCOPROTEIN IIb/IIIa ANTAGONISTS

Mechanism

Inhibition of platelet function is an important strategy in the prevention and treatment of ischemic stroke. Platelet function is regulated by three categories of substances. The first group are agents generated outside the platelet that interact with platelet membrane receptors, for example, catecholamines, collagen, thrombin, and prostacyclin. The second group are agents generated within the platelet that interact with the membrane receptors, for example, adenosine diphosphate (ADP), prostaglandin D2, prostaglandin E2, and serotonin. The third group contains agents generated within the platelet that act within the platelet, for example, prostaglandin endoperoxides and thromboxane A2, cAMP, and cGMP.[22] Glycoprotein IIb/IIIa (GP IIb/IIIa) antagonists fall into the third group targeting the platelet IIb/IIIa receptor complex.

Platelets adhere to damaged foci on the vascular endothelium and become activated. They undergo a conformational change, exposing phospholipids and GP IIb/IIIa receptors and express mediators such as thromboxane A2 (TXA2) and ADP, which further stimulate platelet aggregation by promoting the binding of fibrinogen to GP IIb/IIIa receptors. GP IIb/IIIa antagonists have the advantage of inhibiting platelet adhesion via this nonselective "final common pathway."

GP IIb/IIIa antagonists may be broadly classified as monoclonal antibodies or cyclic peptides. Earlier drugs were intravenously administered hybrid murine/human monoclonal antibody Fab fragments directed against the GP IIb/IIIa receptor, including abciximab, eptifibatide, and tirofiban. More recently, cyclic peptides based on the Arg-Gly-Asp sequence common to many GP IIb/IIIa receptor ligands have been developed (e.g., lotrafiban, xemilofiban, sibrafiban). These agents are orally administered as a prodrug, which is converted by plasma and liver esterases to a peptidomimetic on the Arg-Gly-Asp amino acid sequence.

Trials of GP IIb/IIIa Antagonists in Acute Ischemic Stroke

The abciximab in Acute Ischemic Stroke trial was a randomized, placebo-controlled dose-escalation study to examine the safety of abciximab in acute stroke.[23] It randomized 74 patients within 24 hours of stroke onset to receive one of four doses of abciximab (by bolus with or without additional infusion, 54 patients) or placebo (20 patients). The median baseline National Institute of Health Stroke Scale (NIHSS) score was 15. The rates of asymptomatic ICH were 19% in the intervention group compared to 5% in the placebo group ($p = 0.07$). Most (9 of 11) of the asymptomatic ICH patients had more severe stroke (NIHSS >14). No cases of symptomatic ICH or major systemic bleeding occurred. There was a trend toward a lower rate of stroke recurrence (2% vs. 5%) and a higher rate of functional recovery at 3 months in the group treated with abciximab than with placebo.

Based on these findings, the Abciximab Emergent Stroke Treatment Trial (AbESTT) randomized 400 patients with stroke within 6 hours of onset to receive abciximab or placebo.[24] The abciximab dose chosen was the highest of the four strata studied in the previous dose-escalation study (i.e., 0.25 μg/kg intravenous bolus followed by 0.125 μg/kg/min infusion for 12 hours). No difference in the primary safety outcome of symptomatic ICH within 5 days was detected, but a trend toward a higher rate was detected in the intervention arm (3.6% vs. 1%, $p = 0.09$). Eighty-eight percent (seven of eight) of abciximab-treated patients with sICH had severe strokes (NIHSS >14). Although this phase 2 trial was not powered to detect efficacy, a nonsignificant shift in favorable outcomes on mRS score at 3 months was observed ($p = 0.33$).

Following this trial, AbESTT-II was initiated as a phase 3 randomized trial, which aimed to recruit 1800 patients, 1200 within 4.5 hours of onset, and a further 600 later than 4.5 hours or within 2.5 hours of waking with stroke symptoms.[25] Due to an excess of hemorrhages in the abciximab group, AbESTT-II was discontinued in 2005 upon the recommendation of the Safety and Efficacy Monitoring Committee, initially for patients waking with stroke, and later for all patients. Eight hundred and eight patients had been recruited at this point.

The Safety of Tirofiban in Acute Ischemic Stroke (SaTIS) trial examined 250 patients 6–22 hours after stroke onset treated with tirofiban infusion or placebo for 48 hours.[26] No increase in ICH was reported in the active group. Although no benefit in early functional recovery was observed, 5–6-month mortality was lower in the tirofiban-treated group (relative risk reduction (RRR) 27%, 95% CI 0.08–0.95, $p = 0.03$).

Combination GP IIb/IIIa and rt-PA Therapy for Acute Stroke The combination of antiplatelet and thrombolytic drugs has proven efficacy in the setting of myocardial ischemia where an additive effect is seen. In acute stroke thrombolysis with a very narrow time window and less than 50% optimal reperfusion rates,[27] adjunctive therapy with antiplatelets may be a promising approach. However, MAST-I concluded that the group of patients receiving streptokinase plus aspirin had a marked increase in 10-day mortality.

Early studies indicate that combined GP IIb/IIIa inhibition with rt-PA thrombolysis may improve clinical and MRI outcomes after acute ischemic stroke, with an acceptable safety profile. The dual targeting of platelets and fibrin by combination therapy may provide synergistic benefits, including increased arterial recanalization, reduced microvascular thrombosis, reduced arterial reocclusion, and less rt-PA-mediated blood–brain barrier injury and secondary activation of the coagulation system.

In 2004, the abciximab and rt-PA in Acute Ischemic Stroke Treatment trial treated five patients with abciximab and half dose of rt-PA within 3 hours of symptom onset.[28] The primary aim was to examine the frequency of SICH at 24 hours. This occurred in one of the five patients. The median NIHSS improvement was 6.

In another study of 19 patients with complete or near-complete (TIMI grade 0 or 1) middle cerebral artery (MCA) occlusion, combination therapy with reduced-dose rt-PA and tirofiban infusion was associated with recanalization in 68% of patients, significant reductions of MRI ischemic lesion volumes, and substantial clinical improvement (median NIHSS change from 17 at baseline to 2 after treatment, $p = 0.002$).[29] No cases of sICH occurred.

The same investigators found significant improvements in clinical outcomes and reduction in ischemic lesion volumes on MRI in 13 patients treated with tirofiban and reduced-dose rt-PA compared to 16 patients treated with standard rt-PA therapy.[30]

Further carefully designed trials incorporating a range of clinical and surrogate measures are required to further examine the potential of GP IIb/IIIa antagonist monotherapy for selected (e.g., large artery disease) and unselected patients with acute stroke. Equally, further trials of combination therapy with GP IIb/IIIa antagonists and fibrinolytic agents are needed. Ongoing trials, such as the Reopro Retavase Reperfusion of Stroke Safety Study-Imaging Evaluation (ROSIE)[31] and ROSIE-2[32] are designed to determine the optimal dose of abciximab (combined with rt-PA reteplase 3–24 hours after onset) and epifibatide (combined with ASA/LMWH/rt-PA within 3 hours).

ACUTE STROKE THERAPY WITH OTHER ANTIPLATELET AGENTS

The use of other antiplatelet agents in the acute setting has not been extensively investigated.

Dipyridamole

Dipyridamole exerts its effect by inhibition of platelet phosphodiesterase E5, increasing cyclic guanosine monophosphate and cyclic adenosine monophosphate (cAMP).[33] By inhibiting its uptake and metabolism by erythrocytes, dipyridamole also increases the availability of adenosine within blood vessels, promoting inhibition of platelet aggregation and local vasodilatation.[34] Dipyridamole may also inhibit cAMP phosphodiesterase in platelets, which further increases cAMP levels[35] and may enhance endothelial nitric oxide production, contributing to its antithrombotic effect. Existing trials of dipyridamole in stroke have focused on secondary prevention and will be discussed briefly.

The European Stroke Prevention Study 2 (ESPS-2) trial examined four treatment arms—extended-release dipyridamole (ER-DP) 200 mg twice daily alone, aspirin 25 mg twice daily alone, ER-DP 200 mg twice daily + aspirin 25 mg twice daily, or placebo.[36] In comparison with placebo the overall reduction in stroke risk was 16% with ER-DP alone and 18% with aspirin alone. The combination of ER-DP and aspirin led to a 37% reduction in stroke risk compared to placebo. Compared with aspirin alone, the combination of ER-DP with aspirin reduced the risk of stroke by 23%.

The European/Australian Stroke Prevention in Reversible Ischaemia Trial (ESPRIT)[37] confirmed the finding of ESPS 2, showing that the combination of aspirin and dipyridamole is more effective than aspirin alone in the prevention of new vascular events in patients with nondisabling cerebral ischaemia of presumed arterial origin. Adding the ESPRIT data to the meta-analysis of previous trials resulted in an overall risk ratio for the composite of vascular death, stroke, or MI of 0.82 (95% CI 0.74–0.91).

PROFESS is an ongoing large randomized trial examining combination ER-DP plus aspirin therapy compared with clopidogrel (each group also with or without telmisartan, an angiotensin receptor antagonist) for the secondary prevention of early and late recurrent stroke, and other vascular events.

Thienopyridine Derivatives

Ticlopidine inhibits the $P2Y_{12}$ platelet ADP receptor, thus inhibiting ADP-dependent activation of the GP IIb/IIIa receptor. It has a slow onset of action and takes 3–7 days to reach its maximal antiplatelet effect. It is inactive *in vitro* and must undergo activation by the hepatic cytochrome p450 enzyme system. Secondary prevention trials have found that ticlopidine-treated patients have an estimated RRR of 33% for the composite endpoint of stroke, myocardial infarction, or vascular death after ischemic stroke.[38,39] Significant adverse effects include bone marrow depression, rash, diarrhea, and thrombotic thrombocytopenic purpura. No clinical trials have studied ticlopidine for the treatment of stroke in the acute phase.

Clopidogrel also inhibits the $P2Y_{12}$ ADP receptor following hepatic activation *in vivo*.[40,41] Clopidogrel's antiplatelet effect is maximal after 3–5 days of therapy.[42] Administration of a loading dose of 150–300 mg produces a more rapid inhibitory effect than seen with the 75 mg daily dose.[43]

The CAPRIE trial found that compared to aspirin (325 mg daily), clopidogrel (75 mg daily) was associated with RRR of 8.7% ($p = 0.043$) for the composite endpoint of ischemic stroke, MI, or vascular death among 19,185 subjects with stroke, MI, or peripheral arterial disease, but no significant reduction in the composite endpoint in the subgroup with stroke (RRR 7.3%, $p = 0.26$). No comparison of clopidogrel with aspirin in the acute stroke period was performed. Furthermore, stroke as an endoint was not significantly reduced in the stroke patients entered in this trial (RRR 8.0%, $p =$ NS).

The Management of Atherothrombosis with Clopidogrel in High risk patients (MATCH) trial compared combination therapy with aspirin (75 mg) and clopidogrel (75 mg) to clopidogrel (75 mg) alone for prevention of recurrent stroke and other vascular events in patients with TIA or ischemic stroke.[44] No additional reduction in risk was achieved by combination therapy compared with clopidogrel alone (RRR 6.6%, CI −7.0 to 18.5, $p = 0.324$). Further, 3% of patients receiving combination therapy had life-threatening bleeding compared to 1% in the clopidogrel alone group ($p < 0.0001$). MATCH was also a secondary prevention trial and provided no analysis of the acute stroke period.

ACUTE ANTITHROMBOTIC TREATMENT OF STROKE SUBTYPES

Although several approaches to stroke classification have been described, the most common mechanism-based classification in current use is the system described by the TOAST investigators.[45] This classification describes five major subtypes of ischemic stroke based on the results of neuroimaging and other medical investigations, namely (1) LAA, (2) cardioembolism, (3) small-vessel occlusion, (4) stroke of other determined etiology, and (5) stroke of undetermined etiology. Inter-rater reliability of the TOAST scheme has been reported as moderate-to-substantial (K 0.5–0.7).

Antithrombotic Therapy for Acute Cardioembolic Stroke

Early Recurrence Rates in Cardioembolic Stroke The primary rationale for acute antithrombotic therapy in cardioembolic stroke, including that associated with AF, is prevention of early recurrence secondary to further embolism.

Data from patients with AF who are treated with aspirin or placebo in the IST, HAEST, and CAST trials indicate that the risk of early stroke recurrence is approximately 5% in the first 14 days.[46] Differences exist between trials for parameters, such as the definition of recurrence, distinction from progressing stroke, degree of investigator blinding, and control group assignment. However, the recurrence rates from clinical trials are broadly comparable to 1-month rates (ranging from 2.4% to 10.8%) observed with TOAST-defined cardioembolic stroke in four large population studies.[47] The mechanism of initial and recurrent stroke associated with AF may not always be cardiogenic embolism. In IST, the risk of early recurrence associated with AF was only slightly higher than that in patients with sinus rhythm, suggesting that other mechanisms may have supervened in a significant proportion of cases. The degree to which other mechanisms may account for stroke in patients with AF has not been well studied. One study found that late recurrence rates of lacunar stroke in patients with AF were not different in those treated with anticoagulation than in those treated with aspirin.[48]

Acute Aspirin Therapy for AF-associated Stroke A combined analysis of the IST and CAST trials indicated a 21% RRR (95% CI −5 to 41) in the frequency of early recurrent stroke associated with acute aspirin therapy compared to placebo in patients with AF. No difference in early mortality or sICH was found. This finding was largely driven by the relatively large (about 25% RRR) benefit observed in the unblinded IST, compared to the smaller benefit (5% RRR) observed in the double-blinded CAST.

Acute Anticoagulation for AF-associated Stroke HAEST and IST provided valuable data on relatively large numbers (449 in HAEST, 3169 in IST) of patients with AF-associated ischemic stroke treated with acute anticoagulation (danaparoid in HAEST, UFH in IST). HAEST found no reduction in early stroke recurrence or effect on late functional outcome in the LMWH arm. In contrast, IST found a dose-dependent reduction in early recurrence rates, but no late functional benefit associated with UFH. However, this was offset by an increase in rates of sICH among patients with AF receiving UFH, with no net benefit in the composite outcome of recurrence stroke and sICH combined. The reasons for the discrepancy between trials is unclear.

Acute Anticoagulation for All Cardioembolic Stroke No benefit in early recurrence or late functional outcome in all cardioembolic stroke was observed in the TOAST or FISS[49] trials, both placebo-controlled trials that randomized patients to acute LMWH therapy (daltaparin and fraxiparine, respectively) in the active arms. A small reduction in early stroke recurrence was observed in the Cerebral Embolism Study Group trial, which compared IV adjusted-dose UFH to no UFH.[50] However, the absolute numbers were small (45 patients included, 2 recurrences in the UFH compared to none in the control arm), which precludes reliable interpretation of this finding. TAIST found no efficacy in using heparin in the management of patients with presumed cardioembolic stroke.

It is generally believed that the rates of embolization from left ventricular thrombus occurring with acute myocardial infarction, left ventricular aneurysm formation, and idiopathic dilated cardiomyopathy are higher than those from the left atrial appendage associated with AF.[51] However, few precise data exist on rates in these settings, and no randomized trials have been performed to determine the role of acute anticoagulation. Empirically, many experienced physicians will treat with UFH or LMWH following identification of left ventricular thrombus, with or without clinical evidence of acute stroke, provided that a large cerebral infarct has not occurred which would increase sICH risk.

Antithrombotic Treatment of Acute Stroke Due to Large Artery Atherosclerosis

Early Recurrence Rates in Large Artery Disease Stroke due to LAA has been associated with a higher risk of early recurrence compared to cardioembolic, undetermined, and lacunar subtypes. A meta-analysis of population studies found a 4.5% recurrent stroke risk associated with LAA at 7 days and 9.4% recurrence at 1 month, a threefold increase in adjusted risk as compared to other subtypes.[52] Patients with strokes caused by LAA appear to be at the greatest risk of worsening and recurrence in the early poststroke period. In the National Institute of Neurological Disorders and Stroke (NINDS) stroke database, patients with LAA had a 30% risk of worsening during acute hospitalization and a 7.9% risk of stroke recurrence within 30 days.

Clinical trials and meta-analyses have demonstrated that early carotid endarterectomy (CEA) is the preferred treatment for most patients with severe symptomatic internal carotid artery (ICA) stenosis and selected patients with moderate disease.[53] However, CEA is often delayed in clinical practice, or may not be appropriate in some patients due to an unfavorable risk–benefit profile. In these settings, it is reasonable to consider acute antithrombotic treatment to prevent early recurrent stroke.

The relationship between LAA and early recurrence is likely to be largely mediated by arterial embolism from atherosclerotic plaque, although recurrent low-flow stroke may also occur due to severe vessel stenosis or occlusion. In recently symptomatic individuals with moderate-or-severe ICA stenosis, platelet-fibrin embolic signals (ES) are commonly detected in the MCA using transcranial Doppler (TCD) ultrasound and have been reported to independently predict a five-fold increase in 90-day recurrence.[54]

Antiplatelet Agents in LAA Disease No large randomized trials comparing acute antiplatelet agents with placebo in patients with LAA have been performed. The CARESS trial compared dual antiplatelet therapy (clopidogrel 300 mg loading dose followed by 75 mg daily, plus aspirin 75 mg daily) with aspirin monotherapy in 107 recently symptomatic patients with >50% ICA stenosis, using TCD ES detection as a surrogate marker of efficacy.[55] A 40% reduction (95% CI 13.8–58, $p = 0.005$) in the proportion of ES-positive patients was detected at 7 days with reduced ES frequency per hour in the dual therapy group ($p = 0.001$). Although not powered for clinical endpoints, four recurrent strokes and seven TIAs occurred in the monotherapy group compared to no strokes and four TIAs in the combination therapy group.

Junghans and Siebler[56] reported a series of 24 patients with recent stroke or TIA due to LAA and detected ES on TCD who were treated acutely with intravenous tirofiban, a GP IIb/IIIa receptor antagonist. Median ES rate at baseline was 38 signals per hour. ES were abolished by tirofiban in all patients, and returned following cessation of infusion. Although preliminary, these data support the rationale for trials of acute GP IIb/IIIa receptor blockade in patients with recently symptomatic LAA awaiting CEA.

Subgroup analyses of the MATCH data suggested a 12% risk reduction in recurrent vascular events at 18 months in patients with large vessel disease who were given combination aspirin and clopidogrel compared with clopidogrel alone.

Finally, a Cochrane review of antiplatelet therapy following CEA found no evidence of a difference in mortality when antiplatelets were compared with placebo. However, treatment with antiplatelet agents following CEA decreased the risk of postoperative stroke (OR 0.58, 95% CI 0.34–0.98).[57]

Anticoagulation in Stroke Due to LAA Disease Few clinical trials have been performed in this population. In the TOAST trial, a secondary analysis in patients with stroke due to LAA found favorable outcomes at 7 days in 54% of danaparoid-treated patients, compared to 38% of the placebo-treated group ($p = 0.02$). At 3 months, 68% of patients in the danaparoid group compared to 53% of those in the placebo group had favorable outcomes ($p = 0.02$).

Stroke Due to Small Vessel Occlusion

Lacunar stroke is characterized by occlusion of a small penetrating artery creating a small deep infarct. Lacunar strokes have the lowest early recurrence risk and best survival rates, but may still cause significant functional morbidity. Although subgroup analyses are available from secondary prevention trials in lacunar stroke, few clinical trial data are available regarding nonthrombolytic antithrombotic therapy for lacunar stroke in the acute setting.

Stroke Due to Other Determined Etiology

This category includes patients with rare causes of strokes such as nonatherosclerotic vasculopathies, cerebral venous thrombosis, hypercoagulable states, or hematologic disorders. Two such disorders are discussed below.

Arterial dissection

Dissection of the internal carotid and vertebral arteries is a common cause of stroke, particularly in young patients. Although many occur due to trauma, it is estimated that over half occur spontaneously.[58] The mechanism of stroke following arterial dissection is either by artery-to-artery embolism, by thrombosis *in situ*, or by dissection-induced lumenal stenosis with secondary cerebral hypoperfusion and low-flow "watershed" infarction.[59] Occasionally, dissection may lead to the formation of a pseudoaneurysm as a source of thrombus formation. Vertebrobasilar dissections that extend intracranially have a higher risk of rupture leading to subarachnoid hemorrhage (SAH).[60,61]

Acute anticoagulation is widely used in the acute setting of arterial dissection. Once again, the rationale is to prevent propagation of local thrombosis and formation of new thrombus at the site of the injured arterial wall, which is believed to reduce the likelihood of early stroke recurrence.[62–65] This practice, while rational, is based on anecdotal evidence and case series, as randomized controlled trials have not been performed. If SAH is present, heparin is contraindicated. In patients with dissection without SAH, the risk of heparin causing hemorrhagic transformation is less than 5%.

In the absence of evidence to the contrary, some experienced physicians prescribe antiplatelet agents for acute management and secondary prevention. Case series have reported outcomes following treatment with antiplatelet agents that are comparable to those in patients treated with anticoagulation.[66,67] A case series published in 2000 looked at 116 patients, 71 treated with anticoagulation and 23 with aspirin. It found that the rate of TIA, recurrent stroke, or death in those treated with anticoagulation was 8.3% and in those treated with aspirin was 12.4%, a difference that was not statistically significant. They concluded that a further multicenter trial involving about 2000 patients is needed to provide adequate power for comparison of the two treatment options.[68]

Endovascular stent insertion is emerging as another possible treatment modality. Although it is likely that intra-arterial stenting will have a role in carotid atherosclerotic disease, the role of stenting in the management of craniocervical dissection is less clearly defined. One view is that the stent may act as a filter, trapping thrombus within pseudoaneurysms and preventing embolism from mural or intraaneurysmal thrombus.[69]

Stent placement may also decrease the degree of vessel stenosis and may prevent extension of the dissection.[70–73] Until randomized trials are performed, stenting for craniocervical dissection should be considered experimental and unproven.

Cerebral venous sinus thrombosis

Cerebral venous sinus thrombosis (CVST) is frequently a challenging diagnosis due to the highly variable clinical manifestations.[74,75] Risk factors include inherited or acquired hypercoaguable states, pregnancy/postpartum state, use of estrogen-containing oral contraceptive pills, and infection adjacent to the cerebral sinuses. Cerebral venous infarctions are frequently hemorrhagic and may be associated with considerable vasogenic edema.

Two small trials of heparin therapy for treatment of CVST have been performed. In the first, intravenous adjusted-dose UFH was compared to placebo.[76] The trial was terminated early after only 20 patients were enrolled because of the superiority of UFH ($p < 0.01$). In the heparin group, 8 out of 10 patients had recovered fully after 3 months, while the remaining 2 patients had only mild neurological deficits. In the placebo group, only one patient had recovered completely and three had died. Although this study represents an advance in clinical knowledge and provides some support for the use of UFH, it must be acknowledged that there was a significant delay before treatment was initiated (33 days in the heparin group and 25 days in the placebo group) and the authors used their own unvalidated "sinus venous thrombosis severity scale" to assess clinical outcome.

A historical cohort of 102 patients with CVT (43 of whom had an ICH) was also retrospectively examined in this study to estimate the safety of UFH. Twenty-seven patients with ICH received dose-adjusted intravenous heparin. Of these four died and two suffered permanent severe neurological deficit. Of the 13 patients with ICH who did not receive heparin, 9 died. The authors concluded that heparin is effective for the treatment of CVST, and the presence of hemorrhagic venous infarction is not a contraindication for its use.

The second trial compared a LMWH, nadroparin, to placebo.[77] Sixty patients were randomized to receive weight-adjusted nadroparin (180 anti-factor Xa units/kg per 24 hours) or matching placebo for 3 weeks (double-blind part of trial), followed by 3 months of oral anticoagulants for patients allocated nadroparin (open part). All patients with clinically suspected cerebral venous sinus thrombosis confirmed by cerebral angiography or by MRI were eligible. Thirty patients received nadroparin and 29 received placebo. In the nadroparin group, patients were randomized within 10 days and in the placebo group patients were randomized within 11.2 days. The two groups were matched for cerebral hemorrhage rates, clinical severity at baseline, age, and sex. At 3 weeks, six patients in the nadroparin group and seven controls had a poor outcome, defined as death or BI <15 (risk difference −4%; 95% CI −25 to 17). After 12 weeks, four patients in the active group and six in the placebo group had a poor outcome (risk difference −7%; 95% CI −26 to 12). Two patients in the heparin group died while four died in the placebo group. No new sICH occurred in either group.

Although more data are required, particularly in the setting of hemorrhagic venous infarction, based on the current evidence it seems reasonable to conclude that anticoagulation with UFH and LMWH is safe and probably effective in CVST. The optimal duration of therapy has not been well studied.

For patients who demonstrate continued neurological deterioration despite anticoagulation, local intrathrombus thrombolysis may be beneficial.[78,79] In case series in which most patients received urokinase, favorable outcome with no major therapeutic morbidity has been described.[80–86] In one study, 29 patients with angiogram-proven CVST were reviewed retrospectively. Of the 18 who received local urokinase, 17 recovered completely, and 1 was left with a mild neurological deficit. Heparin was given to four patients, three of whom made a complete recovery. Six presented in a comatose state with severe CVST and only supportive measures were used. It is difficult to draw conclusions from these data, as only patients with mild or moderately severe disease were selected for thrombolytic treatment.

Frey et al.[87] treated 12 patients with clinically disabling and nonresolving or worsening CVST with both IV UFH and endovascular rt-PA. Seven patients had hemorrhage visible on pretreatment MRI. Six patients (50%) achieved recanalization—of these five made a complete recovery and one had visual impairment from prolonged papilledema. Three patients achieved partial recanalization—of these, two recovered completely and one had a permanent language disorder. In three patients, blood flow was not restored—of these, one became independent, one had a residual right hemiparesis, and one developed epilepsy. In two patients, sICH occurred or was exacerbated after treatment. Another study reported no exacerbation of ICH following urokinase treatment in 13 patients despite pretreatment ICH in 4 patients.[87]

Randomized trials comparing acute anticoagulation to thrombolysis for selected patients with moderate and severe CVT are needed.

GUIDELINES

A number of evidence-based guidelines exist to help choose appropriate acute stroke therapy.

Guidelines for the Early Management of Patients With Ischemic Stroke: A Scientific Statement From the Stroke Council of the American Stroke Association: 2005[88]

- Aspirin should be given within 24–48 hours of stroke onset in most patients (grade A evidence).
- The administration of aspirin as an adjunctive therapy, within 24 hours of the use of thrombolytic agents, is not recommended (grade A evidence).
- Aspirin should not be used as a substitute for other acute interventions, especially intravenous administration of rt-PA, for the treatment of acute ischemic stroke (grade A evidence).
- No recommendation is made about the urgent administration of other antiplatelet aggregating agents (grade C evidence).
- Urgent routine anticoagulation with the goal of improving neurological outcomes or preventing early recurrent stroke is not recommended for the treatment of patients with acute ischemic stroke (grade A).
- More studies are required to determine if certain subgroups (large vessel atherothrombosis or patients perceived to be at high risk of recurrent embolism) may benefit from urgent anticoagulation.
- Urgent anticoagulation is not recommended for treatment of patients with moderate-to-severe stroke because of a high risk of serious intracranial bleeding complications (grade A).
- Initiation of anticoagulant therapy within 24 hours of treatment with intravenously administered rt-PA is not recommended (grade A).

Antithrombotic and Thrombolytic Therapy for Ischemic Stroke: The Seventh ACCP Conference on Antithrombotic and Thrombolytic Therapy: 2004[89]

- For patients with Acute Ischemic Stroke they recommend clinicians *not* to use full-dose anticoagulation with IV, subcutaneous, or low-molecular-weight heparins or heparinoids (*grade 2B evidence*).
- Some experts recommend early anticoagulation for various specific stroke subgroups, including cardioembolic stroke, progressing stroke, stroke

due to LAA stenosis, documented intraluminal thrombus, or arterial dissections.

- Clinical trials have not, however, adequately evaluated adjusted-dose IV anticoagulation in these selected stroke patients.
- No trials have evaluated the role of very early anticoagulation (12 hours after stroke onset) in any stroke population.
- For patients with ischemic stroke who are not receiving thrombolysis, they recommend early aspirin therapy, 160–325 mg/day (*grade 1A evidence*).
- Aspirin should be started within 48 hours of stroke onset and may be used safely in combination with low doses of subcutaneous heparin for DVT prophylaxis.
- For acute stroke patients with restricted mobility, they recommend prophylactic low-dose subcutaneous heparin or low-molecular-weight heparins or heparinoids (*grade 1A*).
- Low-dose heparin should be restricted for 24 hours after administration of thrombolytic therapy. Low-dose heparin may be used safely in combination with aspirin.

They defined their grading of recommendations as follows: grade 1 recommendations are strong and indicate that the benefits do, or do not, outweigh risks, burden, and costs; grade 2 suggests that individual patients' values may lead to different choices.

European Stroke Initiative Recommendations: 2003[90]

- Aspirin (100–300 mg/day) may be given within 48 hours after ischemic stroke (Level of Evidence I).
- If thrombolytic therapy is planned, no aspirin should be given.
- Aspirin is not allowed for 24 hours after thrombolytic therapy.
- There is no recommendation for general use of heparin, low-molecular-weight heparin, or heparinoids after ischemic stroke (Level of Evidence I).
- Full-dose heparin may be used when there are selected indications, such as cardiac sources with a high risk of recurrent embolism, arterial dissection, or high-grade arterial stenosis prior to surgery (Level of Evidence IV).
- Administration of low-dose heparin or low-molecular-weight heparin in an equivalent dose is always recommended in bedridden patients to reduce the risk of DVT and PE (Level of Evidence II).

Used levels of evidence

- Level I: Highest level of evidence. Primary endpoint of RCT with adequate sample size or meta-analysis of qualitatively outstanding RCTs.
- Level II: Intermediate level of evidence. Small randomized trials or predefined secondary endpoints of large RCTs.

- Level III: Lower level of evidence. Prospective case series with concurrent or historical cohort or post hoc analyses of large RCTs.
- Level IV: Undetermined level of evidence. Small uncontrolled case series of general agreement despite lack of evidence.

REFERENCES

1. Choay J. Structure and activity of heparin and its fragments: an overview. *Semin Thrombosis Haemostasis* 1989:15;359–364.
2. Sobel M, McNeill PM, Carlson P, Kermode JC, Adelman B, Conroy R, Marques D. Heparin inhibition of von Willebrand factor *in vitro* and *in vivo. J Clin Invest* 1991;87:1787–1793.
3. Sobel M, Soler DF, Kermode JC, Harris RB. Localization and characterization of a heparin binding domain peptide of human von Willebrand factor. *J Biol Chem* 1992;267:8857–8862.
4. Gordon DL, Linhardt R, Adams HP. Low molecular-weight heparins and heparinoids and their use in acute or progressing ischemic stroke. *Clin Neuropharmacol* 1990;13: 522–543.
5. Cella G, Scattolo N, Luzzato G, Stevanato E, Vio C, Girolami A. Effects on platelets and on the clotting system of four glycosaminoglycans extracted from hog mucosa and one extracted from aortic intima of the calf, *J Med* 1986;17:331–346.
6. Meuleman DG. Orgaran (Org 10172): its pharmacological profile in animal models. *Haemostasis* 1992;22:58–65.
7. Maffrand JP, Herbert JM, Bernat A, Defreyn G, Delebassee D, Savi P, Pinot JJ, Sampol J. Experimental and clinical pharmacology of pentosan polysulphate. *Semin Thrombosis Haemostasis* 1991;17 (Suppl. 2):186–198.
8. International Stroke Trial Collabarative Group. The International Stroke Trial (IST): a randomised trial of aspirin, subcutaneous heparin , both, or neither among 19435 patients with acute ischemic stroke. *Lancet* 1997;349:1569–1581.
9. Camerlingo M, Salvi P, Belloni G, Gamba T, Mario Cesana B, Mamoli A. Intravenous heparin started within the first 3 hours after onset of symptoms as a treatment for acute nonlacunar hemispheric cerebral infarctions. *Stroke* 2005;36:2415–2420.
10. Publications Committee for the Trial of Org 10172 in Acute Stroke Treatment (TOAST) Investigators. Low molecular weight heparinoid ORG 10172 (Danaparoid) and outcome after acute ischemic stroke. *JAMA* 1998;279:1265–1272.
11. Bath P, Iddenden R, Bath F. Low-molecular-weight heparins and heparinoids in acute ischemic stroke, a meta-analysis of randomised controlled trials. *Stroke* 2000;31: 1770–1778.
12. The Cochrane Collaboration. Anticoagulants for acute ischemic stroke 2006; [Review].
13. Berge E, Abdelnoor M, Nakstad PH, Sandset PM, on behalf of the Haest Study Group. Low molecular-weight heparin versus aspirin in patients with acute ischemic stroke and atrial fibrillation: a double blind randomised study. *Lancet* 2000;335:1205–1210.
14. Bath P, Lindenstrom E, Boysen G, De Deyn P, Friis P, Leys D, Marttila R, Olsson J-E, O'Neill D, Orgogozo J-M, Ringelstein B, Van der Sande J-J, Turpie A for the TAEST

Investigators. Tinzaparin in acute ischemic stroke (TAIST): a randomised aspirin-controlled trial. *Lancet* 2001;358:702–710.

15. Sandercock P, Counsell C, Stobbs SL. Low-molecular-weight heparins or Heparinoids versus standard Unfractionated heparin for acute ischemic stroke (Review). The Cochrane Collaboration; 2006.
16. Diener H-C, Ringelstein EB, von Kummer R, Landgraf H, Koppenhagen K, Harenberg J, Rektor I, Csányi, A, Schneider D, Klingelhöfer J, Brom J, Weidinger G for the PROTECT Trial Group. Prophylaxis of thrombotic and embolic events in acute ischemic stroke with the low-molecular-weight heparin certoparin: results of the PROTECT Trial. *Stroke* 2006;37:139–144.
17. Berge E, Sandercock P. Anticoagulants versus antiplatelet agents for acute ischemic stroke (Review). The Cochrane Collaboration; 2006.
18. International Stroke Trial Collabarative Group. The International Stroke Trial (IST): a randomised trial of aspirin, subcutaneous heparin , both, or neither among 19435 patients with acute ischemic stroke. *Lancet* 1997;349:1569–1581.
19. CAST (Chinese Acute Stroke Trial) Collaborative Group. CAST: randomised placebo-controlled trial of early aspirin use in 20,000 patients with acute ischemic stroke. *Lancet* 1997;349(9066):1641–1649.
20. Multicentre Acute Stroke Trial–Italy (MAST-I) Group. Randomised controlled trial of streptokinase, aspirin, and combination of both in treatment of acute ischemic stroke. *Lancet* 1995;346(8989):1509–1514.
21. Antiplatelet Trialist' Collaboration. Collaborative overview of randomised trials of antiplatelet treatment. Part I: prevention of death, myocardial infarction and stroke by prolonged antiplatelet therapy in various categories of patients. *BMJ* 1994;308: 81–106.
22. Katzung BG. Basic and clinical pharmacology. 8th ed.; 2001.
23. The Abciximab in Ischemic Stroke Investigators. Abciximab in acute ischemic stroke : a randomized, double-blind, placebo-controlled, dose-escalation study. *Stroke* 2000;31: 601–609.
24. Abciximab Emergent Stroke Treatment Trial Investigators. Emergency administration of abciximab for treatment of patients with acute ischemic stroke: results of a randomized phase 2 trial. *Stroke* 2005;36:880–890.
25. Stroke Trials Registry. Abciximab in Emergent Stroke Treatment Trial - II. www.strokecenter.org/trials. Accessed on July 15, 2007.
26. Juttler E, Kohrmann M, Schellinger PD. Therapy for early reperfusion after stroke. *Nat Clin Prac Cardiovasc Med* 2006;3:656–663.
27. Sasaki O, Shigekazu T, Koike T, Koizumi T, Tanaka R. Fibrinolytic therapy for acute embolic stroke: intravenous, intracarotid, and intra-arterial local approaches. *Neurosurgery* 1995;36:246–253.
28. Abciximab and rt-PA in acute ischemic stroke treatment. Presented at the 28th International Stroke Conference; February 2003. *Acad Emerg Med* 2003;10(12):1396–1399.
29. Straub S, Junghans U, Jovanovic V, Wittsack HJ, Seitz RJ, Siebler M. Systemic thrombolysis with recombinant tissue plasminogen activator and tirofiban in acute middle cerebral artery occlusion. *Stroke* 2004;35;705–709.
30. Seitz RJ, Meisel S, Moll M, Wittsack JH, Junghans U, Seibler M. The effect of combined thrombolysis with rtPA and tirofiban on ischemic brain lesions. *Neurology* 2004;62:2110–2112.

31. Dunn B, Davis LA, Todd JW, Chalela JA, Warach S, NINDS/NIH, Bethesda, MD; for the ROSIE Investigators. Reperfusion of Stroke Safety Study Imaging Evaluation (ROSIE). *Ongoing* Clinical Trials Session, 29th International Stroke Conference; 2004.

32. Reperfusion of Stroke Safety Study Imaging Evaluation-2: Adjunctive Treatment to Standard Alteplase Therapy of Ischemic Stroke. Presented at the 29th International Stroke Conference; February 2004.

33. Diener HC, Cunha L, Forbes C, Sivenius J, Smets P, Lowenthal A. European Stroke Prevention Study. 2. Dipyridamole and asetylsalicylic acid in the secondary prevention of stroke. *J Neurol Sci* 1996;143:1–13.

34. Cote R, Battista RN, Abrahamowicz M, Langlois Y, Bourque F, Mackey A. Lack of effect of aspirin in asymptomatic patients with carotid bruits and substantial carotid narrowing. The Asymptomatic Cervial Bruit Study Group. *Ann Intern Med* 1995;123: 649–655.

35. Fitzgerald GA. Dipyridamole. *N Engl J Med* 1987;316:1247–1257.

36. European Stroke Prevention Study. 2. Dipyridamole and acetylsalicylic acid in the secondary prevention of stroke. *J Neurol Sci* 1996;143(1–2):1–13.

37. ESPRIT Study Group, Halkes PH, van Gijn J, Kappelle LJ, Koudstaal PJ, Algra A. Aspirin plus dipyridamole versus aspirin alone after cerebral ischaemia of arterial origin (ESPRIT): randomised controlled trial. *Lancet* 2006;367(9523):1665–1673.

38. Antiplatelet Trialists' Collaboration. Collaborative overview of randomised trials of antiplatelet therapy. I:prevention of death, myocardial infarction, and stroke by prolonged antiplatelet therapy in various categories of patients. *BMJ* 1994;308: 81–106.

39. Gent M. A systematic overview of randomised trials of antiplatelet agents for the prevention of stroke, myocardial infarction and vascular death. In: Hass WK, Easton JD, editors. Ticlopidine, platelets and vascular disease. New York: Springer-Verlag; 1993 p99–116.

40. Gachet C. ADP receptors of platelets and their inhibition. *Thromb Haemost* 2001;86:222–232.

41. Savi P, Pereillo JM, Uzabiaga MF, Combalbert J, Picard C, Maffrand JP, Pascal M, Herbert JM. Identification and biological activity of the active metabolite of clopidogrel. Thromb Haemost 2000;84:891–896.

42. Quinn MJ, Fitzgerald DJ. Ticlopidine and clopidogrel. *Circulation* 1999;100:1667–1672.

43. A randomised, blinded, trial of clopidogrel versus aspirin in patients at risk of ischemic events (CAPRIE). CAPRIE Steering Committee. *Lancet* 1996;348(9038):1329–1339.

44. Diener HC, Bogousslavsky J, Brass LM, Cimminiello C, Csiba L, Kaste M, Leys D, Matias-Guiu J, Rupprecht HJ; MATCH investigators. Aspirin and clopidogrel compared with clopidogrel alone after recent ischemic stroke or transient ischemic attack in high-risk patients (MATCH): randomised, double-blind, placebo-controlled trial. *Lancet* 2004;364(9431):331–337.

45. Adams HP Jr, Bendixen BH, Kappelle LJ, Biller J, Love BB, Gordon DL, Marsh EE. Classification of subtype of acute ischemic stroke. Definitions for use in a multicenter clinical trial. TOAST. Trial of Org 10172 in Acute Stroke Treatment. *Stroke* 1993;24; 35–41.

46. Hart RG, Palacio S, Pearce LA. Atrial fibrillation, stroke, and acute antithrombotic therapy. Analysis of randomized clinical trials. *Stroke* 2002;33;2722–2727.

47. Lovett JK, Coull AJ, Rothwell PM. Early risk of recurrence by subtype of ischemic stroke in population-based incidence studies. *Neurology* 2004;62;569–573.

48. Evans A, Perez I, Yu G, Kalra L. Should stroke subtype influence anticoagulation decisions to prevent recurrence in stroke patients with atrial fibrillation? *Stroke* 2001;32;2828–2832.
49. Kay R, Wong KS, Yu YL, Chan YW, Tsoi TH, Ahuja AT, Chan FL, Fong KY, Law CB, Wong A. Low-molecular-weight heparin for the treatment of acute ischemic stroke. *N Engl J Med* 1995;333(24):1588–1593.
50. Cerebral Embolism Study Group. Immediate anticoagulation of embolic stroke: a randomized trial. Cerebral Embolism Study Group. *Stroke* 1983;14:668–676.
51. Cardiogenic brain embolism: cerebral embolism task force. *Arch Neurol* 1986;43:71–84.
52. Lovett JK, Coull AJ, Rothwell PM. Early risk of recurrence by subtype of ischemic stroke in population-based incidence studies. *Neurology* 2004;62:569–573.
53. Barnett HJ, Taylor DW, Eliasziw M, Fox AJ, Ferguson GG, Haynes RB, Rankin RN, Clagett GP, Hachinski VC, Sackett DL, Thorpe KE, Meldrum HE, Spence JD. Benefit of carotid endarterectomy in patients with symptomatic moderate or severe stenosis. North American Symptomatic Carotid Endarterectomy Trial Collaborators. *N Engl J Med* 1998;339(20):1415–1425.
54. Markus H, Mac Kinnon A. Asymptomatic embolization detected by Doppler ultrasound predicts stroke risk in symptomatic carotid artery stenosis. *Stroke* 2005;36; 971–975.
55. Dittrich R, Ritter M, Kaps M, Sieber M, Lees K, Larrue V, Nabavi D, Ringelstein E, Markus H, Droste D. The use of embolic signal detection in multicenter trials to evaluate antiplatelet efficacy: signal analysis and quality control mechanisms in the CARESS trial. *Stroke* 2006;37;1065–1069.
56. Junghans U, Siebler M. Cerebral microembolism is blocked by tirofiban, a selective nonpeptide platelet glycoprotein IIb/IIIa receptor antagonist. *Circulation* 2003;107:2717.
57. Antiplatelet therapy for acute ischemic stroke. The Cochrane review; 2003.
58. Bassi P, Lattuada P, Gomitoni A. Cervical cerebral artery dissection: a multicenter prospective study (preliminary report). *Neurol Sci* 2003;24 (Suppl.1):S4–S7.
59. Lucas C, Moulin T, Deplanque D, Tatu L, Chavot D. Stroke patterns of internal carotid artery dissection in 40 patients. *Stroke* 1998;29:2646–2648.
60. Endo S, Nishijima M, Nomura H, Takaku A, Okada E. A pathological study of intracranial posterior circulation dissecting aneurysms with subarachnoid hemorrhage: report of three autopsied cases and review of the literature. *Neurosurgery* 1993;33:732–738.
61. Han DH, Kwon OK, Oh CW. Clinical characteristics of vertebrobasilar artery dissection. *Neurol Med Chir (Tokyo)* 1998;38(Suppl.):107–113.
62. Bassi P, Lattuada P, Gomitoni A. Cervical cerebral artery dissection: a multicenter prospective study (preliminary report). *Neurol Sci* 2003;24 (Suppl.1):S4–S7.
63. Jacobs A, Lanfermann H, Neveling M, Szelies B, Schroder R, Heiss WD. MRI- and MRA-guided therapy of carotid and vertebral artery dissections. *J Neurol Sci* 1997;147:27–34.
64. Engelter S, Lyrer P, Kirsch E, Steck AJ. Long-term follow-up after extracranial internal carotid artery dissection. *Eur Neurol* 2000;44:199–204.
65. Schievink W. The treatment of spontaneous carotid and vertebral artery dissections. *Curr Opin Cardiol* 2000;15:316–321.
66. Engelter S, Lyrer P, Kirsch E, Steck AJ. Long-term follow-up after extracranial internal carotid artery dissection. *Eur Neurol* 2000;44:199–204.

67. Lyrer P, Engelter S. Antithrombotic drugs for carotid artery dissection. *Cochrane Database Syst Rev* 2003.
68. Beletsky V, Nadareishvili Z, Lynch J, Shuaib A, Woolfenden A, Norris JW, for the Canadian Stroke Consortium. Cervical arterial dissection: time for a therapeutic trial? *Stroke* 2003;34:2856–2860.
69. Lu CJ, Kao HL, Sun Y, Liu HM, Jeng JS, Yip PK, Lee YT. The haemodynamic effects of internal carotid artery stenting: a study with color-coded duplex sonography. *Cerebrovasc Dis* 2003;15:264–269.
70. Cohen JE, Leker RR, Gotkine M, Gomori M, Ben-Hur T. Emergent stenting to treat patients with carotid artery dissection: clinically and radiologically directed therapeutic decision making. *Stroke* 2003;34:e254–e257.
71. Lylyk P, Cohen JE, Ceratto R, Ferrario A, Miranda C. Angioplasty and stent placement in intracranial atherosclerotic stenoses and dissections. *AJNR Am J Neuroradiol* 2002;23:430–436.
72. Malek AM, Higashida RT, Phatouros CC, Lempert TE, Meyers PM, Smith WS, Dowd CF, Halbach VV. Endovascular management of extracranial carotid artery dissection achieved using stent angioplasty. *AJNR Am J Neuroradiol* 2000;21: 1280–1292.
73. Muller BT, Luther B, Hort W, Neumann-Haefelin T, Aulich A, Sandmann W. Surgical treatment of 50 carotid dissections: indications and results. *J Vasc Surg* 2000;31:980–988.
74. Kalbag RM, Woolf AL. *Cerebral venous thrombosis*. London: University Press; 1967.
75. Ameri A, Bousser M. Cerebral venous thrombosis. *Neurol Clin* 1992;10:87–111.
76. Einhäupl KM, Villringer A, Meister W, Mehraein S, Garner C, Pellkofer M, Haberl RL, Pfister HW, Schiedek P. Heparin treatment in sinus venous thrombosis. *Lancet* 1991;338:597–600.
77. de Bruijn, SFTM, Stam J. Randomized, placebo-controlled trial of anticoagulant treatment with low-molecular-weight heparin for cerebral sinus thrombosis. *Stroke* 1999;30:484–488.
78. Bousser MG. Cerebral venous thrombosis: nothing, heparin, or local thrombolysis? *Stroke* 1999;30:481–483.
79. Frey JL, Muro GJ, McDougall CG, Dean BL, Jahnke HK. Cerebral venous thrombosis: combined intrathrombus rtPA and intravenous heparin. *Stroke* 1999;30:489–494.
80. Smith AG, Cornblath WT, Deveikis JP. Local thrombolytic therapy in deep cerebral venous thrombosis. *Neurology* 1997;48:1613–1619.
81. Tsai FY, Wang AM, Matovich VB, Lavin M, Berberian B, Simonson TM, Yuh W. MR staging of acute dural sinus thrombosis: correlation with venous pressure measurements and implications for treatment and prognosis. *Am J Neuroradiol* 1995;16: 1021–1029.
82. Horowitz M, Purdy P, Unwin H, Carstens G, Greenlee R, Hise J, Kopitnik T, Batjer H, Rollins N, Samson D. Treatment of dural sinus thrombosis using selective catheterization and urokinase. *Ann Neurol* 1995;38:58–67.
83. Di Rocco C, Iannelli A, Leone G, Moschini M, Valori VM. Heparin-urokinase treatment in aseptic dural sinus thrombosis. *Arch Neurol* 1981;38:431–435.
84. Holder CA, Bell DA, Lundell AL, Ulmer JL, Glazier SS. Isolated straight sinus and deep cerebral venous thrombosis:successful treatment with local infusion of urokinase. *J Neurosurgery* 1997;86:704–707.

85. Smith TP, Higashida RT, Barnwell SL, Halbach VV, Dowd CF, Fraser KW, Teitelbaum GP, Hieshima GB. Treatment of dural sinus thrombosis by urokinase infusion. *Am J Neuroradiol* 1994;15:801–807.

86. Spearman MP, Jungreis CA, Wehner JJ, Gerszten PC, Welch WC. Endovascular thrombolysis in deep venous thrombosis. *Am J Neuroradiol* 1997;18:502–506.

87. Frey JL, Muro GJ, McDougall CG, Dean BL, Jahnke HK. Cerebral venous thrombosis: combined intrathrombus rtPA and intravenous heparin. *Stroke* 1999;30:489–494.

88. Adams H, Adams R, Del Zoppo G, Goldstein LB. Guidelines for the early management of patients with ischemic stroke: 2005 guidelines update a scientific statement from the stroke Council of the American Heart Association/American Stroke Association. *Stroke* 2005;36;916–923.

89. Albers GW, Amarenco P, Easton JD, Sacco RL, Teal P. Antithrombotic and thrombolytic therapy for ischemic stroke, The Seventh ACCP Conference on Antithrombotic and Thrombolytic Therapy. *Chest* 2004;126:483S–512S.

90. European stroke initiative recommendations for stroke management—update 2003. Cerebrovasc Diseases 2003;16:311–337.

8

INTENSIVE CARE MANAGEMENT OF ACUTE ISCHEMIC STROKE

KEVIN N. SHETH AND DAVID M. GREER

INTRODUCTION

Ischemic stroke patients may present with, or later develop, characteristics that require intensive levels of care. Dedicated Neurointensive Care Units have advanced the care and improved the outcome of patients with severe brain injuries, including ischemic stroke.[1] Silva et al.[2] compared the effect of intensive care monitoring versus standard medical therapy in patients with ischemic stroke or intracerebral hemorrhage; patients admitted to the intensive care unit (ICU) were those with a higher severity of stroke. They found that mortality at 1 year was significantly reduced in the patients admitted to the ICU, although level of dependency was not significantly influenced. Cavallini et al.[3] prospectively studied 268 patients who underwent admission based on bed availability to a specialized stroke ICU or a routine care unit, and found that patients who underwent more intensive monitoring in the stroke ICU had improved detection of adverse changes in monitoring parameters, improved treatment of these parameters, and improved outcomes. However, Rordorf et al.[4] found that stroke patients with higher APACHE II scores, signifying a more severe physiological state, had a higher risk of death.

Depending upon the location and severity of the stroke at admission, patients may have cardiac and/or respiratory instability at the time of presentation to the emergency department (ED). They may need to be stabilized hemodynamically or intubated for airway protection or respiratory distress. Blood pressure management is often a crucial management issue, and the use of vasopressor or antihypertensive medications is common. In stroke patients at risk for malignant cerebral

Acute Ischemic Stroke: An Evidence-based Approach, Edited by David M. Greer.

edema, multiple general measures may be taken, and intracranial pressure (ICP) monitoring is sometimes necessary. In more severe situations, osmotic agents or other more invasive techniques are needed to prevent herniation. These therapeutic strategies, and the evidence to support their use, will be the topic of this chapter.

INITIAL STABILIZATION

In stroke patients presenting to the ED, the first goal of treatment is immediate cardiac and respiratory stabilization. The systemic blood pressure is most often elevated in the setting of an acute stroke as the result of a catecholamine surge, and if the patient is hypotensive, the clinician should consider a concomitant cardiac process, such as myocardial infarction (MI), congestive heart failure (CHF), or pulmonary embolism (PE).

Stroke patients commonly have airway compromise, either secondary to a depressed level of consciousness or due to mechanical dysfunction of the airway from the stroke itself. Either mechanism can increase the risk for aspiration in the acute setting. Furthermore, patients with large hemispheric strokes or lesions involving the brainstem may be particularly prone to emesis, another predisposing factor for aspiration. The emergency physician must weigh the risks of the patient aspirating in this setting versus the loss of aspects of the neurological exam when the patient does require intubation, since medications used during intubation will nearly always influence the neurological examination. In addition, an endotracheal tube will preclude spoken language. Certainly, if the patient is considered unstable or imminently unsafe in the physician's judgment, then elective intubation should ensue, but a cursory neurological examination should be performed first when possible.

Stroke patients who require mechanical ventilation are not necessarily destined for a poor outcome. In a study by Santoli et al.,[5] 58 patients underwent mechanical ventilation and 16 survived. Eleven achieved a Barthel Index (BI) score of 60, indicating a good outcome. Within this study population, those patients with bilaterally absent corneal and pupillary reflexes had uniformly poor outcomes, underscoring the need for careful assessment of brainstem reflexes in intubated stroke patients. Other factors that have been associated with poor outcome in intubated stroke patients are advanced age and lower Glasgow Coma Score (GCS) at the time of intubation,[6] as well as seizures and pulmonary edema.[7]

Once intubated, the patient should be placed on the most minimal settings that will allow for normocarbia and adequate oxygenation. The positive end-expiratory pressure (PEEP) should be kept <10 cm H_2O (optimally as low as 5 cm H_2O), as higher levels of PEEP may impair venous return to the heart and theoretically increase the ICP. Georgiadis et al.[8] evaluated the effect of different inspiratory:expiratory (I:E) ratios on patients with stroke and subarachnoid hemorrhage who were undergoing intracranial monitoring. They did not find any significant variation in the cerebral perfusion pressures (CPP) with varying I:E ratios, but it should be noted that their study did not include patients who had elevated ICPs, and thus the effect in patients with significant cerebral edema should remain in question.

It is difficult to predict if a neurologically injured patient will successfully be extubated. Salam et al.[9] studied 88 patients prospectively, measuring cough peak flow (CPF), endotracheal secretions, and the ability to complete four simple tasks prior to extubation. In patients who failed extubation, they had a lower CPF ($p = 0.03$), higher amount of secretions (RR 3.0, 95% CI 1.0–8.8), and diminished ability to complete the four simple tasks (RR 4.3, 95% CI 1.8–10.4).

If a stroke patient receives intravenous (IV) thrombolysis, care often continues in the ED until the patient arrives in the ICU. Close monitoring must continue during this time, with special attention to the blood pressure. The blood pressure is most commonly checked via an arm cuff, since the placement of invasive lines (e.g., arterial catheterization) is relatively contraindicated once the patient has received intravenous thrombolysis (unless the situation is emergent and mandates such treatment). The systolic pressure must not exceed 185 mm Hg, and the diastolic pressure limit should be 110 mm Hg. Should the blood pressure exceed these limits, IV antihypertensive agents should be administered. IV pushes of labetolol (10–20 mg over 1–2 minutes) may be effective, but if patients are refractory to these initial measures then a continuous infusion of labetolol (0.5–2.0 mg/minute), nicardipine (5–15 mg/hour), or nitroprusside (0.25–10 mg/kg/minute) may be necessary to keep the patient's blood pressure within the range. There will be a more detailed discussion of these antihypertensive agents, including their side effect profiles, later in this chapter.

GENERAL ICU MEASURES

Stroke patients who require ICU admission most commonly do so because of concerns of cerebral edema and possible neurological deterioration, and several general measures may be undertaken to minimize the likelihood of developing these complications. Head of bed elevation to 30° helps to reduce ICP and allows for more unimpeded return of venous blood to the heart. Some of the earliest work on head of bed elevation in brain injured patients was by Rosner and Coley,[10] who studied 18 patients with ICP elevations, and found that for every 10° of head elevation above the horizontal position the ICP decreased by an average of 1 mm Hg; however, the CPP also decreased by an average of 2–3 mm Hg. Adequate hydration and systemic blood pressure are essential to maintaining adequate CPP in this setting. Fan[11] systematically reviewed studies of head of bed elevation with brain injuries, showing a consistent reduction in ICP across most studies. Meixensberger et al.[12] evaluated the effect of head elevation on tissue perfusion, measuring local tissue p_{O_2} by a parenchymal microcatheter. They found that ICP could be significantly improved without compromising the regional cerebral oxygenation. The head should also be kept in the midline as much as possible, as significant head turning may cause venous compression in the neck, thereby increasing ICP. This was studied in neonates by Goldberg et al.,[13] who found significant elevations in ICP when their heads were in the side position versus midline.

However, in patients with a flow-dependent state (e.g., basilar stenosis with a fluctuating exam), sometimes the head of bed should be kept flat, or even in the

Trendelenberg position, in order to help perfuse the ischemic brain regions. Wojner-Alexander et al.[14] studied 20 stroke patients with transcranial Doppler (TCD) of the middle cerebral artery (MCA), measuring mean flow velocities (MFV) at 30°, 15°, and 0° head of bed elevation. The MFV improved in all patients by lowering the head of bed, and three patients demonstrated immediate neurological improvement when lowered to 0°.

The patient should be kept calm as much as possible, but this may be difficult if they are delirious, and sometimes the use of sedating medications is necessary. This carries with it the risk of confounding the neurological exam, which is vital to follow during this acute period when the patient is at risk for deterioration. Thus, short-acting medications in the lowest effective doses should be administered.

Fluid and electrolyte status requires special attention, and care should be given to avoid hypotonic fluids. In general, judicious fluid restriction should be used, as this will minimize cerebral edema. However, since stroke patients may present in a dehydrated state, which may predispose them to thrombosis, adequate isotonic fluids should be administered. Typical hydration orders include normal saline, with or without potassium supplementation, at a rate of 50–100 cm^3/hour. The patient's serum sodium should optimally be kept in the 140–145 mmol/L range in the first few days following the stroke; the sodium may be manipulated to higher ranges later in the ICU course, should the patient require osmotic therapy. Glycemic control is of great importance, and fluids containing dextrose should generally be avoided. Continuous insulin infusions are more commonly being utilized in the Neurointensive Care Unit setting, often with a target serum glucose range of 80–120 mg/dL. Hyperglycemia has been associated with increased volumes of stroke (both in experimental animal models and in humans), increased cerebral edema, and worse neurological outcomes after stroke.[15] An increased rate of hemorrhagic transformation following intravenous thrombolysis has also been found in association with hyperglycemia.[16] Proposed mechanisms of injury include acidosis,[17] increased excitotoxic amino acids,[18] increased cerebral edema, and breakdown of the blood–brain barrier (BBB).[19]

Other electrolytes of importance include calcium (especially if the patient is receiving a calcium channel blocker, such as nicardipine) and magnesium, as hypomagnesemia may predispose the patient to seizures, further complicating the ICP management. If the patient received intravenous iodinated contrast as part of their stroke evaluation, then careful monitoring of the blood urea nitrogen (BUN) and creatinine levels is necessary to detect contrast nephropathy.

Other general measures should be employed to prevent the development of common ICU complications. Stroke patients are at high risk for developing deep venous thrombosis (DVT), and prophylaxis should begin immediately upon admission to the ICU with compression stockings and pneumatic compression devices. Low-grade anticoagulation with subcutaneous heparin or low-molecular-weight heparin has also become a mainstay of treatment,[20] but should be delayed for 24 hours after a patient has received intravenous recombinant tissue-plasminogen activator (rt-PA). In the setting of a rapid platelet drop, vigilant attention is needed to diagnose heparin-induced thrombocytopenia and thrombosis, and heparin-containing products may need to be avoided. H2-antagonists or proton pump inhibitors should be given to prevent gastritis/ulcer formation. Enteral feeding should begin as early as possible, either orally if the patient is able to swallow, or by the use of a nasogastric tube. However, if the patient is at high risk for possible respiratory decompensation with the need for intubation, or if invasive surgical procedures are planned, then feeding should be withheld. All stroke patients should have a formal swallowing evaluation to reduce the risk of aspiration pneumonia, the most common infectious complication in stroke patients. Frequent chest physical therapy and repositioning are also useful techniques. The second most common infectious complication is a urinary tract infection, and the use of indwelling catheters should be limited as much as possible in the individual patient. Finally, bed-bound stroke patients are at high risk for constipation and bowel obstruction, and stool softeners and bowel motility agents may be helpful in preventing these complications. Table 8.1 shows commonly used orders in the admission of stroke patients to the ICU.

Brain-injured patients commonly experience fever, and hyperthermia may correlate with poor outcome in these patients, although a direct causative link has yet to be established. The impact of fever on patients in a neurocritical care unit has been evaluated, and after controlling for severity of illness, diagnosis, age, and complications, increased body temperature was found to strongly associate with an increased length of ICU and hospital stay, as well as higher mortality and

TABLE 8.1 General Admission Orders for Stroke Patients to the ICU.

System	Order
Neurology	1. Head CT 24 hours after IV rt-PA 2. Neuro checks every 1–2 hours 3. Avoid invasive procedures including blood draws for 24 hours 4. Head of bed elevation to 30°
Cardiology	1. Troponin, CK, CK-MB every 8 hours with EKG 2. Transthoracic ECHO (sometimes with agitated saline contrast) 3. Hold antihypertensive medications 4. Cardiac telemetry
Pulmonary	1. Admission chest X-ray 2. Aspiration precautions 3. Incentive spirometry as appropriate 4. If ventilated, use minimal settings, especially PEEP
Infectious disease	1. U/A, urine C&S, sputum and blood cultures with initial temperature >101.0°C
Endocrine	1. Sliding scale insulin 2. Insulin infusion if serum glucose >180 3. Hold Metformin as patient may need further dye exposure
Renal/fluids/ electrolytes	1. Isotonic fluids only 2. Replace potassium, calcium, magnesium
Prophylaxis	1. H_2 blocker/PPI 2. Stockings and pneumatic compression boots in lower extremities 3. Subcutaneous unfractionated or low molecular weight heparin

worse overall outcome.[21] Patients with brain injury may become febrile from a host of different causes, most commonly including pneumonia, urinary tract infection, medications, and DVT, and these entities may contribute to worse outcomes for non-neurological reasons. The term "neurogenic fever" is reserved for situations in which patients with a primary cerebral insult experiences fever, but no secondary causes are found. The severity and duration of the fever appear to directly correlate with the degree of brain injury, as well as with the presence of intracerebral hemorrhage. It is important to remember that neurogenic fever is a diagnosis of exclusion.

Excellent biological arguments exist for a direct impact of fever specifically on neurological outcome. On a local level, fever produces increased levels of excitatory amino acids (e.g., glutamate and dopamine), free radicals, lactic acid, and pyruvate.[22] There is an increase in cell depolarizations and BBB breakdown. Enzymatic function is impaired and cytoskeletal stability reduced. These events lead to increased cerebral edema, with a possible reduction in CPP as well as larger volumes of ischemic injury.[23,24]

A variety of brain injuries may be impacted by fever, including ischemic stroke,[25–28] subarachnoid hemorrhage,[29,30] intracerebral hemorrhage,[31,32] traumatic brain injury,[33] and global ischemic injury from cardiac arrest.[34] Furthermore, the neuroprotective effects of hypothermia have been demonstrated for cardiac arrest patients[35] and show promise in ischemic stroke patients as well.[36]

It appears that fever may worsen brain injury from any etiology, although it has yet to be shown that neurological outcome is directly influenced by hyperthermia. If such a link were established, it would further the case for aggressive fever control in neurologically injured patients. Although induced hypothermia has been shown to be effective in certain populations, it carries with it potential additional risks, including infection,[37] coagulopathy, electrolyte imbalances,[38] and cardiac dysrhythmias.[39] Until hypothermia is proven to be effective, the goal of therapy should be maintenance of normothermia during the acute period of brain injury, thereby avoiding the potential harms of hyperthermia in this vulnerable time.

BLOOD PRESSURE MANAGEMENT

Manipulation of blood pressure becomes necessary in many ischemic stroke patients, as patients with ongoing ischemia and fixed stenotic arterial lesion(s) may require blood pressure management to feed the ischemic penumbra. Conversely, patients with cerebral edema may require blood pressure lowering to reduce the detrimental effect of increased cerebral blood flow (CBF). In the normal human brain, CBF is kept relatively constant by the mechanism of cerebral autoregulation. This applies throughout a range of CPP from approximately 40 to 140 mm Hg. Beyond this range, the autoregulatory capacity is overwhelmed, and at pressures below 40 mm Hg further ischemia ensues. At pressures above 140 mm Hg, cerebral edema often worsens. Both of these circumstances assume an *intact* autoregulatory capacity, which may be significantly impaired in acute stroke patients. Older patients, or patients with chronic hypertension, often have poor vasoreactivity of the cerebral resistance vessels, perhaps secondary to morphometric changes with sympathetic denervation within the vessels themselves.[40] Consequently, they may be more susceptible to worsening ischemia due to an impaired ability to vasodilate, even in the setting of diminished cerebral perfusion. Alternatively, patients with a large ischemic stroke, by definition, have an impaired BBB, and with relatively higher blood pressures they may lose their ability to appropriately vasoconstrict, leading to more profound cerebral edema.

Blood pressure lowering in the setting of an acute ischemic stroke can be detrimental. Oliveira-Filho et al.[41] found that the degree of systolic blood pressure reduction in the first 24 hours strongly correlated with poor outcome at 3 months in acute stroke patients (odds ratio (OR) 1.89 per 10% decrease, 95% CI 1.02–3.52, $p = 0.047$). In contrast, there is much debate regarding the efficacy of induced hypertension in stroke patients. In a pilot study by Rordorf et al.,[42] controlled augmentation of the systolic blood pressure by 20% in the acute setting resulted in significant clinical improvement in 7 out of 13 acute stroke patients. Marzan et al.[43] retrospectively evaluated 34 acute stroke patients who underwent induced hypertension (10–20% of the initial value) for a median of 26 hours, and found that cardiac arrhythmias occurred in one patient, and intracerebral hemorrhage in two patients (one fatal). They concluded that the process is feasible and safe in patients with acute stroke. Koenig et al.[44] performed a retrospective analysis of 100 acute stroke patients, 46 of whom underwent induced hypertension, aiming for a mean arterial pressure (MAP) target of 10–20% higher than the patient's baseline value. There was no difference in adverse events between the induced hypertension group and the group that received standard medical therapy, although the length of stay was significantly increased in patients who underwent induced hypertension.

The most commonly used intravenous vasopressor agent is phenylephrine, which is a preferential α-1 agonist, with little or no activity on the intracranial cerebral vasculature. Its use must be weighed against the potential risks, including the possibility for exacerbating underlying coronary artery disease (CAD) or causing hemorrhagic conversion of an ischemic stroke. Induced hypertension therapy for acute ischemic stroke is discussed further in Chapter 5. Table 8.2 provides a summary of the commonly used vasopressor agents and their side effects.

For patients with massive cerebral infarction, induced hypertension is relatively contraindicated, as this may exacerbate cerebral edema. However, the clinician must also be wary of reducing the blood pressure too aggressively, as relative hypotension may induce a reflexive increase in the CBF by cerebral vasodilation and thereby exacerbate cerebral edema. Multiple intravenous antihypertensive agents are available for use, the most common being beta-blockers, calcium channel blockers, and nitrates. Labetolol is typically well tolerated, and may be protective against cardiac ischemia. However, it may also exacerbate asthma/COPD and may be ineffective in treating refractory, severe hypertension. Nicardipine is a recommended alternative; it is a potent vasodilator that is well tolerated, but more costly. It does have negative inotropic effects and may cause left ventricular dysfunction. Nitroprusside should be used with great caution, as it can cause cerebral vasodilation and impair autoregulation, thereby increasing ICP. It can also cause excessive

TABLE 8.2 Vasopressor Medications.

Agent	Dosing (μg/minute)	Onset of Action	Side Effects	Misc
Phenylephrine	10–1000 μg/minute	Seconds	Bradycardia, coronary vasoconstriction, decreased renal perfusion, metabolic acidosis	Alpha-1, increased cardiac output (CO), decreased systemic vascular resistance (SVR)
Norepinephrine	2–100 μg/minute	Seconds to minutes	Bradycardia, arrhythmia	Alpha-1, beta-1, increased CO, decreased SVR
Epinephrine	1–12 μg/minute	Seconds	Increased myocardial demand, flushing, arrhythmia, decreased renal perfusion	Alpha-1, beta-1, beta-2, increased CO, variable SVR
Dopamine	10–1000 μg/minute	Up to 5 minutes	Ectopy, tachycardia, headache	Alpha-1, beta-1, dopamine, increased CO, SVR
Dobutamine	10–1000 μg/minute	1–10 minutes	Tachycardia, hypotension, nausea, dyspnea	Beta-1, beta-2, increased CO, decreased SVR
Isoproterenol	0.1–20 μg/minute	Seconds	Arrhythmia, headache, hyperglycemia, hypokalemia	Beta-1, beta-2, increased CO, decreased SVR
Vasopressin	0.04–10 units/minute	1–5 minutes	Arrhythmia, chest pain, headache, nausea, H_2O retention, seizures	Increased CO
Milrinone	50 μg/kg over 10 minute bolus then 0.375–0.75 μg/kg/minute	5–15 minutes	Arrhythmia, headache	Increased CO, decreased SVR

hypotension in elderly or hypovolemic patients, and can be associated with rebound hypertension upon withdrawal. It also carries the potential for cyanide and thiocyanate toxicity with prolonged use. Table 8.3 provides an explanation of different available IV antihypertensive agents.

TABLE 8.3 Intravenous Antihypertensive Agents.

Drug	Duration	Onset	Dosing	Side Effects	Miscellaneous
Nicardipine	2–4 hour	5–10 minute	2.5–15 mg/hour	Tachycardia, headache, heart failure, flushing, peripheral edema	Long half-life, precluding rapid titration
Labetalol	3–6 hour	5–10 minute	10–120 mg/hour	Conduction block, heart failure, bradycardia, bronchospasm, exacerbate underlying pulmonary disease	Rapid onset of action
Esmolol	10–20 minute	<5 minute	2–21 mcg /minute	Conduction block, hypotension, bronchospasm	Rapid onset, short half-life
Sodium nitroprusside	1–4 hour	<1 minute	10–800 mcg /minute	Cyanide or thiocyanate toxicity, hypotension, headache	Can increase ICP, should not be given in pregnancy
Nitroglycerin	<5 minute	<5 minute	1–1000 mcg/ minute	Headache, tachycardia	Useful in cardiac ischemia
Enalaprilat	4–6 hour	Up to 30 minute	1.25–40 mg q6 hour	Hyperkalemia, renal failure, cough, anaphylaxis	Useful in left ventricular dysfunction, variable response, should not be given in pregnancy
Hydralazine	4–8 hour	Up to 30 minute	5–40 mg prn dosing	Headache, tachycardia, lupus like syndrome, potential nephrotoxicity	Often given with beta-blocker to counter reflex sympathetic drive, may increase ICP
Phentolamine	<10 minute	<3 minute	5–20 mg IV	Tachycardia	Used in states of excess adrenergic tone (e.g., pheochromocytoma)
Diazoxide	Up to 24 hour	<5 minute	1–3 mg/kg up to 150 mg	Hypernatremia, dizziness, vomiting	Avoid in patients with sulfa allergies; also used in patients with hypoglycemia

MANAGEMENT OF CEREBRAL EDEMA ASSOCIATED WITH ISCHEMIC STROKE

There are three types of ischemic strokes that are more commonly associated with an increased risk of morbidity and mortality: moderate-to-large cerebellar strokes, large cerebral hemispheric strokes, and moderate-to-large strokes in the middle cranial fossa, where a theoretical compartment exists that may lead to early herniation if untreated. Kasner et al.[45] evaluated 201 patients with large MCA strokes, and found several factors to be associated with the development of malignant or fatal brain edema. In a multivariable analysis, these factors included a history of hypertension (OR 3.0) or CHF (OR 2.1), increased white blood cell (WBC) count at admission (OR 1.08 per 1000 WBC/μL), hypodensity on computed tomography (CT) scan involving >50% of the MCA territory (OR 6.3) and involvement of additional vascular territories (anterior cerebral artery, posterior cerebral artery, or anterior choroidal artery, OR 3.3). In a bivariable analysis, initial level of consciousness, National Institutes of Health Stroke Scale (NIHSS) score, early nausea and vomiting, and elevated serum glucose were also associated with fatal brain edema. An analysis of 24 complete MCA infarcts by Maramattom et al.[46] found a higher rate of malignant edema in female patients (72% vs. 20%) and those with additional territories of infarction (72% vs. 0%) (Fig.8.1).

Qureshi et al.[47] evaluated the timing of deterioration in patients with massive MCA strokes in a multicenter retrospective chart review. They found that 68% of patients manifested clinical deterioration by 48 hours, and nearly another 20% did so by 72 hours. Thus, the first 3–5 days appears to be the most crucial time for detecting patients at high risk for deterioration, although there was a small minority of patients who had deterioration at greater than 5 days from symptom onset. Early impairment in consciousness was also found to be predictive of mortality in one cohort of patients within a randomized clinical trial.[48] One postmortem study of 192 patients found features in 45 patients that they postulate led to "malignant"

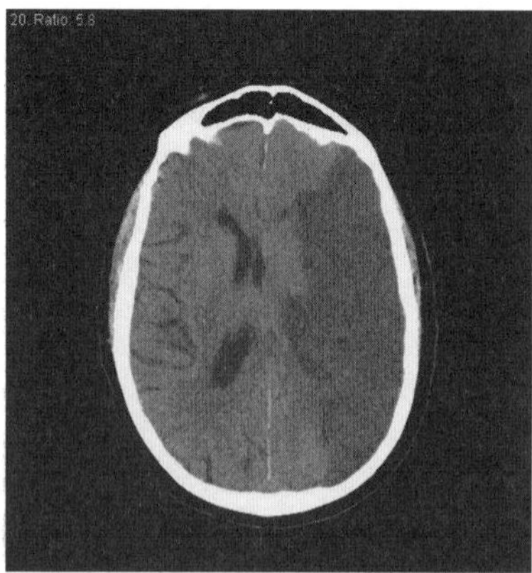

FIGURE 8.1 Massive middle cerebral artery infarction.

infarction.[49] These included larger volumes of infarction (including areas in addition to the MCA territory), hemorrhagic transformation, Duret hemorrhages, carotid occlusion, and ipsilateral abnormalities of the circle of Willis ($p < 0.5$). In a multivariable analysis, younger age, female sex, absence of stroke history, higher heart rate, carotid artery occlusion, and an abnormal ipsilateral circle of Willis all also correlated with malignant infarction ($p < 0.3$). CT features have been evaluated in a retrospective analysis of 135 patients from seven centers, and in a multivariable analysis the features associated with poor outcome included an anteroseptal shift of $\geq$5 mm and infarction beyond the MCA territory.[50]

Another important factor to consider is the patient's age. Younger patients are at higher risk of early neurological deterioration from cerebral edema associated with strokes, as they have less overall brain atrophy, and thus less tolerance for swelling within the cranial vault. Older patients, however, are more susceptible to poor outcomes, as clinicians may be less likely to be aggressive in their management, excluding them from potentially life-saving procedures. This may lead to a self-fulfilling prophesy for poor outcome in older aged patients. Older patients who do survive massive cerebral infarctions also have been shown to have less rehabilitation capacity, likely secondary to decreased "neuroplasticity" in the older brain.

Medical Measures to Control Cerebral Edema

Hyperventilation reduces ICP by reducing CBF. Carbon dioxide is a potent cerebral vasodilator, and thus vasoconstriction is induced by rapidly decreasing the p_{CO_2} (thereby concomitantly increasing the CSF pH), subsequently reducing the entry of blood into the cerebral circulation and lowering the ICP. The effect is almost immediate, reducing ICP typically within minutes. However, it is short lived, and may theoretically result in worsening of the cerebral infarction volume secondary to vasoconstriction affecting the ischemic penumbrum. Furthermore, there is also a risk of rebound vasodilation and worsening ICP when the p_{CO_2} returns to normal, and thus the use of hyperventilation should be seen as a bridge at best, used toward a more definitive treatment in an acutely herniating patient. There have been no recent clinical trials, but evidence from the 1970s did not reveal an effect on outcome. Furthermore, there is growing evidence that hyperventilation is not always used according to guidelines, and may lead to worse outcomes.[51] Hyperventilation is not a technique that lends itself to adequate clinical study, as most clinicians, recognizing its acute effectiveness, would not consider it ethical to randomize decompensating patients to hyperventilation versus no hyperventilation.

Osmotherapy employs agents such as mannitol, glycerol, and hypertonic saline to create an osmotic gradient between the brain (optimally, the edematous infarcted tissue) and the bloodstream, such that water is drawn out from the brain, thereby reducing edema. Each of these agents has been shown to be effective, and may be used alone or in combination with a diuretic, such as furosemide. Their action, however, depends upon an intact blood-brain barrier (BBB), and concerns have been raised for possible paradoxical worsening when one is absent. In this hypothesis, mannitol extravasates from the vessel into the interstitial tissue and water follows a new osmotic gradient.[52] Furthermore, even with an intact BBB, mannitol may concentrate in the CSF, also paradoxically increasing the ICP hours after administration.[53]

Mannitol is an extracellular, non metabolizable sugar, acting to create a gradient between the intravascular, intracellular, and interstitial spaces. It is also felt to have rheological effects, increasing blood flow in the cerebral microcirculation by decreasing red blood cell deformity, and thus decreasing serum viscosity.[54] It should be administered in a weight-based fashion, 1–1.5 g/kg intravenously, with repeated doses every 6 hours as needed for refractory ICP.[55] However, its use may be limited by the potential for nephrotoxicity, especially when there is inadequate clearance between doses. A generally employed technique is the measurement of the serum osmolarity (osms), holding the administration of the next dose of mannitol if the serum osms exceed 320. However, this may be an insensitive measure of the clearance of mannitol, and many now advocate the measurement of the osmolar gap. Multiple formulations have been evaluated for measuring the osmolar gap, and

$$1.86(\mathrm{Na} + \mathrm{K}) + (\mathrm{glucose}/18) + (\mathrm{BUN}/2.8)$$

appears to have a high correlation with serum mannitol levels.[56] However, it has yet to be determined what the appropriate osmolar gap should be for the ischemic stroke patient, and thus the repeated administration of mannitol may depend upon what the treating clinician feels is the appropriate gap for that patient, or when they feel that the osmolar gap gives the best approximation for the volume status in the individual patient. In a nonrandomized head-to-head trial of mannitol with hypertonic saline, mannitol appeared to be significantly more effective in improving CPP.[57] To date, mannitol has not been subjected to a prospective, randomized trial in space-occupying cerebal infarction, either versus placebo or versus any other osmotic agent.

Glycerol is also a nonmetabolizable sugar and is touted to have potential neuroprotective qualities as well. It is not felt to be as potent an osmotic agent as mannitol. Prior animal studies suggested an effect for rheology and edema minimization.[58] Human studies in acute stroke have suggested a benefit for glycerol in short-term but not long-term outcomes, and a Cochrane review did not support its routine use in controlling cerebral edema.[59] One significant concern raised in a cerebral microdialysis study of 7 large MCA infarct patients with 16 ICP elevations was the short-lived ICP lowering effect of glycerol (only 70 minutes), as well as the rapid accumulation of glycerol in the brain tissue itself, which may ultimately worsen edema with cumulative doses.[60]

Hypertonic saline is actively excluded from an intact BBB and also acts to draw water into the intravascular space by the creation of a sodium gradient. Various concentrations have been evaluated, with continuous sodium chloride infusions ranging from 3% to 9%, and bolus infusions up to 23.4% administered over 20 minutes in a 30 mL solution.[61] When a continuous infusion is used, the serum sodium is typically titrated to the 155–160 range. Sodium levels above this range raise the concern for seizures and other toxic side effects. Hypertonic saline may hold an advantage over mannitol, as it has been found in animal models to decrease edema in both the affected and unaffected hemispheres.[62] It also has a higher reflection coefficient, a marker of the relative selectivity of the BBB to a particular substance.[63] Hypertonic saline has also been shown to be effective in cases of cerebral edema that are refractory to mannitol therapy.[64] Systemic effects include transient volume expansion, hemodilution, natriuresis, and improved pulmonary gas exchange. However, repeated use may lead to electrolyte abnormalities, congestive heart failure (CHF), bleeding, and phlebitis. To date, there have been no randomized trials of the use of hypertonic saline in hemispheric cerebral infarction, either versus placebo or versus other osmotic agents. One study by Bhardwaj et al.[65] suggested that infarct volumes were increased by hypertonic saline in an animal model of transient focal cerebral ischemia, but this has not been observed in any human studies to date.

Barbiturates, including pentobarbital, have been evaluated in clinical studies of a variety of cerebral insults with ICP elevation, including traumatic brain injury, cerebral aneurysm rupture, and ischemic stroke. They are effective in reducing ICP by lowering the cerebral metabolic rate,[66] and may have neuroprotective qualities by being free radical scavengers.[67] Their use, however, is complicated by the side effects of hypotension and sedation, as well as an increased infection risk with prolonged use. The ability to follow the neurological exam is lost, and this is a vital tool in monitoring a patient's clinical status following a stroke. Hypotension may compound ischemia by reducing the CPP, thereby collapsing any collateral vessels that may have been feeding ischemic but not yet infarcted tissue, or by causing global ischemia in a patient with high ICP who is dependent upon a higher MAP to maintain their CPP. Thus, although there have been no randomized studies of barbiturates in cerebral infarction, their use is generally not recommended.

Tris-hydroxymethyl-aminomethane (*THAM*) has been evaluated in ischemic stroke to reduce mass effect and ICP. It acts as a buffer, neutralizing acidosis on a local level, including in the brain parenchyma. It has been studied in animal models of stroke, showing an effect in reducing the size of[68] and swelling from[69] cerebral infarction. To date, however, THAM has not been studied in a controlled fashion in humans with ischemic stroke.

Corticosteroids have been evaluated in several types of cerebral injury, including cerebral infarction. Corticosteroids reduce vasogenic edema, such as that associated with neoplasms, but not cytotoxic edema, the type associated with ischemic stroke. A large meta-analysis found no benefit to the use of corticosteroids in ischemic stroke (or intracerebral hemorrhage),[70] and their use is not recommended, except to treat concomitant conditions that mandate it (e.g., COPD flare).

Hypothermia for Ischemic Stroke

Early clinical data have shown promise for induced hypothermia for the treatment of acute ischemic stroke. Hypothermia acts by decreasing the cerebral metabolic rate, stabilizing cell membranes, preserving the integrity of the BBB, reducing the release of destructive enzymes, reducing the inflammatory response, and decreasing the release of excitotoxic neurotransmitters, such as glutamate and dopamine. Early treatment with hypothermia may reduce total infarct volume, and may prevent the development of cerebral edema. However, its use is associated with several potential adverse side effects, including an increased risk of infection, coagulopathy, hypokalemia, hyperglycemia, and cardiovascular suppression. Furthermore, when hypothermia is discontinued, a rebound elevation of ICP has also been noted, which may be fatal. The timing, degree, and duration of hypothermia in ischemic stroke have not been fully worked out, nor has the safest rate of re-warming.

Numerous small studies have been conducted for hypothermia in ischemic stroke, but most of these were feasibility phase II studies, and often did not include control patients.[71] Schwab et al.[72] found hypothermia to be useful and feasible in 25 patients with severe MCA strokes, cooling them to 33°C for 48–72 hours, with a significant reduction in ICP. However, this study poignantly demonstrated the problems with re-warming, as fatal herniation occurred in a significant proportion of patients as they returned to normothermia. Pneumonia also occurred in 40% of patients, perhaps higher than would be expected from the natural history of large MCA stroke patients. Controlled rewarming was then evaluated, and appeared to be more effective in controlling the ICP in a more graduated and safe fashion.[73]

The COOL AID study[36] randomized 40 patients within 12 hours of ischemic stroke, 18 to hypothermia with a target temperature of 33°C for 24 hours, and 22 to standard medical management. The two groups had similar clinical outcomes, as well as similar lesion growth as measured on magnetic resonance imaging (MRI). They concluded that induced hypothermia for ischemic stroke appears safe, but could make no conclusions regarding efficacy. The Nordic Cooling Stroke Study (NOCSS), currently in progress, is a multicenter, multinational trial planning to enroll 1000 patients at 25 centers. Patients with ischemic stroke within 6 hours will be eligible, but they must have moderate-to-severe hemispheric strokes. Patients will be randomized to standard medical management or induced hypothermia to 35°C with surface cooling methods, using meperidine to control shivering. Table 8.4 provides a review of the randomized studies of hypothermia in stroke patients.

Multiple methods of inducing hypothermia are currently available. Traditional methods, such as the use of ice packs, cooling blankets, or mattresses that deliver cold air, are often ineffective and difficult to control. Overshooting of the target temperature is not uncommon with these techniques, and with lower temperatures comes a higher rate of complications, including dangerous cardiac dysrhythmias. More advanced methods include the use of intravenous cooling catheters,[74] external cooling vests,[75] and selective head cooling via a helmet device[76] or local brain cooling used in conjunction with surgical management.[77] The advantage of these techniques is that they are more effective at bringing the patient to the target temperature and do not have significant overshoot. However, they are more expensive, and the intravenous catheters pose the additional risk of infection and DVT.

Shivering is common with the induction of hypothermia, and may inhibit the ability to get the patient to the target temperature. Multiple agents have been evaluated in the prevention of shivering. Tylenol is only modestly effective, and is complicated by significant hypotension.[78] Other agents that may be effective include buspirone, meperidine, and dexmedetomidine, the last two of which may be highly effective when used in combination.[79] These agents have mild sedating effects and may affect the neurological exam in stroke patients.

TABLE 8.4 Trials of Hypothermia in MCA Infarction.

Author	Publication	Design	Number of Patients	Clinical Question	Outcome
Els et al.	*Cerebrovasc Diseases* 2006; 21 (1–2): 79–85	Prospective, randomized; hemicraniectomy vs. hemicraniectomy plus cooling	12 of 25 tx with hypothermia plus surgery	Hypothermia to 35°C on safety and outcome in pts with >2/3 MCA infarct	Overall mortality 12% with no group differences. Increased pressor need in combined group. Nonsignificant trend by NIHSS at 6 months in combined group
De Georgia et al.	*Stroke* 2004; 63:312–317	Prospective, randomized; cooling vs. standard therapy for feasibility and safety	18 of 40 tx with hypothermia	Hypothermia to 33°C with endovascular catheter on safety in pts with anterior circulation stroke and NIHSS ≥8	Similar clinical outcomes and lesion growth as measured on DWI MRI. Nonsignificant reduction in DWI volume in patients who cooled well.
Georgiadis et al.	*Stroke* 2002; 33(6): 1584–1588	Nonblinded prospective; hemicraniectomy for nondominant and cooling for dominant hemisphere	19 of 36 tx with hypothermia	Hypothermia to 33°C with cooling blankets or endovascular technique on clinical course in pts with >2/3 MCA infarct	12% vs. 47% mortality for surgery vs. hypothermia. Hypothermia with increased complications of hypotension and electrolyte abnormalities. Both tx with longer ICU course
Schwab et al.	*Stroke* 1999; 30(5): 1153	Prospective pilot study; moderate hypothermia in severe stroke and ICP	25 of 25 tx with hypothermia	Hypothermia to 33–34°C with cooling blankets in pts with compete MCA infarct and ICP monitor	44% mortality, all by herniation after secondary rise in ICP after rewarming period. Good control of ICP during hypothermia period. Forty percent rate of pneumonia

Hemicraniectomy for Refractory Edema

Surgical management of ischemic stroke is discussed in further detail in Chapter 6, but worth brief mention here is the use of hemicraniectomy for massive hemispheric cerebral infarction. In patients who are at high risk for herniation, or who are refractory to maximal medical therapy, decompressive hemicraniectomy (DC), with or without partial temporal lobectomy, may be useful in selected patients. DC alleviates tissue shifts and rapidly reduces ICP, allowing for an adequate CPP to perfuse adjacent tissues. DC requires an adequate bone window and duraplasty, as inadequacy of either will leave the patient with a continued restrictive process, and thus continued risk for herniation. Jaeger et al.[80] demonstrated a dramatic improvement in brain tissue oxygenation ($PtiO_2$) in patients undergoing craniotomy with decompression for cerebral edematous states, including patients with MCA infarction. Wagner et al.[81] found that patients with inadequate hemicraniectomy windows were significantly more likely to have parenchymal hemorrhages (41.6%) and additional areas of infarction (28.4%). The timing of surgery is crucial, as patients who are already showing signs of herniation may already be incurring secondary ischemic injury to other brain regions. ICP monitors may be helpful, but it is a matter of some debate as to which side is the correct one to place the monitor, as theoretical compartments within the cranium may impair the correct assessment of the ICP when measured contralateral to the lesion (Fig. 8.2).

To date, only nonrandomized studies of hemicraniectomy in massive hemispheric stroke have been performed. Rieke et al.[82] found that mortality was reduced from 79% in control patients to 34% in those who underwent DC, with a concomitant reduction in poor functional outcome from 95% to 50%. The mean time interval from stroke to surgery was 39 hours in this study, relatively early in the time course, which may have prevented the patients from having secondary injury due to herniation. Schwab et al.[83] reduced mortality with DC to 16%. Both of these studies, however, found that functional outcome was consistently less improved in the elderly population. The Swedish Malignant Middle Cerebral Artery Infarction Study[84] looked at the long-term (median 3.4 years) outcome

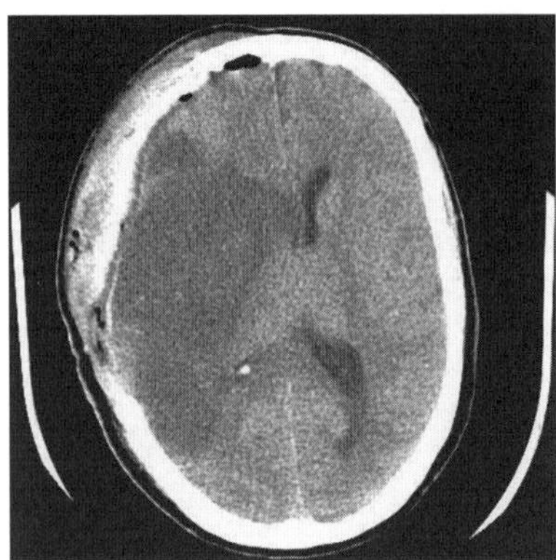

FIGURE 8.2 Massive stroke with inadequate hemicraniectomy, showing continued edema with midline shift.

of 30 patients who underwent DC, finding 6 patients achieving an mRS score of 2 or less, and 15 with mRS score of 3–5, with 43% of survivors becoming ambulatory. A history of hypertension has also been suggested to be a factor predictive of poor outcome, perhaps secondary to an impaired autoregulatory capacity in chronic hypertensive patients.[85] Gupta et al.[86] performed an analysis of 12 studies of DC, involving a total of 129 patients, to which they added 9 patients from their own institution to the analysis. After a minimum follow-up time of 4 months, they found that 7% were functionally independent, 35% were mildly to moderately disabled, and 58% died or were severely disabled. They found only age >50 years to be strongly correlated with poor outcome; in their analysis, there was no correlation of outcome with side of infarct (dominant vs. nondominant hemisphere), timing of surgery, signs of herniation before surgery, or involvement of other vascular territories.

Many clinicians are concerned about the use of DC for dominant hemisphere strokes, but Kastrau et al.[87] found in a retrospective review of 14 dominant hemisphere stroke patients with aphasia that significant improvement (13/14 patients) was achieved in these preselected younger patients who underwent early poststroke DC. In contrast, a retrospective study by Foerch et al.[88] found that older patients fared quite poorly in terms of functional outcome and quality of life, especially in those with severe neurological deficit at admission. These results were replicated by Curry et al.,[89] who also found that younger patients also were more likely to require reoperations for continued herniation. Uhl et al.[90] found no prognostic value to the side of infarction in their analysis of 188 patients who underwent DC for massive hemispheric infarction.

Decompressive hemicraniectomy was indirectly compared with moderate hypothermia (33°C) in a series of 36 patients from Georgiadis et al.[91] They found a lower mortality rate for the patients who underwent hemicraniectomy (47% vs. 12%), as well as a lower complication rate. However, this was not a randomized study, and there was no comparison arm of patients who did not undergo either experimental therapy.

Finally, decompressive hemicraniectomy used in *combination* with mild hypothermia was compared with hemicraniectomy alone in a small study of 25 patients by Els et al.[92] This was a prospective, randomized study of patients with infarction of greater than two thirds of a cerebral hemisphere, with 12 patients undergoing hemicraniectomy alone and 13 undergoing hemicraniectomy with induced hypothermia to 35°C. Surgery was performed 15 ± 6 hours after stroke, and hypothermia instituted immediately after surgery. Adverse events and mortality were not significantly different between the two groups, and although there was a suggestion of better clinical outcomes in the combined therapy group, the results were not significant due to low patient numbers in the trial, and thus all that can be established from this study is that combined therapy appears safe, and may be effective. Table 8.5 lists the hemicraniectomy trials to date in massive hemispheric infarction.

Several randomized trials of DC in massive hemispheric stroke are currently underway. These include Hemicraniectomy and Durotomy for Deterioration From Infarction Relating Swelling Trial (HeaDDFIRST), which enrolled 75 patients at 25 North American Centers (results not yet published); Hemicraniectomy After MCA infarction with Life-threatening Edema Trial (HAMLET),[93] a German study that plans to enroll 112 patients, requiring a decreasing level of consciousness with space-occupying MCA

TABLE 8.5 Trials of Hemicraniectomy in Massive Hemispheric Stroke.

Author	Publication	Design	Number of Patients	Clinical Question	Outcome
Pillai et al.	*J Neurosurg* 2007; 106(1): 59–65	Prospective study; decompression with durplasty various stages of mass occupying MCA infarct	26 patients with mean age of 48 and mean preop GCS of 9.9	Immediate and long-term intervention by survival and functional outcome	73% survival at 1 year; 33% independent, and 55% partially independent by Barthel Index. No patients in PVS
Malm et al.	*Acta Neurol Scand* 2006;113 (1):25–30	Prospective study of hemicraniectomy and neurointensive care in patients with hemicraniectomy	30 patients taken to surgery if transition was awake to response to painful stimuli with mean age of 49	Survival and independence at various time points	Nine patients died within one month. No further deaths in 3.4 years. Forty three percent survivors could walk with minimal aid
Harscher et al.	*Acta Neurochir (Wien)* 2006;141 (1):31–37	Retrospective study of patients based on charts and telephone interviews	30 patients mean age of 59 who underwent craniectomy for space occupying MCA infarction	Survival and functional outcome at various time points	16 patients survived mean time of 2.1 years
Curry et al.	*Neurosurgery* 2005;56(4): 681–692	Retrospective chart, operative report, and imaging review	38 patients treated with hemicraniectomy for large hemispheric infarcts (average volume 407 cm^3)	Survival and surgical selection of patients	32 patients survived at 1 year. Age but not time to surgery, volume of infarction or craniectomy size correlated with ability to walk and Barthel score
Kastrau et al.	*Stroke* 2005; 36(4): 825–829	Retrospective evaluation of aphasia in patients with hemicraniectomy for dominant sphere infarcts	14 patients with surgery evaluated with psychometric quantification twice over 470 days	Evolution of aphasic symptoms	13/14 patients with improved scores and increased ability to communicate from baseline in 13 patients. Young age and early decompressive surgery were main predictors of recovery

infarction; DEcompressive Craniectomy In MALignant Middle Cerebral Artery Infarcts (DECIMAL), a French study at 13 centers, planning to enroll 60 patients, requiring an NIHSS >15, altered LOC, CT changes involving >50% of the MCA territory, or a diffusion-weighted image (DWI) lesion volume >145 cm^3; and Hemicraniectomy for Malignant Middle Cerebral Artery Infarcts (HeMMI), a study from the Philippines, an open, randomized trial planning to enroll 56 patients. A recent pooled analysis of three of these trials suggested a beneficial effect of DC on functional outcome.[124]

Table 8.6 provides a summary of techniques that may be utilized to treat cerebral edema in patients with massive MCA infarction.

Special Circumstances: Cerebellar Infarction

Cerebellar infarction poses a particularly dangerous situation, as the posterior fossa acts as its own compartment, creating the possibility of brainstem compression, early herniation or obstructive hydrocephalus for ischemic strokes that swell, conditions that can develop suddenly and be fatal if not treated expeditiously. Certainly, patients with progressive brainstem signs from a compressive lesion should be considered at risk for fatal herniation and nearly always warrant a surgical decompression.[94] The exact volume of infarction that will have the potential for life-threatening mass effect is unclear, but cerebellar hemispheric strokes that involve greater than one third of the cerebellar hemisphere should be considered for early surgical management. It is also important to look at the appearance of the fourth ventricle, as increasing degrees of effacement are associated with a higher risk of hydrocephalus and herniation.[95] Other neuroimaging features that have correlated with deterioration after cerebellar stroke include hydrocephalus, brainstem deformity, and basal cistern compression.[96] The mode of neuroimaging here becomes crucial, as CT imaging may be incompletely sensitive to the volume of infarction due to the bony anatomy at the skull base, and thus MRI is a more reliable indicator of true lesion volume.[97] Figure 8.3 shows a cerebellar stroke with significant mass effect.

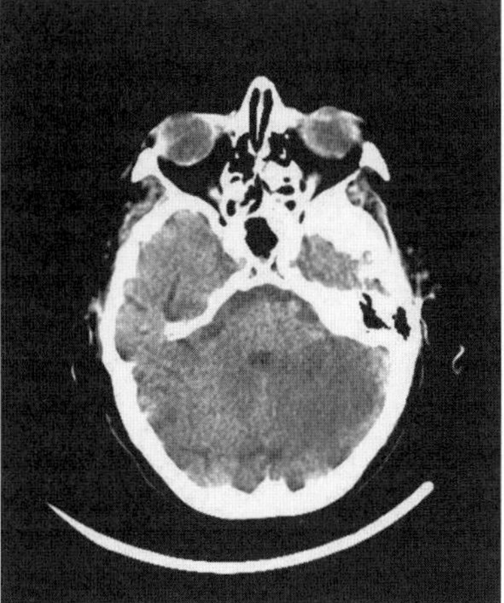

FIGURE 8.3 Massive cerebellar stroke with herniation.

TABLE 8.6 Guidelines for the Management of Cerebral Edema in Patients with Massive Hemispheric Cerebral Infarction.

	MOA	Dose/Administration	Monitoring	Adverse Effects
Emergent Tx Hyperventilation	Reduction of CO_2 causing cerebral vasoconstriction and reduction of CBV	Ambubag/ventilator rate of 30–40 breaths/minutes to increase minute ventilation by 15–20 L/minutes, wean slowly over 12–24 hours to prevent rebound cerebral edema. Effective only for a few hours. Avoid prolonged (>6 hours) or prophylactic use	$PaCO_2$ to keep at 26–30 mm Hg ABG monitoring Q15 minutes to avoid overshoot. $SjvO_2$ and/or $PbtO_2$ monitoring suggested	Cerebral ischemia, Rebound cerebral edema if stopped suddenly
Decompressive surgery	Expansion of cranial vault releasing pressure and improvement in CBF. Evacuation of mass effect	Wide craniectomy with duraplasty and evacuation of mass lesion, done as early as possible	ICP monitoring recommended Brain imaging as clinically indicated	Death, ICH, stroke, bleeding, infection
External ventricular drainage	Drainage of CSF to improve cerebral compliance and reduce ICP	Usually inserted in the nondominant frontal horn of lateral ventricle, EVD at 10–15 cm above external auditory meatus and open 5–10 mL CSF drainage every 30–60 min as needed for ICP >20 mm Hg	ICP monitoring Brain imaging as clinically indicated	CNS infection (ventriculitis), Bleeding, EVD malfunction
First tier Mannitol	Reduces brain water content. Reduces serum viscosity, Increases CBF Free radical scavenger. Reduces CBV. Reduced CSF production	1–2 g/kg IV bolus every 4–6 hours Taper dose if continued use for >24 hours alternate with 23.4% NaCl if with partial response	Serum Na, K, BUN, Glu, Osm, Osm gap before each dose Hold for Osmolar gap >5 (using formula: 1.86(Na + K) + BUN/2.8 + Glu/18 + 10) If baseline Osm Gap >5, hold for change in Osm Gap >5	Renal failure, Electrolyte abnormality, CHF. Rebound effect

Hypertonic saline	Reduces brain water content. Reduces serum viscosity Increases CBF, Improves CO Increased CSF absorption	23.4% NaCl IV bolus over 15–30 minutes @ 0.5–1 mL/kg /dose given every 4–6 hours alternate with or in between mannitol doses	Serum Na, Osm Do not exceed Na rise > 0.5 mEq/L per hr if with history of chronic hyponatremia	Renal failure CHF Electrolyte abnormalities Rebound effect
Second tier Barbiturates	Reduction of metabolic demand Reduces CBF and ICP Free radical scavenger Neuroprotective (anti-apoptotic?)	Thiopental 1–5 g IV loading dose as 500 mg IV bolus Q15–30 minutes over 1–5 hours until ICP response. If complete response (ICP <20), return to first tier agents, or repeat bolus doses as necessary. If incomplete response (ICP >20 but reduction >25%), start IV infusion at 1–8 mg/kg and adjust dose every 30–60 minutes to ICP goal <20 or until burst suppression EEG pattern at 1–2 burst/minutes Duration of treatment between 12 and 18 hours with gradual weaning over 24 hours	Continuous EEG Keep CPP >60 using vasopressors as necessary. $SjvO_2$ or $PbtO_2$ recommended Blood culture Q 24–48 hours Serum lytes, CBC, coags, LFTs daily	Systemic hypotension, systemic infection, respiratory complications, renal and hepatic dysfunction

(continued)

TABLE 8.6 *(Continued)*

	MOA	Dose/Administration	Monitoring	Adverse Effects
Hypothermia	Reduction of metabolic activity. Reduces CBF and ICP. Reduces release of excitatory neurotransmitters	Target temperature of 32–34°C Duration of treatment between 24 and 72 hours, followed by passive/controlled rewarming over 12–24 hours	Bladder temperature Surveillance cultures Coagulation parameters	Shivering Sepsis Hypotension Electrolyte abnormalities
Third tier Surgery	Expansion of cranial vault releasing pressure and improvement in CBF. Evacuation of mass effect	Most effective if done in patients who failed medical management, but do not have an overt herniation syndrome yet	ICP monitoring by EVD or bolt $SjvO_2$ or $PbtO_2$ recommended	Death, ICH, stroke, bleeding, infection

Coma in cerebellar stroke patients can develop from primary compression of the brainstem from the infarct acting as a mass lesion, brainstem compression from hemorrhage into the infarct, primary brainstem ischemic injury, or acute hydrocephalus.[98] A ventriculostomy should be considered as an adjunct to surgery, but generally should not be used in isolation, as relieving pressure from above may theoretically increase the possibility of upward herniation of the cerebellum through the tentorium. Some physicians, however, prefer to use the ventriculostomy in a staged fashion, perhaps holding off on surgery if there is significant clinical improvement. The definitive procedure is a decompressive suboccipital craniotomy. Postoperatively, use of the ventriculostomy should be continued, as swelling and/or bleeding in the posterior fossa may pose a continued risk for mass effect. Serial CT imaging may be useful to evaluate for resolution of the posterior fossa process. Raco and colleagues[99] advocate the use of conservative treatment, favoring clinical monitoring alone whenever possible, reserving the use of a ventriculostomy for a worsening clinical status, and then subsequently reserving suboccipital craniectomy for those who continue to worsen despite the placement of the ventriculostomy. The concern with this approach, however, is that the patient may suffer additional injury, either by compressing the brainstem or from acute hydrocephalus, and thus many favor early surgical intervention in patients with large cerebellar strokes. Furthermore, this study was a retrospective analysis of patients at a single institution, with significant variations in patient factors, including the size of the stroke.

In a multicenter study, Jauss et al.[100] evaluated the clinical features of 84 cerebellar infarction patients, and found that poor outcome was associated with a decreasing level of consciousness after clinical deterioration. Half of the patients in this study who deteriorated to coma had a meaningful recovery after undergoing ventricular drainage or suboccipital decompression, but unfortunately the trial was not randomized or controlled.

An alternative method of managing patients with cerebellar infarction causing obstructive hydrocephalus is endoscopic third ventriculostomy. Baldauf et al.[101] reviewed 10 cases managed by the use of endoscopic third ventriculostomy, 8 of whom had clinical improvement (measured as an improvement in the level of consciousness). This therapy is still experimental, and improvement in outcome has not been demonstrated.

MONITORING OF INTRACRANIAL PRESSURE IN ISCHEMIC STROKE PATIENTS

Patients with massive cerebral infarction may require ICP monitoring, as this may help to guide therapy and predict outcome. Schwab et al.[102] evaluated 48 patients with massive hemispheric infarctions and clinical signs of elevated ICP. They found that ICP measurements correlated well with the patient's clinical status, CT findings and outcome, although they did not find a significant effect of their therapies for elevated ICP on patient outcomes. Multiple methods of monitoring ICP are available for stroke patients at risk for herniation, each with advantages and disadvantages. Unfortunately, noninvasive techniques have not proven to be sufficiently reliable for detecting elevations in ICP, and thus clinicians are left with a host of invasive techniques.

The clinical examination is a valuable tool for monitoring the patient's status and should be performed frequently during the time of concern for swelling. Clinical signs to follow include the patient's mental status and level of alertness, cranial nerve function (particularly the pupillary reaction in patients at risk for uncal herniation), motor strength, and signs of increased ICP, such as worsening headache and nausea/vomiting. Patients developing hydrocephalus often lose their upgaze (assuming that adequate upgaze was present at baseline, which is not always the case with older patients) and develop more sluggish pupillary responses. Neuroimaging, such as CT and MRI, can be performed to assess for progression of cerebral edema, but it is not feasible or safe to perform repeat imaging more frequently than twice a day, at most. Neurosonology with TCD examination may provide clues to the development of increasing ICP, as compression of the basal arteries causes a narrowing of the vessel lumen, thereby increasing the flow velocity and the pulsitility index.[103]

For more invasive ICP monitoring, the gold standard is an external ventricular drain (EVD), which is a hollow catheter inserted directly into the ventricle, providing a direct measurement of the ICP as transmitted through the CSF.[104] It also allows for CSF drainage, thereby alleviating pressure within the cranial vault. However, it is also the most invasive monitor, having to transverse not only the epidural and subdural spaces but also the brain parenchyma *en route* to the ventricle, and thus it poses a risk of intracerebral hemorrhage in approximately 2–6% of patients.[105] It is also associated with an increased risk of infection, especially if left in place for >5 days,[106] although this risk can be minimized with the use of a tunneling technique beneath the scalp.[107] The prophylactic use of antibiotics remains unproven, but is considered standard of care in most Neurointensive Care Units.[108]

Other methods for ICP monitoring include Camino ICP monitors, which are positioned into the brain parenchyma, but do not transverse the hemisphere nearly to the degree that EVDs do, and are associated with a lower risk of intracerebral hemorrhage. The ICP is measured by a fiberoptic transducer at the tip of the catheter.[109] ICP monitors, however, are subject to inaccuracy over time, so-called "drift," and thus may become less reliable after the first few days post-insertion. Epidural and subarachnoid bolts/catheters are the least invasive, placed external to or just within the dura, thereby carrying a much lower risk of hemorrhage and infection, but with unfortunately compromised accuracy.[110]

Newer techniques include monitors capable of performing microdialysis, or measuring brain oxygenation and lactate, which may be useful in monitoring penumbral tissue adjacent to a large area of infarction.[111] No randomized studies have been performed to clearly document their impact on patient outcomes to date.

EEG monitoring may be useful in acute stroke patients. Seizures are not uncommon following stroke, occurring in 6–9% of patients in the acute setting.[112] The possibility of seizures in the patient with a massive stroke with cerebral edema is concerning, given that it could contribute to ICP elevations and worsen herniation effects. In one study of two groups of stroke patients, with ($n = 110$) and without ($n = 275$) seizures, the patients with seizures were significantly more likely to exhibit periodic lateralized epileptiform discharges (PLEDs) and frontal intermittent rhythmic delta activity (FIRDA).[113] Some endorse the use of continuous EEG monitoring in patients with acute ischemic stroke, perhaps adding value to outcome prediction, clinical management, and seizure detection,[114] but its use has not become routinely incorporated. Although it is reasonable to institute antiepileptic drug (AED) therapy in patients with ischemic stroke who have had a clinical or electrographic seizure, the prophylactic administration of AED therapy in patients who have not had a seizure has not been rigorously studied and cannot be routinely recommended.

CARDIAC COMPLICATIONS IN ISCHEMIC STROKE PATIENTS

Acute stroke patients are at high risk for cardiac events, including myocardial infarction (MI) and dysrhythmias from autonomic derangement, particularly with strokes involving the insular cortex. Although the precise mechanisms and triggers for this have yet to be elucidated, it appears that there is a predominance of sympathetic activity associated with strokes involving the right hemisphere.[115] Seizures that originate from the left temporal lobe may be more commonly associated with bradycardia and even cardiac asystole.[116,117] In stroke patients, however, involvement of the *right* hemisphere appears to correlate most strongly with cardiac autonomic derangements. Colivicci et al.[118] evaluated 103 patients with 24-hours Holter monitoring, and found a significantly higher rate of complex arrhythmias in patients with infarction of the right insular cortex. Meyer et al.[119] assessed sympathetic function in acute stroke patients by measuring plasma epinephrine and norepinephrine levels. They found that patients with involvement of the insular cortex, particularly on the right side, had significantly higher levels of plasma catecholamines. This group also separately studied blood pressure, heart rate, cardiac output, and transcranial flow velocities in the MCAs during the first 5 days after stroke, and found strong evidence for autonomic dysfunction in patients with insular stroke, again predominantly on the right side.[120] Although this remains an area of continued research, the insular cortex, particularly on the right side, may have a special association with cardiac pathology in acute stroke patients. Occasionally, these patients will have stunned myocardium, and pathology may reveal contraction band necrosis (Fig. 8.4).

MI in the setting of acute stroke is not uncommon, and may be the result of the catecholamine surge in response to the stroke. Most stroke patients are greater than 65 years of age, and intrinsic CAD is quite common in this age category. It thus becomes vital, especially in stroke patients who are unable to communicate symptoms of angina, to evaluate for the presence of MI in all acute stroke patients. Furthermore, it appears that, again, certain brain regions again appear to correlate

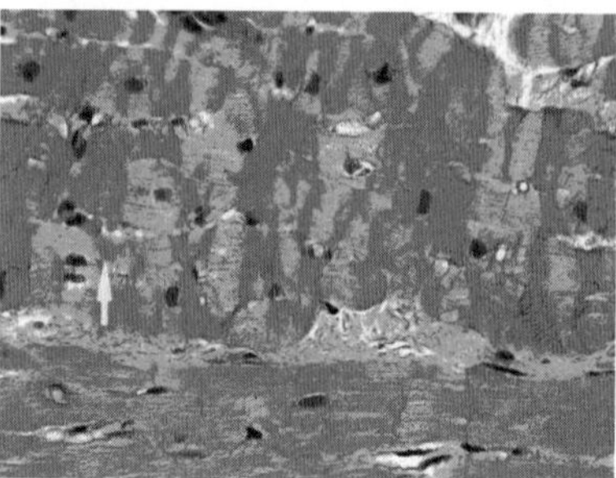

FIGURE 8.4 Contraction band necrosis.

with the risk for developing an MI. Ay et al.[121] performed a case–control study of 50 stroke patients with serum cardiac troponin T elevation, and found that patients with infarctions in the right hemisphere, specifically those with involvement of the insular cortex and inferior parietal lobule, had a troponin elevation rate of 88%, compared with 33% of patients who were without involvement of these areas (OR 15.00, 95% CI 2.65–84.79). Cardiac dysrhythmias have been noted in the acute stages of stroke, both ischemic and hemorrhagic. Orlandi et al.[122] evaluated 44 acute stroke patients with 24-hour cardiac monitors, finding significant dysrhythmias in 75% of hemorrhage patients and 69% of ischemic stroke patients.

Interestingly, not all patients develop significant autonomic activation with stroke. Sander and Klingelhofer[123] evaluated 42 stroke patients with essential hypertension and 45 normotensive patients. The normotensive patients with insular cortex stroke showed significantly reduced circadian blood pressure variations and a higher frequency of nocturnal blood pressure increases, as well as higher plasma norepinephrine levels and more frequent electrocardiographic abnormalities. Although life-threatening cardiac arrhythmias do not occur in the great majority of stroke patients in the acute setting, the clinician should be aware of the increased risk in patients with stroke involving certain brain regions.

CONCLUSIONS

Patients with acute stroke commonly warrant ICU level of care. The care of the stroke patient in the acute setting is paramount, as they are at high risk for cardiac and pulmonary, and infectious complications, a risk that continues during their ICU stay. Neurocritical Care Units have greatly advanced the care of patients with cerebellar stroke and massive hemispheric stroke, with advances in the evidence to support the use of ICP monitoring, osmotic agents, and hypothermia to treat cerebral edema. Several studies of surgical management of hemispheric stroke are underway, and this technique may prove to be quite useful in certain patient populations. With advances in our understanding of cerebral pathophysiology, our ability to care for critically ill acute stroke patients is likely to improve greatly in the years to come.

REFERENCES

1. Suarez JI. Outcome in neurocritical care: advances in monitoring and treatment and effect of a specialized neurocritical care team. *Crit Care Med* 2006;34: s232–s238.
2. Silva Y, Puigdemont M, Castellanos M, Serena J, Suner RM, Garcia MM, Davalos A. Semi-intensive monitoring in acute stroke and long-term outcome. *Cerebrovasc Dis* 2005;19(1):23–30.
3. Cavallini A, Micieli G, Marchesilli S, Quaglini S. Role of monitoring in management of acute ischemic stroke patients. *Stroke* 2003;34(11):2599–2603.
4. Rordorf G, Koroshetz W, Efird JT, Cramer SC. Predictors of mortality in stroke patients admitted to an intensive care unit. *Crit Care Med* 2000;28(5):1301–1305.
5. Santoli F, De Johghe B, Hayon J, Tran B, Piperaud M, Merrer J, Outin H. Mechanical ventilation in patients with acute ischemic stroke: survival and outcome at one year. *Intensive Care Med* 2001;27(7):1141–1146.
6. Bushnell CD, Phillips-Bute BG, Laskowitz DT, Lynch JR, Chilukuri V, Borel CO. Survival and outcome after endotracheal intubation for acute stroke. *Neurology* 1999;52(7):1374–1381.
7. Wijdicks EF, Scott JP. Causes and outcome of mechanical ventilation in patients with hemispheric ischemic stroke. *Mayo Clin Proc* 1997;72(3):210–213.
8. Georgiadis D, Schwarz S, Kollmar R, Baumgartner RW, Schwab S. Influence of inspiration:expiration ratio on intracranial and cerebral perfusion pressure in acute stroke patients. *Intensive Care Med* 2002;28(8):1089–1093.
9. Salam A, Tilluckdharry L, Amoateng-Adjepong Y, Manthous CA. Neurological status, cough, secretions and extubation outcomes. *Intensive Care Med* 2004;30(7): 1334–1339.
10. Rosner MJ, Coley IB. Cerebral perfusion pressure, intracranial pressure, and head elevation. *J Neurosurg* 1986;65(5):636–641.
11. Fan JY. Effect of backrest position on intracranial pressure and cerebral perfusion pressure in individuals with brain injury: a systematic review. *J Neurosci Nurs* 2004;36(5):278–288.
12. Meixensberger J, Baunach S, Amschler J, Dings J, Roosen K. Influence of body position on tissue-p_{O_2}, cerebral perfusion pressure and intracranial pressure in patients with acute brain injury. *Neurol Res* 1997;19(3):249–253.
13. Goldberg RN, Joshi A, Moscoso P, Castillo T. The effect of head position on intracranial pressure in the neonate. *Crit Care Med* 1983;11(6):428–430.
14. Wojner-Alexander AW, Garami Z, Chernyshev OY, Alexandrov AV. Heads down: flat positioning improves blood flow velocity in acute ischemic stroke. *Neurology* 2005;64(8):1354–1357.
15. Pulsinelli WA, Waldman S, Rawlinson D, Plum F. Moderate hyperglycemia augments ischemic brain damage: a neuropathologic study in the rat. *Neurology* 1982;32(11):1239–1246.
16. Demchuk AM, Morgenstern LB, Krieger DW, Linda Chi T, Hu W, Wein TH, Hardy RJ, Grotta JC, Buchan AM. Serum glucose level and diabetes predict tissue plasminogen activator-related intracerebral hemorrhage in acute ischemic stroke. *Stroke* 1999;30(1):34–39.

17. Anderson RE, Tan WK, Martin HS, Meyer FB. Effects of glucose and PaO2 modulation on cortical intracellular acidosis, NADH redox state, and infarction in the ischemic penumbra. *Stroke* 1999;30(1):160–170.

18. Li PA, Shuaib A, Miyashita H, He QP, Siesjo BK, Warner DS. Hyperglycemia enhances extracellular glutamate accumulation in rates subjected to forebrain ischemia. *Stroke* 2000;31(1):183–192.

19. Kawai N, Keep RF, Betz AL. Effects of hyperglycemia on cerebral blood flow and edema formation after carotid artery occlusion in Fischer 344 rats. *Acta Neurochir Suppl* 1997;70:34–36.

20. Kamphuisen PW, Agnelli G. What is the optimal pharmacological prophylaxis for the prevention of deep-vein thrombosis and pulmonary embolism in patients with acute ischemic stroke? *Thromb Res* 2007;119(3):265–274.

21. Diringer MN, Reaven NL, Funk SE, Uman GC. Elevated body temperature independently contributes to increased length of stay in neurological intensive care unit patients. *Crit Care Med* 2004;32(7):1489–1495.

22. Stocchetti N, Protti A, Lattuada M, Magnoni S, Longhi L, Ghisoni L, Egidi M, Zanier ER. Impact of pyrexia on neurochemistry and cerebral oxygenation after acute brain injury. *J Neurol Neurosurg Psych* 2005;76(8):1135–1139.

23. Morimoto T, Ginsberg MD, Deitrich WD, Zhao W. Hyperthermia enhances spectrin breakdown in transient focal cerebral ischemia. *Brain Res* 1997;746(1–2):43–51.

24. Baena RC, Busto R, Dietrich WD, Globus MY, Ginsberg MD. Hyperthermia delayed by 24 hours aggravates neuronal damage in rat hippocampus following global ischemia. *Neurology* 1997;48(3):768–773.

25. Hajat C, Hajat S, Sharma P. Effects of poststroke pyrexia on stroke outcome: a meta-analysis of studies in patients. *Stroke* 2000;31(2):410–414.

26. Reith J, Jorgensen HS, Pedersen PM, Nakayama H, Raaschou HO, Jeppesen LL, Olsen TS. Body temperature in acute stroke: relation to stroke severity, infarct size, mortality and outcome. *Lancet* 1996;347(1999):422–425.

27. Kammersgaard LP, Jorgensen HS, Rungby JA, Reith J, Nakayama H, Weber UJ, Houth J, Olsen TS. Admission body temperature predicts long-term mortality after acute stroke: the Copenhagen Stroke Study. *Stroke* 2002;33(7):1759–1762.

28. Boysen G, Christensen H. Stroke severity determines body temperature in acute stroke. *Stroke* 2001;32(2):413–417.

29. Wartenberg KE, Schmidt JM, Claassen J, Temes RE, Frontera JA, Ostapkovich N, Parra A, Connolly ES, Mayer SA. Impact of medical complications on outcome after subarachnoid hemorrhage. *Crit Care Med* 2006;34(3):617–623.

30. Oliveira-Filho J, Ezzedine MA, Segal AZ, Buonanno FS, Chang Y, Ogilvy CS, Rordorf G, Schwamm LH, Koroshetz WJ, McDonald CT. Fever in subarachnoid hemorrhage: relationship to vasospasm and outcome. *Neurology* 2001;56(10):1299–1304.

31. Schwartz S, Häfner K, Aschoff A, Schwab S. Incidence and prognostic significance of fever following intracerebral hemorrhage. *Neurology* 2000;54(2):350–354.

32. Leira R, Dávalos A, Silva Y, Gil-Peralta A, Tejada J, Garcia M, Castillo J; Stroke Project, Cerebrovascular Diseases Group of the Spanish Neurological Society. Early neurological deterioration in intracerebral hemorrhage: Predictors and associated factors. *Neurology* 2004;63(3):461–467.

33. Stocchetti N, Rossi S, Zanier ER, Colombo A, Beretta L, Citerio G. Pyrexia in head-injured patients admitted to intensive care. *Int Care Med* 2002;28(11):1555–1562.

34. Zeiner A, Holzer M, Sterz F, Schorkhuber W, Eisenburger P, Havel C, Kliegel A, Laggner AN. Hyperthermia after cardiac arrest is associated with an unfavorable neurological outcome. *Arch Intern Med* 2001;161(16):2007–2012.

35. Hypothermia after Cardiac Arrest Study Group. Mild therapeutic hypothermia to improve the neurological outcome after cardiac arrest. *N Engl J Med* 2002;346(8):549–556.

36. De Georgia MA, Krieger DW, Abou-Chebl A, Devlin TG, Jauss M, Davis SM, Koroshetz WJ, Rordorf G, Warach S. Cooling for acute ischemic brain damage (COOL AID): a feasibility trial of endovascular cooling. *Neurology* 2004;63(2):312–317.

37. Clardy CW, Edwards KM, Gay JC. Increased susceptibility to infection in hypothermic children: possible role of acquired neutrophils dysfunction. *Pediatr Infect Dis* 1985;4(4):379–382.

38. Tokutomi T, Mayagi T, Morimoto K, Karukaya T, Shigemori M. Effect of hypothermia on serum electrolyte, inflammation, coagulation, and nutritional parameters in patients with severe traumatic brain injury. *Neurocrit Care* 2004;1(2):171–182.

39. Solomon A, Barish RA, Browne B, Tso E. The electrocardiographic features of hypothermia. *J Emerg Med* 1989;7(2):169–173.

40. Hart MN, Heistad DD, Brody MJ. Effect of chronic hypertension and sympathetic denervation on wall/lumen ratio of cerebral vessels. *Hypertension* 1980;2(4):419–423.

41. Oliveira-Filho J, Silva SC, Trabuco CC, Pedreira BB, Sousa EU, Bacellar A. Detrimental effect of blood pressure reduction in the first 24 hours of acute stroke onset. *Neurology* 2003;61(8):1047–1051.

42. Rordorf G, Koroshetz WJ, Ezzeddine MA, Segal AZ, Buonanno FS. A pilot study of drug-induced hypertension for treatment of acute stroke. *Neurology* 2001;56(9):1210–1213.

43. Marzan AS, Hungerbuhler HJ, Studer A, Baumgartner RW, Georgiadis D. Feasibility and safety of norepinephrine-induced arterial hypertension in acute ischemic stroke. *Neurology* 2004;62(7):1193–1195.

44. Koenig MA, Geocadin RG, de Grouchy M, Glasgow J, Vimal S, Restrepo L, Wityk RJ. Safety of induced hypertension therapy in patients with acute ischemic stroke. *Neurocrit Care* 2006;4(1):3–7.

45. Kasner SE, Demchuk AM, Berrouschot J, Schmutzhard E, Harms L, Verro P, Chalela JA, Abbur R, McGrade H, Christou I, Krieger DW. Predictors of fatal brain edema in massive hemispheric ischemic stroke. *Stroke* 2001;32(9):2117–2123.

46. Maramattom BV, Bahn MM, Wijdicks EFM. Which patient fares worse after early deterioration due to swelling from hemispheric stroke? *Neurology* 2004;63(11):2142–2145.

47. Qureshi AI, Suarez JI, Yahia AM, Mohammad Y, Uzun G, Suri MF, Zaidat OO, Ayata C, Ali Z, Wityk RJ. Timing of neurological deterioration in massive middle cerebral artery infarction: a multicenter review. *Crit Care Med* 2003;31(1):272–277.

48. Cucciara BL, Kasner SE, Wolk DA, Lyden PD, Knappertz VA, Ashwood T, Odergren T, Nordlund A; CLASS-I Investigators. Early impairment in consciousness predicts mortality after hemispheric ischemic stroke. *Crit Care Med* 2004;32(1): 241–245.

49. Jaramillo A, Gongora-Rivera F, Labreuche J, Hauw JJ, Amarenco P. Predictors for malignant middle cerebral artery infarctions: a post-mortem analysis. *Neurology* 2006;66(6):815–820.

50. Barber PA, Demchuk AM, Zhang AM, Zhang J, Kasner SE, Hill MD, Berrouschot J, Schmutzhard E, Harms L, Verro P, Krieger D. Computed tomographic parameters predicting fatal outcome in large middle cerebral artery infarction. *Cerebrovasc Dis* 2003;16(3):230–235.

51. Thomas SH, Orf J, Wedel SK, Conn AK. Hyperventilation in traumatic brain injury patients: inconsistency between consensus guidelines and clinical practice. *J Trauma* 2002(1):52:47–52.

52. Frank JL. Large hemispheric infarction, deterioration, and intracranial pressure. *Neurology* 1995;45(7):1286–1290.

53. Nau R, Desel H, Lassek C, Thiel A, Schinschke S, Rossing R, Kolenda H, Prange HW. Slow elimination of mannitol from human cerebrospinal fluid. *Eur J Clin Pharmacol* 1997;53(3–4):271–274.

54. Hartman A, Dettmers C, Schott H, Beyenburg S. Cerebral blood flow and rheologic alterations by hyperosmolar therapy in patients with brain oedema. *Acta Neurochir Suppl (Wein)* 1990;51:168–169.

55. Cruz J, Minoja G, Okuchi K, Facco E. Successful use of the new high-dose mannitol treatment in patients with Glasgow Coma Scale scores of 3 and bilateral abnormal pupillary widening: a randomized trial. *J Neurosurg* 2004;100(3):376–383.

56. Garcia-Morales EJ, Cariappa R, Parvin CA. Osmole gap in neurosurgical-neurosurgical intensive care unit: its normal value, calculation, and relationship with mannitol serum concentrations. *Crit Care Med* 2004;32(4):986–991.

57. Schwarz S, Schwab S, Bertram M, Aschoff A, Hacke W. Effects of hypertonic saline hydroxyethyl starch solution and mannitol in patients with increased intracranial pressure after stroke. *Stroke* 1998;29(8):1550–1555.

58. Meyer JS, Teraura T, Marx P, Hashi K, Sakamoto K. Brain swelling due to experimental cerebral infarction: changes in vasomotor capacitance and effects of intravenous glycerol. *Brain* 1972;95(4):833–852.

59. Righetti E, Celani MG, Cantisani T, Sterzi R, Boysen G, Ricci S. Glycerol for acute stroke. *Cochrane Database Syst Rev* 2000;CD000096.

60. Berger C, Sakowitz OW, Kiening KL, Schwab S. Neurochemical monitoring of glycerol therapy in patients with ischemic brain edema. *Stroke* 2005;36:e4–e6.

61. Suarez JI, Qureshi AI, Bhardwaj A, Williams MA, Schnitzer MS, Mirski M, Hanley DF, Ulatowski JA. Treatment of refractory intracranial hypertension with 23.4% saline. *Crit Care Med* 1998;26(6):1118–1122.

62. Toung TJ, Hurn PD, Traystman RJ, Bhardwaj A. Global brain water increases after experimental focal cerebral ischemia: effect of hypertonic saline. *Crit Care Med* 2002;30(3):644–649.

63. Qureshi A, Suarez JI. Use of hypertonic saline solutions in treatment of cerebral edema and intracranial hypertension. *Crit Care Med* 2000;28(9):3301–3313.

64. Lee K, Melinosky C, Cacciola J, Bodock M, Guanci M, Rordorf G, Badjatia N. Hypertonic saline therapy for intracranial hypertension refractory to mannitol. *Neurology* 2005;64:S305.

65. Bhardwaj A, Harukuni I, Murphy SJ, et al. Hypertonic saline worsens infarct volume after transient focal ischemia in rats. *Stroke* 2000;31(7):1694–1701.
66. Nordstrom CH, Messeter K, Sundbarg G, Schalen W, Werner M, Ryding E. Cerebral blood flow, vasoreactivity, and oxygen consumption during barbiturate therapy in severe traumatic brain lesions. *J Neurosurg* 1988;68(3):424–431.
67. Smith DS, Rehncrona S, Siesjo BK. Barbiturates as protective agents in brain ischemia and as free radical scavengers *in vitro. Acta Physiol Scand Suppl* 1980;492: 129–134.
68. Kiening KL. Schneider GH, Unterberg AE, Lanksch WR. Effect of tromethamine (THAM) on infarct volume following permanent middle cerebral artery occlusion in rats. *Acta Neurochir* 1997;70:188–190.
69. Wolf AL, Levi L, Marmarou A, Ward JD, Muizelaar PJ, Choi S, Young H, Rigamonti D, Robinson WL. Effect of THAM upon outcome in severe head injury: a randomized prospective clinical trial. *J Neurosurg* 1993;78(1):54–59.
70. Qizilbash N. *Cochrane Database Syst Rev* 2000;CD 000064.
71. Olsen TS, Weber UJ, Kammersgaard LP. Therapeutic hypothermia for acute stroke. *Lancet Neurology* 2003;2(7):410–416.
72. Schwab S, Schwarz S, Spranger M, et al. Moderate hypothermia in the treatment of patients with severe middle cerebral artery infarction. *Stroke* 1998;29(12):2461–2466.
73. Steiner T, Friede T, Aschoff A, Schellinger PD, Schwab S, Hacke W. Effect and feasibility of controlled rewarming after moderate hypothermia in stroke patients with malignant infarction of the middle cerebral artery. *Stroke* 2001;32(12):2833–5.
74. Guluma KZ, Hemmen TM, Olsen SE, Rapp KS, Lyden PD. A trial of therapeutic hypothermia via endovascular approach in awake patients with acute ischemic stroke: methodology. *Acad Emerg Med* 2006;13(8):820–827.
75. Mayer SA, Kowalski RG, Presciutti M, Ostapkovich ND, McGann E, Fitzsimmons BF, Yavagal DR, Du YE, Naidech AM, Janjua NA, Claassen J, Kreiter KT, Parra A, Commichau C. Clinical trial of a novel surface cooling system for fever control in neurocritical care patients. *Crit Care Med* 2004;32(12): 2508–2515.
76. Wang H, Olivero W, Lanzino G, Elkins W, Rose J, Honings D, Rodde M, Burnham J, Wang D. Rapid and selective cerebral hypothermia achieved using a cooling helmet. *J Neurosurg* 2004;100(2):272–277.
77. Wagner KR, Zuccarello M. Local brain hypothermia for neuroprotection in stroke treatment and aneurysm repair. *Neurol Res* 2005;27(3):238–245.
78. Brown G. Acetaminophen-induced hypotension. *Heart Lung* 1996;25(2):137–140.
79. Doufas AG, Lin CM, Suleman MI, Liem EB, Lenhardt R, Morioka N, Akca O, Shah YM, Bjorksten AR, Sessler DI. Dexmedetomidine and meperidine additively reduce the shivering threshold in humans. *Stroke* 2003;34(5):1218–1223.
80. Jaeger M, Soehle M, Meixensberger J. Improvement of brain tissue oxygen and intracranial pressure during and after surgical decompression for diffuse brain oedema and space occupying infarction. *Acta Neurochir Suppl* 2005;95:117–118.
81. Wagner S, Schnippering H, Aschoff A, Koziol JA, Schwab S, Steiner T. Suboptimum hemicraniectomy as a cause of additional cerebral lesions in patients with malignant infarctions of the middle cerebral artery. *J Neurosurg* 2001;94(5):693–696.

82. Rieke K, Schwab S, Krieger D, von Kummer R, Aschoff A, Schuchardt V, Hacke W. Decompressive surgery in space-occupying hemispheric infarction: results of an open, prospective trial. *Crit Care Med* 1995;23(9):1576–1587.

83. Schwab S, Steiner T, Aschoff A, Schwarz S, Steiner HH, Jansen O, Hacke W. Early hemicraniectomy in patients with complete middle cerebral artery infarction. *Stroke* 1998;29(9):1888–1893.

84. Malm J, Bergenheim AT, Enblad P, Hardemark HG, Koskinen LO, Naredi S, Nordstrom CH, Norrving B, Uhlin J, Lindgren A. The Swedish Malignant Middle Cerebral Artery Infarction Study: long-term results from a prospective study of hemicraniectomy combined with standardized neurointensive care. *Acta Neurol Scand* 2006;113(1):25–30.

85. Rabinstein AA, Mueller-Kronast N, Maramattom BV, Zazulia AR, Bamlet WR, Diringer MN, Wijdicks EF. Factors predicting prognosis after decompressive hemicraniectomy for hemispheric infarction. *Neurology* 2006;67(5):891–893.

86. Gupta R, Connolly ES, Mayer S, Elkind MS. Hemicraniectomy for massive middle cerebral artery territory infarction: a systematic review. *Stroke* 2004;35(2):539–543.

87. Kastrau F, Wolder M, Huber W, Block F. Recovery from aphasia after hemicraniectomy for infarction of the speech-dominant hemisphere. *Stroke* 2005;36(4):825–829.

88. Foerch C, Lang JM, Krause J, Raabe A, Sitzer M, Seifert V, Steinmetz H, Kessler KR. Functional impairment, disability, and quality of life outcome after decompressive hemicraniectomy in malignant middle cerebral artery infarction. *J Neurosurg* 2004;101(2):248–254.

89. Curry WT Jr, Sethi MK, Ogilvy CS, Carter BS. Factors associated with outcome after hemicraniectomy for large middle cerebral artery territory infarction. *Neurosurgery* 2005;56(4):681–692.

90. Uhl E, Kreth FW, Elias B, Goldammer A, Hempelmann RG, Liefner M, Nowak G, Oertel M, Schmieder K, Schneider GH. Outcome and prognostic factors of hemicraniectomy for space occupying cerebral infarction. *J Neurol Neurosurg Psychiatry* 2004;75(2): 270–274.

91. Georgiadis D, Schwarz S, Aschoff A, Schwab S. Hemicraniectomy and moderate hypothermia in patients with severe ischemic stroke. *Stroke* 2002;33(6):1584–1588.

92. Els T, Oehm E, Voigt S, Klisch J, Hetzel A, Kassubek J. Safety and therapeutical benefit of hemicraniectomy combined with mild hypothermia in comparison with hemicraniectomy alone in patients with malignant ischemic stroke. *Cerebrovasc Dis* 2006;21(1–2): 79–85.

93. Hofmeijer J, Amelink GJ, Algra A, van Gijn J, Macleod MR, Kappelle LJ, van der Worp HB; the HAMLET Investigators. Hemicraniectomy after middle cerebral artery infarction with life-threatening edema trial (HAMLET). Protocol for a randomised controlled trial of decompressive surgery in space-occupying hemispheric infarction. *Trials* 2006;7:29.

94. Auer LM, Auer T, Sayama I. Indications for surgical treatment of cerebellar hemorrhage and infarction. *Acta Neurochir (Wein)* 1986;79:74–79.

95. Kirollos RW, Tyagi AK, Ross SA, van Hille PT, Marks PV. Management of spontaneous cerebellar hematomas a prospective treatment protocol. *Neurosurgery* 2001;49(6):1378–1387.

96. Koh MG, Phan TG, Atkinson JL, Wijdicks EFM. Neuroimaging in deteriorating patients with cerebellar infarcts and mass effect. *Stroke* 2000;31(9):2062–2067.

97. Saatci I, Baskan O, Cekirge HS, Besim A. Comparison of MR sequences in early cerebral infarction at 0.5 T. *Acta Radiol* 2000;41(6):553–558.

98. Taneda M, Hayakawa T, Mogami H. Primary cerebellar hemorrhage: quadrigeminal cistern obliteration on CT scans as a predictor of outcome. *J Neurosurg* 1987;67(4):545–552.

99. Raco A, Caroli E, Isidori A, Salvati M. Management of acute cerebellar infarction: one institution's experience. *Neurosurgery* 2003;53(5):1061–1065.

100. Jauss M, Krieger D, Hornig C, Schramm J, Busse O. Surgical and medical management of patients with massive cerebellar infarction: results of the German-Austrian Cerebellar Infarction Study. *J Neurol* 1999;246(4):257–264.

101. Baldauf J, Oertel J, Gaab MR, Schroeder HW. Endoscopic third ventriculostomy for occlusive hydrocephalus caused by cerebellar infarction. *Neurosurgery* 2006;59(3):539–544.

102. Schwab S, Aschoff A, Spranger M, Albert F, Hacke W. The value of intracranial pressure monitoring in acute hemispheric stroke. *Neurology* 1996;47(2):393–398.

103. Chan K-H, Miller JD, Dearden NM, Andrews PJ, Midgley S. The effect of changes in cerebral perfusion pressure upon middle cerebral artery blood flow velocity and jugular bulb venous oxygen saturation after severe brain injury. *J Neurosurg* 1992;77(1):55–61.

104. Lyons MK, Meyer FB. Cerebrospinal fluid physiology and the management of increased intracranial pressure. *Mayo Clinic Proc* 1990;65(5):684–707.

105. Lang EW. Chestnut RM. Intracranial pressure monitoring and management. *Neurosurg Clin North Am* 1994;5:573–605.

106. Mayhall CG, Archer NH, Lamb VA, Spadora AC, Baggett JW, Ward JD, Narayan RK. Ventriculostomy-related infections: a prospective epidemiologic study. *N Engl J Med* 1984;310(9):553–559.

107. Khanna RK, Rosenblum ML, Rock JP, Malik GM. Prolonged external ventricular drainage with percutaneous long-tunnel ventriculostomies. *J Neurosurg* 1995;83(5):791–794.

108. Wyler AR, Kelly WA. Use of antibiotics with external ventriculostomies. *J Neurosurg* 1972;37(2):185–187.

109. Crutchfield JS, Narayan RK, Robertson CS, Michael LH. Evaluation of a fiberoptic intracranial pressure monitor. *J Neurosurg* 1990;72(3):482–487.

110. Vries JK, Becker DP, Young HF. A subarachnoid screw for monitoring intracranial pressure: technical note. *J Neurosurg* 1973;39(3):416–419.

111. Johnston AJ, Gupta AK. Advanced monitoring in the neurology intensive care unit: microdialysis. *Curr Opin Crit Care* 2002;8(2):121–127.

112. Lesser RP, Lüders DH, Dinner DS, Morris HH. Epileptic seizures due to thrombotic and embolic cerebrovascular disease in older patients. *Epilepsia* 1985;26(6):622–630.

113. De Reuck J, Goethals M. Claeys I, Van Maele G, De Clerck M, EEG findings after a cerebral territorial infarct in patients who develop early- and late-onset seizures. *Eur Neurol* 2006;55(4):209–213.

114. Jordan KG. Emergency EEG and continuous EEG monitoring in acute ischemic stroke. *J Clin Neurophysiol* 2004;21(5):341–352.

115. Oppenheimer SM, Gelb A, Girvin JP, Hachinski VC. Cardiovascular effects of human insular cortex stimulation. *Neurology* 1992;42(9):1727–1732.

116. Locatelli ER, Varghese JP, Shuaib A, Potolicchio SJ. Cardiac asystole and bradycardia as a manifestation of left temporal lobe complex partial seizure. *Ann Intern Med* 1999;130(7):581–583.

117. Rocamora R, Kurthen M, Lickfett L, Von Oertzen J, Elger CE. Cardiac asystole in epilepsy: clinical and neurophysiologic features. *Epilepsia* 2003;44(2):179–185.

118. Colivicci F, Bassi A, Santini M, Caltagirone C. Cardiac autonomic derangement and arrhythmias in right-sided stroke with insular involvement. *Stroke* 2004;35(9):2094–2098.

119. Meyer S, Strittmatter M, Fischer C, Georg T, Schmitz B. Lateralization in autonomic dysfunction in ischemic stroke involving the insular cortex. *Neuroreport* 2004;15(2):357–361.

120. Strittmatter M, Meyer S, Fischer C, Georg T, Schmitz B, Location-dependent patterns in cardio-autonomic dysfunction in ischemic stroke. *Eur Neurol* 2003;50(1):30–38.

121. Ay H, Koroshetz WJ, Benner T, Vangel MG, Melinosky C, Arsava EM, Ayata C, Zhu M, Schwamm LH, Sorensen AG. Neuroanatomic correlates of stroke-related myocardial injury. *Neurology* 2006;66(9):1325–1329.

122. Orlandi G, Fanucchi S, Strata G, Pataleo L, Landucci Pellegrini L, Prontera C, Martini A, Murri L. Transient autonomic nervous system dysfunction during hyperacute stroke. *Acta Neurol Scand* 2000;102(5):317–321.

123. Sander D, Klingelhofer J. Extent of autonomic activation following cerebral ischemia is different in hypertensive and normotensive humans. *Arch Neurol* 1996;53(9):890–894.

124. Vahedi K, Hofmeijer J, Juettler E, Vicaut E, George B, Algra A, Amelink GJ, Schmiedeck P, Schwab S, Rothwell PM, Bousser M-G, van der Worp HB, Hacke W, for the DECIMAL, DESTINY, and HAMLET Investigators. Early decompressive surgery in malignant infarction of the middle cerebral artery: a pooled analysis of three randomised controlled trials. *Lancet Neurol* 2007;6:215–222.

9

EVALUATION OF ACUTE STROKE ETIOLOGIES

Karen L. Furie, Michael H. Lev, Walter J. Koroshetz, and David M. Greer

INTRODUCTION

Early identification of stroke etiology can improve outcome prediction and help define the approach to subacute management. High-risk conditions, such as atrial fibrillation (AF), acute myocardial infarction, and high-grade carotid stenosis can impact recurrent stroke rates and long-term outcome. Diagnostic imaging and cardiac monitoring can be used to identify the stroke etiology in a large proportion of cases. Early evaluation of stroke mechanisms may help reduce the length of hospitalization, reducing cost and improving outcome.

Although much of the focus of acute stroke management is on early initiation of reperfusion strategies, establishing the pathophysiology of the infarction in the emergency setting may have important implications for the acute and subacute phases of care. The implications for identifying an intracranial large artery occlusion with regard to acute neurointerventional approaches are discussed in Chapter 4. Identification of high-grade symptomatic extracranial carotid stenosis, AF, or other high-risk sources may affect acute management and help predict outcome. Accurate subtyping by stroke mechanism at the time of presentation could guide initial decisions regarding the diagnostic evaluation and treatment, and help with early prognostication.

Acute Ischemic Stroke: An Evidence-based Approach, Edited by David M. Greer.

STROKE SUBTYPES

Ischemic stroke is a heterogeneous disease. A symptom, such as slurred speech, could herald occlusion of the carotid artery with potentially devastating consequences, or the occlusion of a small penetrator vessel only 100 μm in diameter. Cardioembolic strokes can be life threatening if the embolus occludes a major intracranial vessel, or trivial if the embolus is tiny and passes to a small distal branch. Pathologically, ischemic strokes can be classified into subtypes based on the mechanism of infarction. Clinically, the subtype of stroke is derived through analysis of the clinical stroke syndrome, the infarct localization on neuroimaging, and the results of diagnostic studies, such as carotid ultrasound or cardiac echocardiography, which identify the cause of the vascular occlusion.

The most commonly used stroke subtyping scheme, the Trial of Org 10172 in Acute Stroke Treatment (TOAST) classification, separates stroke into five categories: large vessel atherothrombotic, cardioembolic, small vessel/lacunar, undetermined, and "other."[1] More recently, efforts have been made to update and standardize the methodology of subtyping.[2] Advances in diagnostic imaging have facilitated improved discrimination of stroke etiology, even in the setting of multiple competing mechanisms within a single patient. An evidence-based classification algorithm (SSS-TOAST) harmonizes elements of the diagnostic stroke evaluation with the aim of identifying the most likely mechanism in the presence of multiple potential causes (Table 9.1).

TABLE 9.1 Pathophysiologic Mechanisms of Ischemic Stroke.

- Large artery
- Cardioembolic
- Lacunar (small vessel)
- Undetermined
  - Cryptogenic
  - More than one mechanism
  - Incomplete evaluation
- Other

STROKE OUTCOME

The severity of the neurological deficit at the time of stroke onset is a major predictor of stroke outcome. In an analysis of the placebo-treated patients in the National Institute of Neurological Disorders and Stroke (NINDS) recombinant tissue-plasminogen activator (rt-PA) study, the best acute predictor of a poor outcome at 1 year was an National Institute of Health Stroke Scale (NIHSS) score >17 for patients over 70 years. These criteria had a high specificity (98%), but sensitivity was only 31%.[3] The low sensitivity of the acute NIHSS score alone in predicting this "worst-case scenario" indicates the need for additional means to improve prognostication in the acute setting.

Later in the clinical course of stroke, the severity of the neurological deficit is more predictive. In the TOAST study, an NIHSS score measured within 24 hours of onset and the subtype of stroke determined the probability of excellent outcome.[1] Still there was variability, especially in those patients with moderately severe deficits. The group of patients with NIHSS scores between 11 and 15 were almost equally divided among those who had excellent, good, or poor outcomes. Of those with the worst NIHSS scores (>23), 20% had good or excellent outcomes at 3 months. Of those with the best NIHSS scores (<3), 3% had poor outcome or were dead. Others have reported similarly good correlation with 3-month outcomes when the NIHSS was assessed at later times (up to 72 hours from onset of stroke).[4] Currently, no study has prospectively studied physician accuracy in predicting patient outcome in the emergency setting. Despite this, the clinician's intuitive prediction of a patient's ultimate degree of disability probably plays a major role in counseling patients and families, and deciding on an appropriate therapy.

Stroke Subtype Predicts Outcome

Patients with large vessel atherothrombotic stroke have been reported to have worse short- and long-term survival as compared to other subtypes of stroke.[5–11] In a population-based study from Rochester Minnesota, only 24% of patients classified as atherothrombotic were independent during the period of worst deficit and 50% were independent at 1 year.[9] Large vessel atherothrombotic stroke patients also have the highest rate of recurrent stroke.[6,10,11]

Cardioembolic strokes may also have poor outcome, especially with large emboli as in AF.[12,13] In the Rochester population, patients with cardioembolic stroke were the most impaired during the hospitalization: only 14% were independent as compared to 38% with lacunar stroke, 24% with atherosclerotic stroke, and 27% with ischemic stroke of unknown cause.[14] The latter group probably included patients with emboli of unknown origin. As evidence of the proportion of patients with devastating strokes, patients classified as cardioembolic subtype were also least likely to be independent at 1 year (27%).

Small vessel/lacunar strokes have better short- and long-term (1-year) survival as compared to other stroke subtypes.[5–11] In the NINDS trial of rt-PA within 3 hours of onset, patients classified as small vessel stroke on the basis of their clinical syndrome had a 50% chance of a normal NIHSS score at 3 months if they received placebo, increasing to 70% in the treatment group.[15] In the Lausanne cohort, 95% were independent after their first event, as opposed to only 65% of the cardioembolic strokes and 49% with large vessel atherothrombotic infarctions.[16] Eighty-two percent of patients with small vessel stroke were independent at 1 year.[6] Even at the time of maximal deficit, between 38% and 64% of small vessel/lacunar patients were independent, with motor impairment and extent of white matter disease adversely affecting outcomes.[14,17] In TOAST, small vessel/lacunar stroke was the only subtype associated with a favorable outcome, independent of the NIHSS score.[18]

The rate of recurrent clinical stroke is also associated with the stroke subtype, and is lowest in small vessel/lacunar strokes.[6,10,11] Recurrent stroke within 30 days occurred in 4.4% of small vessel/lacunar strokes, compared to 12.5% cardioembolic and 16% atherothrombotic in a Polish population.[19] In the Rochester population-based study, recurrent stroke risk within 7 days was 1.4% for lacunar stroke, 2.4% for cardioembolic stroke, and 8.5% for atherothrombotic stroke. At 30 days, recurrence rates were 1.4% in lacunar, 5.3% in cardioembolic, and 18.5% in atherothrombotic subtypes.[14] Long-term (5-year) recurrence rates are also highest in large vessel atherothrombotic stroke patients.[14,16] Five-year recurrence rates were intermediate (31.7%) in cardioembolic subtypes and lowest (24.8%) in patients with lacunar stroke. Long-term survival was affected by age and the severity of neurological status at the time of the stroke.[8,19] Furthermore, patients with stroke have high mortality rates. In the Rochester study, 5-year mortality reached 80% in the cardioembolic, 32% in the atherothrombotic, and 35% in the lacunar groups.[14]

Neuroimaging, Stroke Subtype, and Outcome

Radiological assessment of ischemic stroke provides an indication of outcome, as the imaging defines the extent and location of permanent brain injury and provides clues as to the stroke subtype. The current recommendation for imaging the patient with an acute stroke-like deficit is a noncontrast computed tomography (CT) scan to be performed within 30 minutes of arrival at an emergency ward.[20] However, standard CT and magnetic resonance imaging (MRI) brain imaging techniques show infarcted regions hours to days after symptom onset. In contrast, recent work has demonstrated that advanced MRI techniques can predict final stroke size in the acute setting.[21] The power of diffusion- and perfusion-weighted MRI techniques in detecting early ischemic injury has raised the question of whether acute diffusion/perfusion MRI should replace CT as the standard imaging technique for emergency stroke evaluation (Table 9.2).[22–26]

Since functional outcome and risk of recurrent stroke are, in part, predictable based on the pathophysiologic subtype of stroke, the ability to accurately classify patients based on emergency clinical and imaging data would provide valuable predictive information. Unfortunately, misclassifications of stroke subtypes based on clinical data and a noncontrast CT scan are common. The final subtyping of stroke is made with all available clinical data, but is heavily influenced by neuroimaging studies that identify the location, size, and vascular distribution of the infarct, or that establish that the arteries supplying the region of stroke are stenotic or occluded.

Using clinical and emergency CT findings, the TOAST investigators found that their initial designation of subtype of stroke matched the final diagnosis in only 62% of patients. No subtype of stroke was more accurately diagnosed than another by initial assessment.[27] In a series of 100 consecutive stroke patients, the accuracy of the initial classification was reported as 70%.[28]

It may be especially difficult to confidently establish the diagnosis of the most benign subtype of stroke, small vessel/lacunar stroke, accounting for 10–29% of all

TABLE 9.2 Recommended Routine Stroke Evaluation.

- I. All Stroke
  - A. Brain imaging with CT or MRI
  - B. Cerebrovascular imaging (using one of the following modalities)
    - CT based: CTA head and neck
    - MR based: MRA head and neck
    - Ultrasound: Carotid non-invasive studies and transcranial Doppler
  - C. ECG and cardiac enzymes
  - D. Risk factor assessment
    - Hypertension
    - Lipids
    - Diabetes
    - Homocysteine (optional)
    - Tobacco and alcohol use
    - Diet and physical activity
    - Toxicology screen
- II. Suspected embolic stroke with patent large arteries
  - A. Transthoracic echocardiography (TTE) with agitated saline contrast
  - B. Cardiac monitor (Holter or ambulatory ECG)
  - C. Transesophageal echocardiogram (optional)

strokes.[1,9,29–34] Overall, the clinical symptoms/signs of a small vessel/lacunar stroke (pure motor hemiparesis, pure sensory stroke, ataxic hemiparesis, sensorimotor stroke, dysarthria/clumsy hand syndrome) have an accuracy of 88%.[34] Toni et al.[35] reported that the clinical findings alone had a positive predictive value (PPV) of 58% for pure motor hemiparesis and 51% for sensorimotor stroke using CT or autopsy as the gold standard. The fallibility is greatest for pure motor strokes.[34] Lack of clinical certainty, coupled with the potential severe consequences of error, leads to unnecessary diagnostic testing and suboptimal treatment. In the Northern Manhattan Stroke Study, 225 patients with stroke symptoms consistent with a small vessel/lacunar syndrome underwent neuroimaging to determine the accuracy of the clinical subtyping. The clinical symptoms/signs had a PPV of 87% for detecting a radiological small vessel/lacunar stroke, highest for pure sensory strokes (100%), and lowest for pure motor hemiparesis (79%). The sensitivity was 71% and specificity 90%. Of the 195 patients in whom the clinical and radiographic evidence supported a small vessel/lacunar mechanism, 25% were ultimately attributed to other mechanisms (i.e., cardioembolic 5%, atherothrombotic 9%, cryptogenic 9%) after the full evaluation (duplex ultrasound, Holter monitor, echocardiogram, etc.) was completed. Conversely, 6% of 336 patients believed to have had a nonsmall vessel/lacunar stroke based on clinical findings were ultimately attributed to a small vessel/lacunar mechanism.[36]

The utility of computed tomography angiography (CTA) in the setting of acute stroke has not been thoroughly explored, but it is an extremely attractive means of identifying large- or medium-sized vessel stenoses or occlusions, which underlie many strokes. One review described a prospective study of 21 patients with acute nonhemorrhagic stroke imaged with both CTA and digital subtraction angiography (DSA). Two raters correctly assessed all trunk occlusions of the basilar artery, internal carotid artery (ICA), and middle cerebral artery (MCA), although assessment of more distal MCA branch occlusions was less reliable. Additionally, there was an 88% agreement rate in judging the degree of collateral vessels and 62% accurate prediction of hemispheric infarct size.[37] In a different study of 145 patients with symptoms of acute stroke, arterial stenoses or occlusions were found to be present on 43% of CTA. For 27 cases in which both CTA and magnetic resonance angiography (MRA) were obtained, findings were in agreement for 98% of the vessels; agreement was 99% for the 28 cases in which both CTA and DSA were acquired.[38] Therefore, current data attest to the accuracy of CTA in detecting lesions in large intracranial vessels.

Because the severity of the vascular lesion contributes to the size of the infarction and thus the clinical outcome, CTA results may be expected to predict outcome. One study assessed the utility of CTA in 40 patients with acute stroke syndromes and an NIHSS score of $\geq$8. The extent of leptomeningeal collaterals on CTA correlated with the outcome from thrombolysis.[39] In 40 hyperacute stroke patients who received rt-PA, those with CTA evidence of poor collaterals, autolysed thrombi, and "T" lesions showed little benefit from treatment.[39]

A growing body of data has shown the ability of advanced MR techniques to aid in predicting stroke subtype and functional outcome. In a recent study, classification of stroke subtype using the TOAST criteria within 24 hours of stroke onset was accurate in only 48% of patients. The addition of MR angiography improved accuracy to 56%; performing diffusion-weighted imaging (DWI) increased correct classification to 94%.[40] In those patients with a final diagnosis of large vessel/atherosclerotic stroke, the pre-MRI diagnosis matched the final diagnosis in 56% before the MRA exam was evaluated, improving to 89% after the MRA. An extremely low accuracy of clinically classifying patients with small vessel stroke (35%) was reported. However, the initial diagnosis matched the final diagnosis in 100% of cases after DWI/MRA. The pre-MRI Oxfordshire classification matched the final diagnosis in only 67%, increasing to 100% after the DWI/MRA. Stroke outcome at 30 days has also been seen to correlate with the volume of the DWI abnormality on scans taken within 24 hours of stroke onset.[41]

These advances in MR imaging of acute stroke have fueled the debate over whether MRI should replace CT as the primary imaging modality in the evaluation of the acute stroke patient. However, MR scanners are extremely costly to build and operate and are not available in most emergency rooms, especially on a 24-hour basis. In addition, there are more contraindications to MR scanning (e.g., pacemaker, cochlear implants, aneurysm clips, claustrophobia, inability to remain still). Medically unstable patients may not be able to enter the magnet safely because many monitoring and treatment devices cannot be brought into the room. Furthermore, it has not been demonstrated that the superior resolution for detecting small strokes meaningfully alters stroke management or outcome.

Implications for Subacute Management Based on Etiology

Cardioembolism Cardioembolism accounts for approximately 30% of all stroke and 25–30% of strokes in the young (age <45 years).[42] [1] AF accounts for a large proportion of these strokes (15–25%). Symptoms may be suggestive, but they are not diagnostic. Repetitive, stereotyped, transient ischemic attacks (TIAs) are unusual in embolic stroke. The classic presentation for cardioembolism is the sudden onset of maximal symptoms. The size of the embolic material determines, in part, the course of the embolic material. Small emboli can cause retinal ischemic or lacunar symptoms. Posterior cerebral artery territory infarcts, in particular, are often due to cardiac embolism. This predilection is not completely consistent across the various cardiac structural abnormalities that predispose to stroke, and may be due to patterns of blood flow associated with specific cardiac pathologies.

An ischemic stroke is considered cardioembolic if the clinical and neuroimaging findings support this diagnosis and a cardiac source of embolism is identified. Other stroke subtypes should be excluded before assigning a cardioembolic etiology by ensuring that there is not a ≥50% stenosis or occlusion of a large artery supplying the ischemic territory, a clinical and radiographic syndrome consistent with a small vessel (lacunar) stroke, an established diagnosis of vasculitis or other unusual cause of stroke, or a >4 mm atheroma of the aortic arch.

Neuroimaging data can support a diagnosis of cardioembolism. Multifocal infarctions that involve more than one vascular territory favor a proximal source of embolism. Recurrent ischemic events in a single vascular territory in the absence of a proximal large artery stenosis may also be due to cardioembolism. Embolic-appearing infarcts on neuroimaging may be clinically "silent."

It is extremely important to exclude infective endocarditis as a cause for cardioembolism. Stroke occurs in 15–20% of infective endocarditis, usually within the first 48 hours. Appropriate antibiotic therapy dramatically reduces the risk of recurrent stroke. Late embolism occurs in less than 5% of cases.[43] An elevated erythrocyte sedimentation rate in the setting of cerebral ischemic symptoms, fever or a new murmur should trigger a diagnostic evaluation, including blood cultures, a transthoracic echocardiogram, and if a high level of suspicion remains, a transesophageal echocardiogram. The most common organisms causing native valve endocarditis are streptococci, staphylococci, and enterococci, although other species of bacteria, fungi, spirochetes, and rickettsiae can infect valves. The risk of subarachnoid hemorrhage from mycotic aneurysms represents a contraindication to the use of anticoagulation in infectious endocarditis.

Event-loop recording and 24–48 hours Holter monitoring are more sensitive than a standard 12-lead ECG for detecting AF in stroke patients. In one study of 465 consecutive patients admitted with a diagnosis of new ischemic stroke, 210 underwent Holter monitoring. The mean duration of monitoring was 22.8 ± 4.0 hours. Previously undiscovered AF was identified in five cases (2.4%), all of which represented nonrheumatic AF. In three cases, the Holter test was negative despite AF documented on an admission electrocardiogram. Thus, the standard 24-hour duration of monitoring probably underestimates the prevalence of paroxysmal AF in this population.[44] Studies from Switzerland have reported similarly low rates of PAF in stroke patients on Holter monitoring (2.7–5%) and slightly higher rates of detection using an ambulatory 7-day monitor (5.7%).[45,46]

Many patients have a rhythm that varies between atrial flutter and AF. Atrial flutter is associated with a 40% higher risk of stroke. Given that the concordance of the AF and atrial flutter is high, anticoagulation should be considered in patients with atrial flutter and coexisting cardiac pathology predisposing to left atrial thrombus.

Transesophageal echocardiography (TEE) has greater sensitivity for detecting abnormalities in the left atrium such as spontaneous echo contrast, left atrial thrombus, reduced left atrial appendage velocity, and complex aortic arch atheroma, which are markers of increased stroke risk. In a study of 227 patients with acute cerebral ischemia and an "undetermined" etiology after TTE and vascular imaging, 8% had a high-risk source requiring anticoagulation identified on TEE. An additional 22% had a possible cardioembolic source (e.g., patent foramen ovale, atrial septal aneurysm, aortic plaque <4 mm identified on TEE).[47] Another similar study found that in 231 patients with ischemic stroke or TIA of unknown mechanism, TTE identified a high-risk source in 16%, but TEE identified a source in an additional 39%, and roughly a third were subsequently anticoagulated for the condition, although warfarin was not proven to be superior to antiplatelet therapy for many of the diagnoses.[48] Left atrial thrombus was the most common abnormality requiring anticoagulation, detected in 16% of TEE subjects. The increased utility of TEE was seen in both young (age <45) and older patients (Table 9.3).

Five randomized primary and secondary prevention trials[49,50] have demonstrated the efficacy and safety of warfarin in preventing AF-related stroke. Pooled data from these trials demonstrated a 68% reduction in ischemic stroke (95% CI 50–79) and an intracerebral hemorrhage rate of <1% per year. The data for aspirin suggested that it had a lesser effect, with a 36% risk reduction (95% CI 4–57).

It is important to obtain a baseline EKG and cardiac enzymes to evaluate the possibility of an acute myocardial infarction. The short-term (2–4 weeks) stroke risk after acute myocardial infarction (AMI) is 2.5%.[51] Stroke is usually an early (within 14 days) complication of AMI and is more common in anterior wall (4–12%) than in inferior wall infarction (1%).[51–53] Approximately 40% of patients with an anterior wall myocardial infarction develop left ventricular thrombus,

TABLE 9.3 Additional Diagnostic Evaluations for Stroke in the Young or Other Unusual Circumstances.

I. TTE with agitated saline

II. Blood cultures and tranesophageal echocardiography (if SBE suspected), ESR

III. Additional hypercoagulable studies

Protein C, protein S, antithrombin III, activated protein C resistance, lipoprotein(a) anticardiolipin antibodies, lupus anticoagulant, prothrombin gene mutation 20210a

IV. Lumbar puncture

V. Conventional angiography (optional)

usually in the first 2 weeks. Patients with low ejection fraction after AMI have a cumulative 5-year stroke risk of 8.1%.

Carotid Stenosis

Carotid artery disease is one of the major causes of ischemic stroke.[1,2] The predominant mechanisms by which it causes stroke are (a) arterial embolism from atherosclerotic plaques; (b) hemodynamic changes, leading to "watershed" infarcts; and (c) distal propagation of thrombus originating from acute carotid occlusion.[3]

The degree of carotid stenosis is a major predictor of subsequent stroke. In the North American Symptomatic Carotid Endarterectomy Trial (NASCET) and in the European Carotid Surgery Trial (ECST), patients with >69% stenosis of a symptomatic carotid had a significant reduction in stroke risk with carotid endarterectomy, provided the surgical risk was less than 3%.[54,55] However, in patients with moderate carotid stenosis, the benefit of surgical treatment is less clear. The NASCET investigators subsequently demonstrated a small but significant reduction in the 5-year rate of ipsilateral stroke in symptomatic patients with 50–69% carotid stenosis when treated with endarterectomy, as compared to patients treated medically; and a nonsignificant reduction in symptomatic patients with <50% carotid stenosis when treated surgically, again compared to patients that received medical therapy.[56]

The noninvasive studies commonly performed to directly image the extracranial carotid disease include:

- Carotid duplex ultrasound (CDUS)
- MRA
- CTA

CTA and MRA are described in more detail in Chapter 2; therefore, this section will focus on CDUS. CDUS is widely available, well-validated, and is free of the risks and complications of radiographic contrast administration. Using ROC analysis, velocity criteria for detecting a residual lumen diameter of <1.5 mm have been developed based on pathological correlation with CEA plaques.[57] In addition, transcranial Doppler can play an adjunctive role in defining the hemodynamic significance of a lesion.[58]

When MRA, CTA, and CDUS were compared in 67 patients, there was good agreement with angiography to predict "surgical" disease.[59] *In vivo* determination of plaque correlates slightly better with ultrasound ($r = 0.8$) than MRA ($r = 0.76$).[60] In the CARMEDAS multicenter study, the concordance rates among ultrasound, contrast-enhanced MRA (89%), ultrasound/CTA (83%), and CTA/MRA (89%) for diagnosing a >50% stenosis were not significantly different.[61] Although this study identified a subgroup of asymptomatic surgical patients in whom ultrasound was more concordant than CTA, the absence of a biological rationale for this suggests that it is a type I error.

Johnston and Goldstein[62] found that compared to DSA, there was a misclassification rate of 7.9% for combined US and time-of-flight (TOF) MRA compared to either alone (CDUS 28%, TOF MRA 18%). They repeated this study with contrast-enhanced MRA (CEMRA) and found that 24% of patients would be misclassified as a surgical candidate with CEMRA and 36% with CDUS as compared to 17% for both CEMRA and CDUS.[63] Other studies have also shown that concordant results between contrast-enhanced MRA and duplex ultrasonography have a high sensitivity (100%) and specificity (81.4%) compared with DSA.[64]

For detecting >70% stenosis, the sensitivity and specificity for MRA alone have been reported as 92.2% (86.2–92.2%) and 75.7% (68.6–82.5%), and for CDUS, 87.5% (82.1–92.9%) and 75.7% (69.3–82.2%), respectively. Combined, they are 96.3% (90.8–99%) and 80.2% (73.1–87.3%).[65] In a later study by the same group comparing CDUS and CEMRA, the sensitivity/specificity were 86% (84–89%)/87% (84–90%) and 95% (92–97%)/90% (86–93%), respectively.[66] In another study, CEMRA had a sensitivity of 94.9% and specificity of 79.1% for identifying a stenosis of 70% or greater.[63] Below 50%, ultrasound is inaccurate in assessing the degree of stenosis.[67]

In the past, conventional ultrasound detected only 27% of pseudo-occlusions, whereas the addition of color flow Doppler increased detection to 94%. The accuracy of color-coded duplex sonography (CCDS) was tested in 401 consecutive patients with CCDS followed by ICA angiography. The sensitivity of CCDS was 88% with a specificity of 99% in preocclusive lesions, as compared to sensitivity of 87% and specificity of 99% for complete occlusions. Of note, in this study, carotid endarterectomies were performed in two of three angiographically occluded vessels deemed to be patent with CCDS. At surgery, they had residual flow confirming the CCDS findings.[68] For detecting occlusion, the sensitivity of CEMRA and CDUS have been reported as 98% (94–100%) versus 100% (99–100%), and a specificity of 96% (94–98%) versus 100% (99–100%), respectively.[66]

There are limitations to ultrasound, however. A high-grade stenosis of the contralateral carotid artery can falsely elevate velocities and overestimate the degree of stenosis.[69] For discriminating between a high-grade stenosis and a total occlusion, ultrasound is imperfect. Calcification is a limiting factor in duplex imaging. Roughly 9–12% of symptomatic patients have >1 cm of calcification that impairs color flow imaging.[70–72] Carotid bifurcations above the mandible, tortuous vessels, and echolucent plaques also pose diagnostic imaging challenges using ultrasound. CDUS is most informative when combined with imaging of the intracranial circulation in order to exclude tandem lesions and identify potentially dangerous intracranial pathology (e.g., cerebral aneurysms) prior to reperfusion interventions. This can be accomplished with ultrasound (transcranial Doppler) or by combining CDUS with computed tomographic or magnetic resonance imaging of the brain and intracranial vessels.

In patients who have not had a large infarction, or who have suffered a TIA, CEA should be undertaken preferably early (within 3–30 days poststroke/TIA) rather than 6–8 weeks after the ictus.[73,74] Patients with non-significant carotid stenosis are not stroke-risk free. Although the risk of having a stroke with <50% stenosis is small, the attributable risk of stroke is high, since the prevalence of low-grade carotid stenosis is elevated in the general population.[75]

Antiplatelet agents have been the mainstay of medical management for secondary prevention of strokes in patients with symptomatic carotid disease. Antiplatelets can reduce the risk of stroke by 11–15%.[76] The combination of antiplatelets, however, increases the risk of major bleeding. In a recent study (Clopidogrel and Aspirin Regimen for the Reduction of Emboli in the Symptomatic Carotid Stenosis (CARESS) Trial), patients with symptomatic carotid disease and microembolic signals (MES) on TCD were randomized to clopidogrel plus aspirin or aspirin monotherapy. Intention-to-treat analysis revealed a significant reduction in MES: 43.8% of dual-therapy patients had MES at day 7, as compared with 72.7% of monotherapy patients (relative risk reduction 39.8%, 95% CI 13.8–58.0, $p = 0.0046$). The risk of ischemic stroke or TIA within the first week postrandomization was also higher in the monotherapy group.[77]

The potential anti-inflammatory role of statins has also been studied. Statins have been shown to reduce stroke risk, due to its effect on multiple predisposing factors.[78] Patients with symptomatic carotid stenosis treated with pravastatin for 3 months prior to carotid endarterectomy had fewer macrophages ($15 \pm 10\%$ vs. $25.3 \pm 12.5\%$), less lipid ($8.2 \pm 8.4\%$ vs. $23.9 \pm 21.1\%$), less oxidized LDL immunoreactivity, greater TIMP-1 immunoreactivity, and higher collagen content than those treated with placebo. ICAM-1, VCAM-1, MMP-1, MMP-9, TIMP-2 immunoreactivity, and nuclear factor-kappa B (NF-κB) immunoreactivity were not significantly different in the two groups.[79] Similarly, 18 patients with asymptomatic aortic and/or carotid plaques and hypercholesterolemia were treated with simvastatin with demonstrable reduction in wall thickness and wall area, but not lumen area, on *in vivo* black-blood MRI scans after 12 months of therapy. There were no changes observable after 6 months of therapy.[80]

CONCLUSION

Individuals presenting with symptoms of cerebrovascular ischemia are at high risk for recurrence. Early diagnostic evaluation is essential to identify high-risk conditions, such as high-grade stenosis of a large artery, acute myocardial infarction, subacute bacterial endocarditis, and AF, which can guide therapeutic decisions and help establish prognosis.

REFERENCES

1. Adams HP Jr, Bendixen BH, Kappelle LJ, Biller J, Love BB, Gordon DL, Marsh EE 3rd. Classification of subtype of acute ischemic stroke. Definitions for use in a multicenter clinical trial. *Stroke* 1993;24:35–41.
2. Ay H, Furie KL, Singhal A, Smith WS, Sorensen AG, Koroshetz WJ. An evidence-based causative classification system for acute ischemic stroke. *Ann Neurol* 2005;58:688–697.
3. Frankel MR, Morgenstern LB, Kwiatkowski T, Lu M, Tilley BC, Broderick JP, Libman R, Levine SR, Brott T. Predicting poor prognosis after acute ischemic stroke: an analysis of the placebo group from the NINDS rt-PA stroke trial. *Neurology* 2000;54:A89.

4. Muir KW, Weir CJ, Murray GD, Povey C, Lees KR. Comparison of neurological scales and scoring systems for acute stroke prognosis. *Stroke* 1996;27:1817–1820.
5. Brainin M, Seiser A, Czvitkovits B, Pauly E. Stroke subtype is an age-independent predictor of first-year survival. *Neuroepidemiology* 1992;11(6):190–195.
6. Nadeau SE, Jordan JE, Mishra SK, Haerer AF. Stroke rates in patients with lacunar and large vessel cerebral infarction. *J Neurol Sci* 1993;114:128–137.
7. Anderson CS, Jamrozik KD, Burvill PW, Chakera TM, Johnson GA, Stewart-Wynne EG. Determining the inicidence of different subtypes of stroke: results from the Perth Community Stroke Study. *Med J Aust* 1993;158:85–89.
8. Anderson CS, Taylor BV, Hankey GJ, Stewart-Wynne EG, Jamrozik KD. Validation of a clinical classification for subtypes of acute cerebral infarction. *J Neurol Neurosurgery Psychiatry* 1994;57:1175–1179.
9. Sacco SE, Whisnant JP, Broderick JP, Phillips SJ, O'Fallon WM. Epidemiological characteristics of lacunar infarcts on a population. *Stroke* 1991;22(10):1236–1241.
10. Salgado AV, Ferro J M, Gouveia-Oliveira A. Long-term prognosis of first-ever lacunar strokes: a hospital-based study. *Stroke* 1996;27(4):661–666.
11. Clavier I, Hommel M, Besson G, Noélle B, Perret JE. Long-term prognosis of symptomatic lacunar infarcts: a hospital-based study. *Stroke* 1994;25:2005–2009.
12. Lin HJ, Wolf PA, Kelly-Hayes M, Beiser AS, Kase CS, Benjamin EJ, D'Agostino RB. Stroke severity in atrial fibrillation. *Stroke* 1996;27:1760–1764.
13. Jørgensen HS, Nakayama H, Reith J, Raaschou HO, Olsen TS. Acute stroke with atrial fibrillation. *Stroke* 1996;27:1765–1769.
14. Petty GW, Brown RD, Whisnant JP, Sicks JD, O'Fallon WM, Wiebers DO. Ischemic stroke subtypes. A population based study of functional outcome, survival, and recurrence. *Stroke* 2000:1062.
15. The National Institute of Neurological Disorders and Stroke rt-PA Stroke Study Group. Tissue plasminogen activator for acute ischemic stroke. *N Engl J Med* 1995;333(24): 1581–1587.
16. Yamamoto H, Bogousslavsky J. Mechanisms of second and further strokes. *J Neurol Neurosurg Psychiatry* 1998;64:771–776.
17. Bamford J, Sandercock P, Dennis M, Burn J, Warlow C. Classification and natural history of clinical identifiable subtypes of cerebral infarction. *Lancet* 1991;337:1521–1526.
18. The Publication Committee for the Trial of ORG 10171 in Acute Stroke Treatment (TOAST) Investigators. Low molecular weight heparinoid ORG 10172 (Danaparoid), and outcome after acute ischemic stroke: a randomized controlled trial. *JAMA* 1998; 279(16):1265–1272.
19. Woo J, Kay R, Yuen YK, Nicholls MG. Factors influencing long-term survival and disability among three-month stroke survivors. *Neuroepidemiology* 1992;11:143–150.
20. Marler JR, Jones PW, Emr M. *Proceedings of a National Symposium on Rapid Identification and Treatment of Acute Stroke*; National Institute of Neurological Disorders and Stroke, National Institutes of Health Bethesda, Maryland; 1997.
21. Sorensen A, Copen WA, Ostergaard L, Buonnano FS, Gonzalez RG, Rordorf G, Rosen BR, Schwamm LH, Weiskoff RM, Koroshetz WJ. Hyperacute stroke: simultaneous measurement of relative cerebral blood volume, relative cerebral blood flow and mean tissue transit time. *Radiology* 1999;210:519–527.

22. Albers GW, Lansberg MG, Norbash AM, Tong DC, O'Brien MW, Woolfenden AR, Marks MP, Moseley ME. Yield of diffusion-weighted MRI for detection potentially relevant findings in stroke patients. *Neurology* 2000;54:1562–1567.
23. Powers W. Testing a test: a report card for DWI in acute stroke. *Neurology* 2000;54: 1549–1551.
24. Zivin JA, Holloway RG. Weighing the evidence on DWI: Caveat emptor. *Neurology* 2000;54:1552–1552.
25. Lansberg MG, Albers GW, Beaulieu C, Marks MP. Comparison of diffusion-weighted MRI and CT in acute stroke. *Neurology* 2000;54:1557–1561.
26. Hacke W, Warach S. Diffusion-weighted MRI as an evolving standard of care in acute stroke. *Neurology* 2000;54:1548–1549.
27. Madden KP, Karanjia PN, Adams HP, Clarke WR. Accuracy in initial stroke subtype diagnosis in the TOAST study. *Nuerology* 1995;45:1975–1979.
28. Bogousslavsky J, Regli F, Besson G, Melo TP, Nater B. Early clinical diagnosis of stroke subtype. *Cerebrovasc Dis* 1993;3:39–44.
29. Mohr JP, Sacco RL. Morbidity and mortality of stroke. In: Moore, WS editor. *Surgery for cerebrovascular disease*. W.B. Saunders Company, 1996; p 9–15.
30. Rothrock JF, Lyden PD, Brody ML, Taft-Alvarez B, Kelly N, Mayer J, Wiederholt WC. An analysis of ischemic stroke in an urban southern California population. *Arch Intern Med* 1993;153:619–624.
31. Lodder J, Boiten J. Incidence, natural history, and risk factors in lacunar infarction. *Adv Neurol* 1993;62:213–227.
32. Yip PK, Jeng JS, Lee TK, Chang YC, Huang ZS, Ng SK, Chen RC. Subtypes in ischemic stroke: a hospital-based stroke registry in Taiwan (SCAN-IV). *Stroke* 1997;28(12):2507–2512.
33. Anderson CS, Jamrozik KD, Broadhurst RJ, Stewart-Wynne EG. Predicting survival for 1 year among different subtypes of stroke: results from the Perth Commnity Stroke Study. *Stroke* 1994;25:1935–1944.
34. Lodder J, Bamford J, Kappelle J, Boiten J. What causes false clinical prediction of small deep infarctions? *Stroke* 1994;25:86–91.
35. Toni D, Del Duca R, Fiorelli M, Sacchetti ML, Bastianello S, Giubilei F, Martinazzo C, Argentino C. Pure motor hemiparesis and sensorimotor stroke: accuracy of very early clinical diagnosis of lacunar strokes. *Stroke* 1994;25(1):92–96.
36. Gan R, Sacco RL, Kargman DE, Roberts JK, Boden-Albala B, Gu Q. Testing the validity of the lacunar hypothesis: the Northern Manhattan Stroke Study experience. *Neurology* 1997;48:1204–1211.
37. Knauth M, von Kummer R, Jansen O, Hahnel S, Dorfler A, Sartor K. Potential of CT angiography in acute ischemic stroke. *Am J of Neurorad* 1997;18:1001–10.
38. Shrier D, Tanaka H, Numaguchi Y, Konno S, Patel U, Shibata D. *CT angiography in the evaluation of acute stroke. Am J Neuroradiol* 1997;18:1011–1020.
39. Wildermuth S, Knauth M, Brandt T, Winter R, Sartor K, Hacke W. Role of CT angiography in patient selection for thrombolytic therapy in acute hemispheric stroke. *Stroke* 1998;29:935–938.
40. Lee LJ, Kidwell CS, Alger J, Starkman S, Saver JL. Impact on stroke subtype diagnosis by diffusion-weighted magnetic resonance imaging and magnetic resonance angiography. *Stroke* 2000;31:1081–1089.

41. Barber PA, Darby DG, Desmond PM, Yang Q. Prediction of stroke outcome with echoplanar perfusion- and diffusion-weighted MRI. *Neurology* 1998;51: 418–426.

42. Petty GW, Brown Jr. RD, Whisnant JP, Sicks JD, O'Fallon WM, Wiebers DO. Ischemic stroke subtypes: a population-based study of functional outcome, survival, and recurrence. *Stroke* 2000;31:1062–1068.

43. Hart RG, Foster JW, Luther MF, Kanter MC. Stroke in infective endocarditis. *Stroke* 1990;21:695–700.

44. Shafqat S, Kelly PJ, Furie KL. Holter monitoring in diagnosis of stroke mechanism. *Inter Med J* 2004;34:305–309.

45. Schaer BA, Zellweger MJ, Cron TA, Kaiser CA, Osswald S. Value of routine hotler monitoring for the detection of paroxysmal atrial fibrillation in patients with cerebral ischemic events. *Stroke* 2004;35:e68–e70.

46. Jabaudon D, Sztajzel J, Sievert K, Landis T, Sztajzel R. Usefulness of amulatory 7 day ECG monitoring for the detection of atrial finrillation and flutter after acute stroke and transient ischemic attack. *Stroke* 2004;35:1647–1651.

47. Harloff A, Handke M, Reinhard M, Geibel A, Hetzel A. Therapeutic strategies after examination by transesophageal echocardiography in 503 patients with ischemic stroke. *Stroke* 2006;37:859–864.

48. de Bruijn SF, Agema WR, Lammers GJ, van der Wall EE, Wolterbeek R, Holman ER, Bollen EL, Bax JJ. Sebastiaan FTM. Transesophageal echocardiography is superior to transthoracic echocardiography in management of patients of any age with transient ischemic attack or stroke. *Stroke* 2006;37:2531–2534.

49. Hart RG, Halperin JL, Pearce LA, Anderson DC, Kronmal RA, McBride R, Nasco E, Sherman DG, Talbert RL, Marler JR. Lessons from the stroke prevention in atrial fibrillation trials. *Ann Intern Med* 2003;138:831–838.

50. Risk factors for stroke and efficacy of antithrombotic therapy in atrial fibrillation. Analysis of pooled data from five randomized controlled trials. *Arch Intern Med* 1994;154:1449–1457.

51. Komrad MS, Coffey CE, Coffey KS, McKinnis R, Massey EW, Califf RM. Myocardial infarction and stroke. *Neurology* 1984;34:1403–1409.

52. Cardiogenic brain embolism. Cerebral embolism task force. *Arch Neurol* 1986;43: 71–84.

53. Cardiogenic brain embolism. The second report of the cerebral embolism task force. *Arch Neurol* 1989;46:727–743.

54. Beneficial effect of carotid endarterectomy in symptomatic patients with high-grade carotid stenosis. North American Symptomatic Carotid Endarterectomy Trial Collaborators. *N Engl J Med* 1991;325(7):445–453.

55. Randomised trial of endarterectomy for recently symptomatic carotid stenosis: final results of the MRC European Carotid Surgery Trial (ECST). *Lancet* 1998;351(9113): 1379–1387.

56. Barnett HJM, Taylor DW, Eliasziw M, Fox AJ, Ferguson GG, Haynes RB, Rankin RN, Clagett GP, Hachinski VC, Sackett DL, Thorpe KE, Meldrum HE, David Spence JD. Benefit of carotid endarterectomy in patients with symptomatic moderate or severe stenosis. North American Symptomatic Carotid Endarterectomy Trial Collaborators. *N Engl J Med* 1998;339(20):1415–1425.

57. Suwanwela N, Can U, Furie KL, Southern JF, Macdonald NR, Ogilvy CS, Hansen CJ, Buonanno FS, Abbott WM, Koroshetz WJ, Kistler JP. Carotid Doppler ultrasound criteria for internal carotid artery stenosis based on residual lumen diameter calculated from en bloc carotid endarterectomy specimens. *Stroke* 1996;27(11):1965–1969.

58. Can U, Furie KL, Suwanwela N, Southern JF, Macdonald NR, Ogilvy CS, Buonanno FS, Koroshetz WJ, Kistler JP. Transcranial Doppler ultrasound criteria for hemodynamically significant internal carotid artery stenosis based on residual lumen diameter calculated from en bloc endarterectomy specimens. *Stroke* 1997;28(10):1966–1971.

59. Patel SG, Collie DA, Wardlaw JM, Lewis SC, Wright AR, Gibson RJ, Sellar RJ. Outcome, observer reliability, and patient preferences if CTA, MRA, or Doppler ultrasound were used, individually or together, instead of digital subtraction angiography before carotid endarterectomy. *J Neurol Neurosurg Psychiatry* 2002;73(1):21–28.

60. Pan XM, Saloner D, Reilly LM, Bowersox JC, Murray SP, Anderson CM, Gooding GA, Rapp JH. Assessment of carotid artery stenosis by ultrasonography, conventional angiography, and magnetic resonance angiography: correlation with ex vivo measurement of plaque stenosis. *J Vasc Surg* 1995;21(1):82–88 [discussion 88–89].

61. Nonent M, Serfaty JM, Nighoghossian N, Rouhart F, Derex L, Rotaru C, Chirossel P, Guias B, Heautot JF, Gouny P, Langella B, Buthion V, Jars I, Pachai C, Veyret C, Gauvrit JY, Lamure M, Douek PC; CARMEDAS Study Group. Concordance rate differences of 3 noninvasive imaging techniques to measure carotid stenosis in clinical routine practice: results of the CARMEDAS multicenter study. *Stroke* 2004;35(3):682–686.

62. Johnston DC, Goldstein LB. Clinical carotid endarterectomy decision making: noninvasive vascular imaging versus angiography. *Neurology* 2001;56(8):1009–1015.

63. Johnston DC, Eastwood JD, Nguyen T, Goldstein LB. Contrast-enhanced magnetic resonance angiography of carotid arteries: utility in routine clinical practice. *Stroke* 2002;33(12):2834–2838.

64. Borisch I, Horn M, Butz B, Zorger N, Draganski B, Hoelscher T, Bogdahn U, Link J. Preoperative evaluation of carotid artery stenosis: comparison of contrast-enhanced MR angiography and duplex sonography with digital subtraction angiography. *AJNR Am J Neuroradiol* 2003;24(6):1117–1122.

65. Nederkoorn PJ, Mali WP, Eikelboom BC, Elgersma OE, Buskens E, Hunink MG, Kappelle LJ, Buijs PC, Wust AF, van der Lugt A, van der Graaf Y. Preoperative diagnosis of carotid artery stenosis: accuracy of noninvasive testing. *Stroke* 2002;33(8):2003–2008.

66. Nederkoorn PJ, Mali WP, Eikelboom BC, Elgersma OE, Buskens E, Hunink MG, Kappelle LJ, Buijs PC, Wust AF, van der Lugt A, van der Graaf Y. Duplex ultrasound and magnetic resonance angiography compared with digital subtraction angiography in carotid artery stenosis: a systematic review. *Stroke* 2003;34(5):1324–1332.

67. Norris JW, Halliday A. Is ultrasound sufficient for vascular imaging prior to carotid endarterectomy? *Stroke* 2004;35(2):370–371.

68. Hetzel A, Eckenweber B, Trummer B, Wernz M, Schumacher M, von Reutern G. Colour-coded duplex sonography of preocclusive carotid stenoses. *Eur J Ultrasound* 1998;8(3):183–191.

69. Henderson RD, Steinman DA, Eliasziw M, Barnett HJ. Effect of contralateral carotid artery stenosis on carotid ultrasound velocity measurements. *Stroke* 2000;31(11):2636–2640.

70. Erickson SJ, Mewissen MW, Foley WD, Lawson TL, Middleton WD, Quiroz FA, Macrander SJ, Lipchik EO. Stenosis of the internal carotid artery: assessment using color

Doppler imaging compared with angiography. *AJR Am J Roentgenol* 1989;152(6):1299–1305.

71. Polak JF, Dobkin GR, O'Leary DH, Wang AM, Cutler SS. Internal carotid artery stenosis: accuracy and reproducibility of color-Doppler-assisted duplex imaging. *Radiology* 1989;173(3):793–798.
72. Steinke W, Kloetzsch C, Hennerici M. Carotid artery disease assessed by color Doppler flow imaging: correlation with standard Doppler sonography and angiography. *AJR Am J Roentgenol* 1990;154(5):1061–1068.
73. Gasecki AP, Ferguson GG, Eliasziw M, Clagett GP, Fox AJ, Hachinski V, Barnett HJ. Early endarterectomy for severe carotid artery stenosis after a nondisabling stroke: results from the North American Symptomatic Carotid Endarterectomy Trial. *J Vasc Surg* 1994;288–295.
74. Ballotta E, Da Giau G, Baracchini C, Abbruzzese E, Saladini M, Meneghetti G. Early versus delayed carotid endarterectomy after a nondisabling ischemic stroke: a prospective randomized study. *Surgery* 2002:287–293.
75. Wasserman BA, Wityk RJ, Trout HH, 3rd, Virmani R. Low-grade carotid stenosis: looking beyond the lumen with MRI. *Stroke* 2005;36(11):2504–2513.
76. Antithrombotic Trialists' Collaboration. Collaborative meta-analysis of randomized trials of antiplatelet therapy for prevention of death, myocardial infarction, and stroke in high risk patients. *BMJ* 2002;324:71–86.
77. Markus HS, Droste DW, Kaps M, Larrue V, Lees KR, Siebler M, Ringelstein EB. Dual antiplatelet therapy with clopidogrel and aspirin in symptomatic carotid stenosis evaluated using doppler embolic signal detection: the Clopidogrel and Aspirin for Reduction of Emboli in Symptomatic Carotid Stenosis (CARESS) trial. *Circulation* 2005;111(17):2233–2240.
78. The Stroke Prevention by Aggressive Reduction in Cholesterol Levels (SPARCL) Investigators: High-dose atorvastatin after stroke or transients ischemic attack. *N Engl J Med* 2006;355:549–559.
79. Crisby M, Nordin-Fredriksson G, Shah PK, Yano J, Zhu J, Nilsson J. Pravastatin treatment increases collagen content and decreases lipid content, inflammation, metalloproteinases, and cell death in human carotid plaques: implications for plaque stabilization. *Circulation* 2001;103(7):926–933.
80. Corti R, Fayad ZA, Fuster V, Worthley SG, Helft G, Chesebro J, Mercuri M, Badimon JJ. Effects of lipid-lowering by simvastatin on human atherosclerotic lesions: a longitudinal study by high-resolution, noninvasive magnetic resonance imaging. *Circulation* 2001;104(3):249.

10

TELESTROKE: APPLICATION OF TELEMEDICINE IN ACUTE ISCHEMIC STROKE

Eric S. Rosenthal and Lee H. Schwamm

INTRODUCTION

The benefit observed in the National Institute of Neurological Disorders and Stroke (NINDS) randomized, controlled trial of intravenous (IV) tissue-type plasminogen activator (rt-PA) in acute ischemic was restricted to patients whose infusion began within 3 hours of symptom onset.[1] Earlier stroke treatment within this 3-hour window was associated with further benefit in clinical outcome.[2] Protocol violations, however, increase the likelihood of intracerebral hemorrhage (ICH) after thrombolysis, and can mitigate its benefit if patients are not properly selected. This risk of adverse events underscores the importance of expert consultation in rapid clinical and radiographic evaluation, identification of contraindications, delivery of rt-PA, and strict adherence to poststroke care guidelines. As a result of strict guidelines recommended for its delivery, rt-PA use has been limited to fewer than 3% of patients presenting with ischemic stroke in the United States.[3]

The disconnect between the efficacy of rt-PA and its infrequent use is a significant problem, one which telemedicine may solve by bringing to the bedside both neurological and imaging expertise, facilitating the appropriate use of this therapy.

Acute Ischemic Stroke: An Evidence-based Approach, Edited by David M. Greer.

CURRENT BARRIERS IN ACUTE STROKE CARE

Pre-Hospital Delays

Fewer than half of all patients with acute stroke are seen in the emergency department (ED) within 3 hours of symptom onset.[4] Patients in remote locations or in hospitals without available stroke expertise may have even more limited access to thrombolysis. In a study of non-urban East Texas communities in the United States, only 1.4% of patients with ischemic stroke received IV rt-PA,[5] versus 14.7% at a university hospital in Houston, the nearest major city.[6] Other studies have linked racial, ethnic, geographic, or socioeconomic differences to low rates of rt-PA utilization,[4,6] suggesting that populations most underserved by stroke expertise may have the lowest rates of rt-PA delivery.

Limited Access to Stroke Expertise

Even when rt-PA is delivered to patients with ischemic stroke, higher rates of adverse outcomes occur when thrombolytic therapy is delivered without consulting physicians with specialized stroke expertise. In one community-based experience, 16% of treated patients developed symptomatic ICH compared to 6% of patients randomized to receive rt-PA in the NINDS trial. Although 96% of treatment decisions involved a neurologist, deviations from the NINDS guidelines were observed in 50% of treated patients.[7] Aggressive corrective measures increased the rate of rt-PA administration while reducing symptomatic ICH to 6% among treated patients at the same hospitals.[8] Other studies have similarly linked increased rates of protocol violations to increased rates of symptomatic ICH or mortality.[9,10]

Unnecessary Interfacility Transfers

Helicopter transport has been employed to shorten the time to presentation at large centers. Results, however, have been mixed. Direct helicopter transport from emergency medical service first responders to a tertiary care facility has permitted improved access to rt-PA but resulted in the costly transfer of patients ineligible for rt-PA (greater than 80% of transported patients).[11] While the average field-to-hospital distance for all patients in this experience was only 29 miles, applying helicopter-based transport on a broad scale may accrue large costs and separate patients from their families even when acute intervention is not required. Up-front transportation limits the benefit of a full neurological consultation to only those patients who receive transport. When patients are transported by helicopter *before* treatment but *after* triage at a community hospital, time delays may become prohibitive.

TELEMEDICINE AS A UNIQUE INTERVENTION

The brain attack coalition (BAC) and more recently the American Heart Association have offered consensus guidelines for criteria designating a primary stroke center, including acute stroke teams, stroke units, written care protocols, an integrated emergency response system, around-the-clock availability, and interpretation of computed tomography (CT) and rapid laboratory testing.[3,12] However, a recent U.S. survey revealed that less than 10% of hospitals met the BAC criteria for a primary stroke center, although 75% of responding neurologists, neurosurgeons, and emergency physicians believed that their own hospital did meet guidelines. This disconnect is not trivial; a community hospital in suburban Maryland is among many to have implemented guidelines, increasing the proportion of patients safely treated with IV rt-PA.[13] Implementation of BAC guidelines in New York State improved the frequency of rt-PA delivery, decreased protocol violations, and shortened pretreatment latency.[14]

If a community hospital cannot provide the radiological and clinical stroke expertise to meet these guidelines, participation in a TeleStroke network may help a hospital to meet guidelines for stroke center designation. As a TeleStroke-networked stroke center, a community hospital can seek to increase the access to and appropriateness of rt-PA delivery, reducing peristroke complications without the costly addition of equipment or personnel. Triage, evaluation, and treatment at local centers prior to transportation would provide rapid management with an efficient use of resources. In a fraction of the time that sick and unstable patients can travel to a center of expertise, telemedicine collapses the boundaries of time and space to permit the expertise itself to travel instantaneously over great distances. Telemedicine-enabled support for the delivery of IV rt-PA to patients had its first success in patients with myocardial infarction; rapid delivery of rt-PA to patients in rural Greece was enabled after the history, physical examination, and an electrocardiogram were reviewed by telephone and fax by physicians in Athens. Door-to-needle times were 20–30 minutes.[15]

The telemedicine-based evaluation of acute stroke is especially challenging. It requires a rapid neurological assessment, CT image acquisition and review, and a detailed history for rt-PA exclusion criteria. Low-cost teleradiology systems are now available for the transmission of compressed CT images viewable on a conventional personal computer (PC) monitor, in accordance with published standards.[16,17] The decreased cost of professional videoconferencing equipment can now empower a physician with clinical and imaging stroke expertise to conduct a remote history, physical exam, and radiological interpretation in real time for the purpose of diagnosing and managing patients with stroke symptoms.[18]

THE ARCHITECTURE OF A TELESTROKE SERVICE

Equipment and Networking

The system in use at the Massachusetts General Hospital is shown diagrammatically in Figure 10.1. A videoconferencing link is established between a community hospital (emergency physician) and a tertiary care hospital (stroke neurologist). All patients are examined on a stretcher in the community hospital's ED using a commercial videoconferencing system on a mobile cart (Polycom, Inc., Austin,

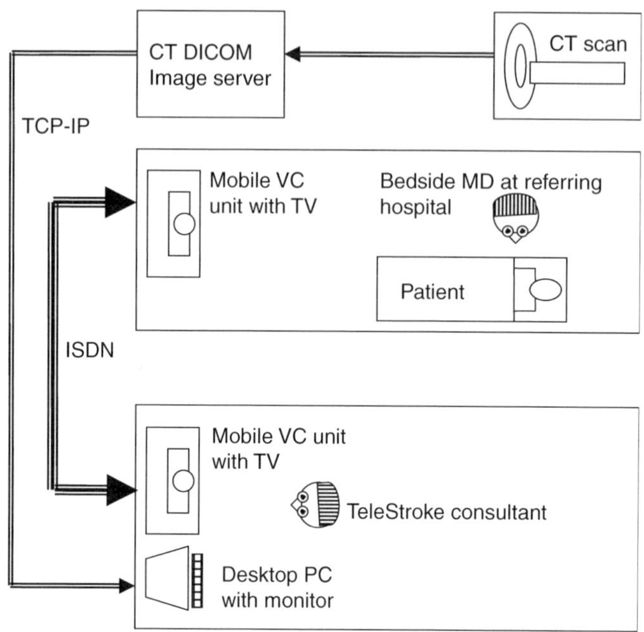

FIGURE 10.1 Schematic representation of the radiological imaging and videoconferencing (VC) links between the remote site and the TeleStroke expert center. CT, computed tomography; DICOM, digital imaging and communications in medicine; ISDN, integrated services digital network; MD, medical doctor; PC, personal computer; TCP-IP, Transmission Control Protocol/Internet Protocol; TV, television. (Reprinted with permission from Rosenthal ES, Schwamm LH. Telemedicine and stroke. Wootton R, Patterson V, editors. *Teleneurology*, London: RSM Press Ltd; 2005; p 53–66.)

TX). Our current system supports multiple users on a single call, which enables supervised consultation, digital archiving, and creation and delivery of medical education content throughout the network. Data are transmitted encrypted over public Internet or multiple ISDN lines at speeds of 384 kbit/s; video transmission occurs at 30 frames/s. Most studies on stroke treatment have used ISDN but some have used Internet Protocol (IP) over a virtual private network. ISDN at a bandwidth of less than 384 kbit/s has not been evaluated for acute neurological management and may not be suitable for clinical applications. The initial capital expense for a commercially available, standards-based videoconferencing infrastructure in a community hospital (i.e., spoke site) is estimated in 2006 at <US $10,000.

In our system, CT scans are transmitted between hospitals in DICOM format and are then evaluated within browser-based image software (AMICAS, Inc.) on a conventional desktop PC connected to a monitor set at $\geq$ 1024 $\times$ 768 pixel resolution. TeleStroke consultations permit side-by-side clinical and radiological evaluation (Fig. 10.2) by the consulting stroke neurologist. For hospitals with a digital picture archiving and communication system (PACS) imaging system, there is no additional capital expense to transmit images; for those without PACS, low

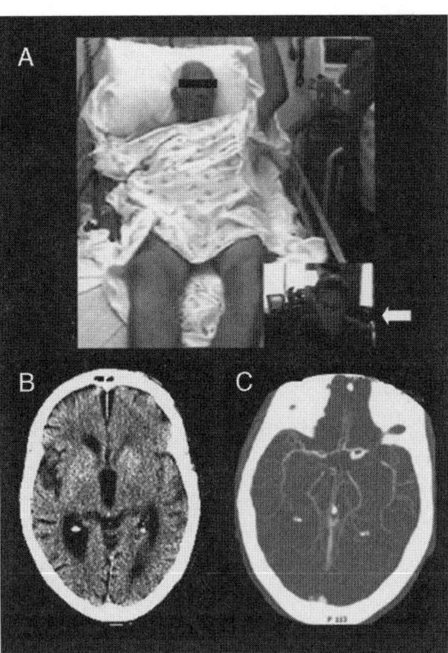

FIGURE 10.2 (**a**) Still frame from the TeleStroke examination by the neurologist at home (inset picture) examining a patient at a remote hospital. Right face and arm weakness were appreciated in the live color video after the patient was asked to raise both arms and look straight ahead. (**b**) Noncontrast wavelet-compressed CT of the brain obtained < 30 minutes after symptom onset viewed from the remote stroke physician's home via teleradiology. Subtle signs of early ischemia included loss of normal contour of the posterior left putamen and insular ribbon. (**c**) Follow-up CT angiography after transfer at 4 hours after symptom onset showed a persistent left middle cerebral artery occlusion. (Reprinted with permission from Rosenthal ES, Schwamm LH. Telemedicine and stroke. Wootton R, Patterson V, editors. *Teleneurology*, London: RSM Press Ltd; 2005; p 53–66.)

cost, secure, HIPAA-compliant, image transmission systems are readily available for under US $5,000.

Performance of a Validated Examination

Studies have directly compared the telemedicine-enabled high bandwidth (384 kbit/s) video observations of a neurologist with the bedside examination of a house officer and the gold standard examination of a panel of six neurologists.[19] The observations of the telemedicine-enabled neurologist were as good as the examination performed in person by the house officer and were in almost perfect agreement with the gold standard panel (κ score 0.81–1.00) for many components of the neurological examination.

Shafqat et al.[20] previously validated the National Institutes of Health Stroke Scale (NIHSS) assessment as a reliable method of evaluating patients with stroke symptoms at a bandwidth of 384 kbit/s comparing a bedside neurologist to a telemedicine-enabled neurologist teamed with a bedside nurse in patients with ischemic stroke and NIHSS scores ranging from 1 to 24. There was an excellent correlation between bedside and remote scores (inter-rater correlation coefficient

0.97, $p < 0.001$) with only minimal increases in the time to perform the evaluation. The inter-rater agreement between telemedicine and bedside examinations was similar to that between any two bedside examinations in previous validation studies of the NIHSS.[21] The remote evaluation of acute ischemic stroke (REACH) project validated the NIHSS in clinical practice with an excellent correlation between bedside and remote NIHSS scores ($r = 0.96, p = 0.0001$).[22] Observational data among stroke patients from Handschu et al.[23] demonstrated weighted κ statistics greater than 0.85 for all aspects of NIHSS scores except for the examination of facial paresis in patients seen within 6 hours of symptom onset.

Accurate Evaluation of Transmitted Radiology Images

The rapid transmission and accurate interpretation of radiological images are essential in determining eligibility for IV thrombolysis among patients with stroke symptoms. Because the accuracy of interpreting these radiological studies affects outcomes after thrombolytic therapy, the person interpreting these images must be able to detect exclusion criteria for the administration of IV rt-PA. Intracranial hemorrhage on initial CT is an absolute contraindication, and the European Cooperative Acute Stroke Study (ECASS) trial and other data suggest that hypodensity on acute brain CT is associated with hemorrhagic transformation after thrombolysis, especially when such a hypodensity occupies greater than one third of the middle cerebral artery territory (>1/3 MCA).[24,25] The contribution to hemorrhagic transformation after thrombolysis of early ischemic changes (EIC), such as edema, lesser hypodensity, sulcal effacement, or ventricular compression, is more controversial. CT protocol violations in thrombolytic trials have been associated with high rates of adverse events,[26] and treatment of patients in the presence of CT exclusion criteria yields excess risk with no observable benefit.[27]

To treat acute stroke patients, CT exclusions to rt-PA eligibility must be accurately identified. A team of experienced acute stroke specialists remotely linked by TeleStroke systems may provide "on call" acute stroke consultation to multiple hospitals without each facility having to maintain its own continuously available stroke consultation service with clinical and imaging expertise.

Convenience sampling of ED physicians, neurologists, and radiologists has suggested that neurologists have near perfect sensitivity for detecting obvious hemorrhage but are less accurate in detecting subtle hemorrhages or hypodensities >1/3 MCA.[28] These studies, however, did not assess vascular neurologists as a separate cohort.

Low-cost teleradiology systems enable the distribution of images without an expensive PACS. A web browser can display images for viewing on a conventional PC monitor located in the hospital or remotely. One pilot study compared stroke neurologists' reading of CT images via teleradiology to gold standard readings of hard-copy film radiographs on a view box. Each neurologist read one half of the CT scans via teleradiology in a blinded fashion, and the other half using a view box. Using the official reading by a neuroradiologist as the gold standard, there was perfect agreement between groups and 100% sensitivity and specificity for the determination of rt-PA eligibility by the stroke neurologist.[29] We also have validated that the stroke neurologist's review by telemedicine of DICOM compressed brain CT images can accurately identify candidates for IV rt-PA; detailed results are shown in Table 10.1.[30] Thus, for a patient with acute stroke symptoms, real-time interpretation of CT scans on a desktop computer during a TeleStroke consultation can favorably compare to image interpretation performed on a view box or on a PACS workstation by a neuroradiologist.

To make the process practical for community hospitals, this technology must be inexpensive and easily operated in the ED. Transmission of CT images to experienced radiologists for formal and final interpretation is essential for quality control and feedback. As a result, systems that permit remote decision-making by expert physicians reduce the manpower needed to provide acute stroke team coverage in ED without around-the-clock access to in-house stroke neurology.

TABLE 10.1 Inter-Rater Agreement Expressed as Kappa (κ) Scores for 26 CT Scans Interpreted by a Stroke Neurologist and a Staff Neuroradiologist.[30]

	SN vs. Stroke-NRAD		SN vs. Staff-NRAD		Staff-NRAD vs. Stroke-NRAD	
CT Finding	κ	95% CI	κ	95% CI	κ	95% CI
Intracranial hemorrhage						
Conventional method	1.00	1.00, 1.00	1.00	1.00, 1.00	1.00	1.00, 1.00
Estimating equations method	1.00	1.00, 1.00	1.00	1.00, 1.00	1.00	1.00, 1.00
Acute hypodensity						
Conventional method	0.63	−0.01, 1.28	0.24	−0.28, 0.75	0.62	−0.04, 1.28
Estimating equations method	0.33*	−0.34, 0.78	0.31	−0.31, 0.75	0.33*	−0.29, 0.76
Subtle signs of acute infarct						
Conventional method	1.00	1.00, 1.00	0.54	0.15, 0.93	0.39	−0.30, 1.08
Estimating equations method	1.00	0.97, 1.00	0.36*	−0.17, 0.73	0.33	−0.27, 0.75
Any early ischemic changes						
Conventional method	0.76	0.32, 1.20	0.29	−0.11, 0.69	0.23	−0.40, 0.86
Estimating equations method	0.82*	0.41, 0.96	0.16*	−0.30, 0.56	0.20*	−0.34, 0.64
Chronic ischemic lesions						
Conventional method	0.88	0.59, 1.13	0.63	0.32, 0.93	0.79	0.41, 1.17
Estimating equations method	0.83	0.42, 0.96	0.62	0.19, 0.85	0.77	0.25, 0.95

A neuroradiologist with stroke expertise reviewed the first 15 of these scans. An asterisk denotes when the use of an adjusted κ score changed the level of agreement. Staff-NRAD, staff neuroradiologist; κ, kappa; SN, stroke neurologist; Stroke-NRAD, neuroradiologist with stroke expertise.

Appropriate Triage and Safe Transportation

Telemedicine consultation has enabled the accurate diagnosis of patients with neurologic syndromes other than stroke or TIA. In 2003, the Telemedic Pilot Project for Integrative Stroke Care (TEMPiS) diagnosed 250 patients with nonvascular diagnoses out of the 2182 telemedicine consultations requested in the first year of operation.[31] However, TeleStroke systems must also enable the safe transfer of patients requiring tertiary care in the form of neurocritical, endovascular, or neurosurgical care. While safe transport has been possible by helicopter, boat, and ambulance, in our personal experience the transport period may be prolonged, requiring attention to organized communication between community hospitals, tertiary care centers, and transport personnel. For example, the TEMPiS investigators documented in 221 transferred patients that helicopter transport saved time over ground transport only when distances exceeded 50 km (31 miles).[32]

Reimbursement and Licensing for Interfacility Consultation

While TeleStroke consultations have often been provided without reimbursement in an investigational setting, transitioning to a system with reimbursement will enable the broad availability of consultation for dedicated clinical practice. Reimbursement policies and licensing restrictions, however, have been slow to change. Currently, federal regulations governing reimbursement for evaluation and management services in the medicare program require that the patient be located in a rural or underserved location, as defined by Metropolitan Statistical Areas or critical access facility designation. These areas do not necessarily correspond to regions of neurologically underserved populations, given the scarcity of vascular neurologists. Further inefficiencies in care delivery occur because many TeleStroke networks in the United States operate with proprietary systems that cannot communicate with other networks, and barriers to interstate consultation remain significant, mostly in the form of regulatory, credentialing, and licensure requirements. As TeleStroke and other telemedicine systems for clinical care become more commonplace, regulation of practice and provision for reimbursement will likely receive further attention. Ideally, all systems will adhere to open standards so that internetwork communication will resemble current mobile phone soltuons that allow seamless interaction between different carriers and technologies.

TELESTROKE IN CLINICAL PRACTICE

Networks of Care

TeleStroke networks (e.g., Fig. 10.3) are now well established in Germany and Ontario, as well as in Georgia, Massachusetts, Texas, California, and Maryland in the United States.

One of the first large series of TeleStroke consultations was described in southern Germany, where seven rural hospitals were linked to a stroke unit in

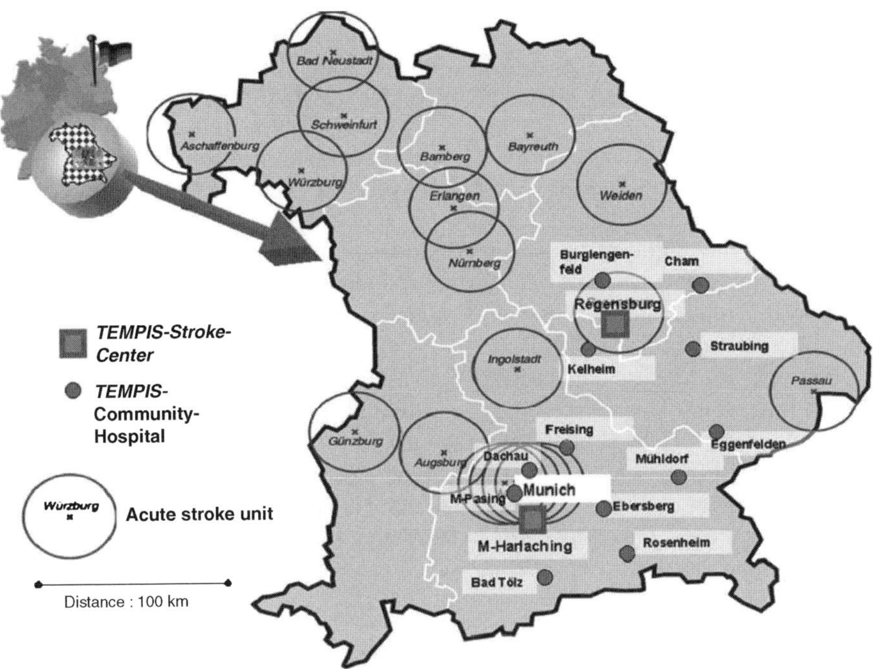

FIGURE 10.3 Regional maps depicting TeleStroke Networks. Two hospitals in the TEMPiS network in Bavaria (Germany) provide acute stroke expertise to 12 community hospitals.[56]

Gunzburg as part of the Telemedicine in Stroke in Swabia (TESS) Project.[33] Of 153 patients examined, 87 were determined to have had an ischemic stroke, but importantly, 40 patients had a diagnosis other than stroke, confirming that telemedicine is also helpful in identifying other emergency neurological conditions that may mimic stroke. The duration of teleconsultation was 15 minutes on average. Thirty-seven percent of the 94 patients with ischemic stroke or TIA reached the hospital within 3 hours, and two received thrombolysis. In the opinion of the referring physicians, relevant contributions were made in over 75% of all cases concerning the diagnostic workup, CT assessment, and therapeutic recommendations.

More recently, thrombolytic therapy was reported in 106 patients as part of the TEMPiS system in Bavaria, Germany. The network consists of two comprehensive and 12 regional centers connected by around-the-clock telemedicine support for stroke care. In the first year following intervention, the number of patients treated with rt-PA increased to 86 patients (2% of all patients admitted with stroke), compared to 10 patients treated in the year preceding intervention. The rate of symptomatic hemorrhage was 8.5%, similar to the NINDS trial.[34]

In the REACH study involving the Medical College of Georgia and five rural hospitals in Georgia,[35] 12 of 75 (16%) patients evaluated received rt-PA, all without intracranial hemorrhagic complications.

We described our own initial experience at the Partners TeleStroke Center in Massachusetts,[30] before expanding this service from 2 to 14 participating community hospitals. In our pilot experience with two community hospitals, six patients were treated with IV rt-PA in the first 27 months. Among the six patients receiving rt-PA, two patients had persistent deficits (one of whom had care withdrawn), two patients had moderate recovery, and two had good recovery (one of whom had initial worsening deficits). There were no violations of NINDS protocol[2] and re-review of the initial CT by a neuroradiologist with stroke expertise did not alter the diagnosis in any case. All patients had follow-up imaging and only one patient developed symptomatic ICH within 36 hours; another developed a small delayed asymptomatic intracerebral hemorrhage.

University of Maryland investigators reported 23 telemedicine consultations and 27 telephone consultations preceding transfer among patients with suspected acute stroke.[36] Of the 23 telemedicine consultations, 2 were aborted because of technical difficulties, but 5 of the 21 patients receiving successful TeleStroke consultation received IV rt-PA. No patient experienced complications. Diagnoses included subarachnoid hemorrhage, intracerebral hemorrhage, seizure, hypoglycemia, and transient ischemic attack as well as acute ischemic stroke (both anterior and posterior circulations).

Patterns of Referral

We have encountered differential rates of utilization of our TeleStroke system among networked community hospitals. A differential rate of referral was also noted in a study of telemedicine for 657 consecutive patients at the University of California, Davis.[37] The TESS project reported that the frequency of teleconsultation in patients with suspected stroke varied from 2% to 86% among seven affiliated community hospitals. Possible reasons for variability include time needed to transport videoconference equipment into the patient room, obtaining written consent in investigational settings, lack of additional medical staff in the local hospitals, different attitudes toward thrombolysis itself as an effective treatment, and underlying variation in how physicians and facilities react to change.

Efficiency of Thrombolytic Administration

In the first 27 months of our own TeleStroke experience,[30] 26 consultations were requested; 12 began within 3 hours of symptom onset. Eight of these 12 patients had acute ischemic stroke, of which 2 were not treated due to mild deficits. Three were diagnosed with TIA or migraine, and one with a subdural hematoma not detected at the local facility. For the 12 acute cases for whom rapid diagnosis and management was essential, we determined the mean times from symptom onset to start of TeleStroke consultation and from consultation start to drug delivery or to determination of rt-PA ineligibility (shown in Fig. 10.4).

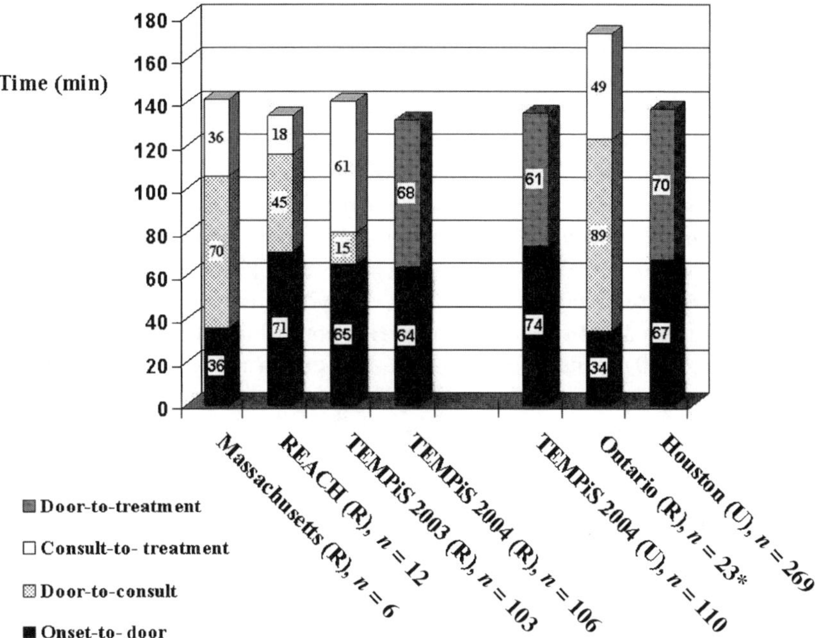

FIGURE 10.4 The mean time (in minutes) among stages of rt-PA administration documented in published studies demonstrates that TeleStroke interventions in community hospitals compare favorably to conventional mechanisms of care in urban (U) and rural (R) patient populations. TeleStroke patients were treated at a community or rural hospital separate over videoconferencing by a remotely located stroke expert, whereas patients presenting through conventional mechanisms were treated by on-site stroke physicians. Interval mean times have been interpolated if not explicitly reported. The "door-to-consult" time in the Ontario study includes interfacility transfer time because patients referred from rural centers were transferred to this rural tertiary care center before the initial stroke consultation. (Adapted with permission from Rosenthal ES Schwamm LH. Telemedicine and stroke. Wootton R, Patterson, V; editors. *Teleneurology*, London: RSM Press Ltd.; 2005; p 53–66.)

The REACH system in southern Georgia (United States) and the TEMPiS system in Germany reported decreased latency to rt-PA delivery on a larger scale. REACH system investigators reported 194 acute stroke consultations delivered via telemedicine. The time from symptom onset to rt-PA delivery decreased from 143 minutes in the first 10 patients treated to 111 minutes in last 20 patients; of 30 patients treated with rt-PA, 23% were treated in 90 minutes or less and 60% were treated within 2 hours without any incidence of post-treatment symptomatic intracerebral hemorrhage.[38] In 2004, the second year of the TEMPiS system, 115 patients in telemedicine-networked community hospitals and 110 patients in stroke centers received rt-PA for acute ischemic stroke or TIA. Patients treated at networked community hospitals encountered shorter mean prehospital latency times than academic stroke centers (onset to admission 64 minutes vs. 74 minutes) and equivalent door-to-treatment times (134 minutes vs. 135 minutes, $p = 0.81$).[39]

TeleStroke consultation can therefore be performed quickly. Its efficiency compares quite favorably to the management of patients in rural Ontario[40] who receive rt-PA *after* transfer from a rural hospital to a tertiary-care center (the so-called "ship and drip" model). The patients located in rural Ontario had a mean total time of 138 minutes between presentation at the rural facility and drug delivery at the tertiary-care center. The door-to-bolus time at the community hospitals linked to our TeleStroke service was 106 minutes, only 36 minutes longer than that measured by the urban acute stroke service in Houston, which permitted a mean door-to-bolus time of 70 minutes.[6] Whereas the door-to-consult time within a telemedicine system may decrease with training and practice, interfacility transfer times, such as those observed in Ontario, are not easily shortened.

Clinical Outcomes Following TeleStroke Intervention

In the TEMPiS TeleStroke system, the probability of a poor outcome (Barthel Index Score <60 or modified Rankin Scale Score >3) was lower in patients networked to telemedicine-enabled consultation.[41] Three thousand one hundred and twenty-two patients with ischemic stroke were examined in a nonrandomized, open-intervention study between two supporting academic hospitals and 10 community hospitals (five non-networked hospitals matched to five networked hospitals). Telemedicine intervention was associated in a multivariate analysis with a reduced probability of poor outcome (death, nursing home placement, or severe disability) after 3 months (OR 0.62, 95% CI 0.52–0.74, $p < 0.0001$). Death or institutionalization alone was not significantly reduced in patients receiving telemedicine intervention (OR 0.88, 95% CI 0.71–1.06 $p = 0.18$). The impact was primarily of reduced probability of severe disability (14% receiving telemedicine intervention vs. 21% of control patients returned home with severe disability). The rate of symptomatic intracerebral hemorrhage was not significantly increased (7.8% vs. 2.7%, $p = 0.14$) in a related comparison of the academic stroke centers to these telemedicine-networked community hospitals, even though these networked hospitals controlled blood pressure more strictly and had similar rates of in-hospital mortality (3.5% vs. 4.5%, $p = 0.74$). This 7.8% rate of symptomatic hemorrhage in networked hospitals nevertheless compares well to the rate found by the NINDS intravenous rt-PA study.[1] Investigators in Texas also found that TeleStroke intervention increased the frequency of rt-PA administration from 0.8% to 4.3% at two community hospitals east of Houston, but without an increased incidence of intracerebral hemorrhage.[42]

User Satisfaction

Videoconferencing in real-time clinical practice has yielded high levels of patient and physician satisfaction in most specialties. A study dedicated to the assessment of telemedicine-based neurology reported high levels of physician and patient satisfaction for technical aspects, process, and effectiveness.[43] These high levels of user satisfaction exist despite the need for rapid evaluation, the potential for technical barriers, and the importance of coordinating clinical teleconferencing with a review of transmitted radiology images. In the TESS project, patients were satisfied with the telemedicine-based examination and commented that it was easy to speak to and cooperate with the remote neurologist. The imaging quality of both patients and CT images was considered good by the stroke neurologists. The audio quality, however, was rated less favorably, especially by the physician on the scene.

MGH Telestroke satisfaction data show excellent patient and physician satisfaction following each of 26 TeleStroke consultations. We rated satisfaction on a Likert scale (1—agree; 2—neutral; 3—disagree) with statements based on those developed by Craig et al.[43] that related to technical quality, process, and efficacy. Full results are depicted in Figure 10.5. Patients felt confident in the quality of a neurological evaluation performed from a distance, and felt that this consultation added value over what would have been locally available. Many expressed the view that it was as good as a face-to-face encounter, suggesting that high-quality videoconferencing does not disrupt the patient–doctor interaction even in an urgent care setting.

Subacute Care and Management

In other experiences, subacute TeleStroke consultation has been shown to improve resource allocation in poststroke management by reducing the length of hospital stays. In one of two small rural hospitals in Ireland, patients were offered a neurological consultation with a neurologist 120 km away using a real-time video link. Hospital stay was significantly shorter for those admitted to the hospital with telemedicine resources ($p = 0.045$). Diagnosis by the teleneurologist was accurate in all cases, although there was no difference in overall mortality between the groups.[44]

In addition to access to acute stroke care, referral to stroke centers may also be important for the comprehensive quality of care in all patients presenting to the hospital with stroke.[45] A study of patterns of care among patients with suspected stroke presenting to the EDs in rural East Texas hospitals revealed that head CT was performed in only 88% and ECG was performed in only 85% of patients; blood pressure lowering was inappropriately aggressive, yielding pressures below current recommendations.[5] Other studies have shown that telephone consultation for cognitive testing may provide a useful method for the diagnosis of poststroke dementia.[46] Even after discharge, telemedicine-enabled family discussions may be helpful for caregivers of stroke survivors.[47] In addition, telemedicine is useful for stroke rehabilitation in the subacute or postdischarge setting.[48]

Emerging Technologies

Improvements in videoconferencing should increase the quality of the received picture, and permit higher quality images over lower bandwidth. Additionally, improvements in mobile or wireless networks (e.g., EDGE network, EVDO

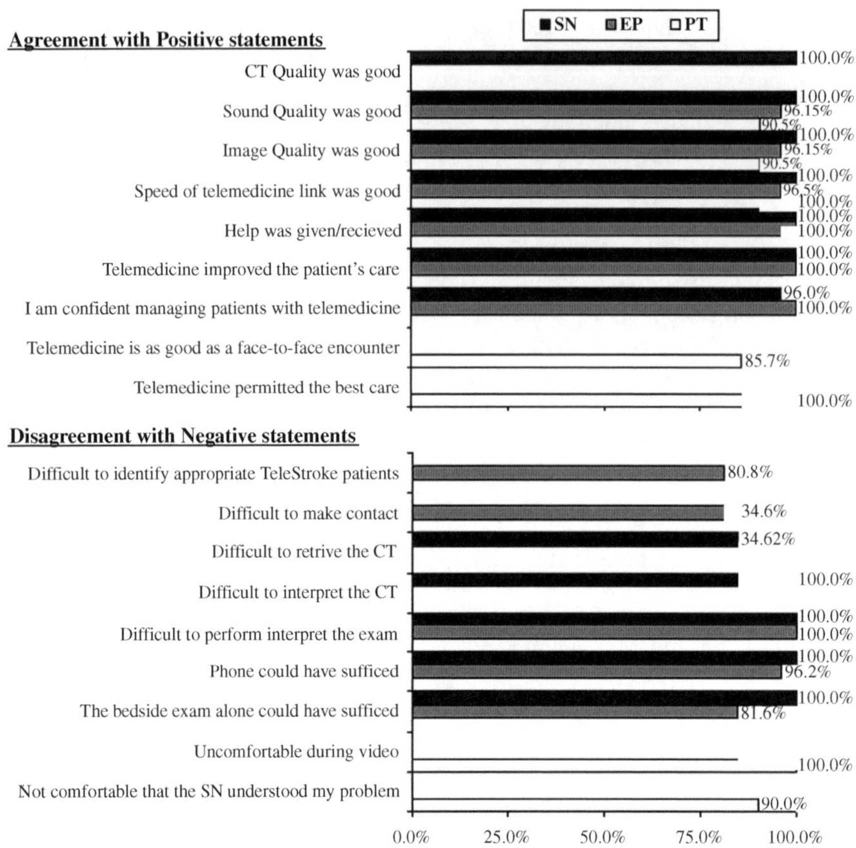

FIGURE 10.5 User satisfaction of the stroke neurologist (SN), emergency physician (EP), and patient or surrogate (PT) shown as the percent of each group noting agreement with positive statements and disagreement with negative statements. (Reprinted with permission from Rosenthal ES, Schwamm LH. Telemedicine and stroke. Wootton R, Patterson V; editors. *Teleneurology*, London: RSM Press Ltd; 2005; p 53–66.)

Revision A) will support earlier diagnosis and management by allowing an interview and clinical examination of a patient in the field or *during* transportation by paramedics in an ambulance. Investigators in San Diego recently presented a case series of 25 patients for whom wireless TeleStroke consultation was completed; they found excellent inter-rater reliability among 82% of modified NIHSS items.[49]

Future Directions

In most investigations, TeleStroke intervention has been compared only to a period of historical control but not concomitantly to other mechanisms of consultation, such as telephone, email, or direct transport. A large-scale, prospective trial with a control arm and standardized time measurements could definitively establish TeleStroke as a safe, efficient, reliable, and effective technology.

Of note, allied health care professionals soon may routinely assume a role as referring TeleStroke providers at spoke hospitals; a recent case report documented the first delivery of rt-PA by an advance practice nurse in the ED at a hospital in rural Texas networked by a TeleStroke system to a stroke center in Houston.[50]

FINANCIAL AND LEGAL CONSIDERATIONS

Opportunities for Community and Rural Hospitals

Financial and legal challenges will help shape the scalability and widespread clinical utility of telemedicine for acute stroke. Smaller hospitals often face a limited supply of local stroke specialists, the recruitment of which is often shaped by available salaries, emergency coverage requirements, opportunities for vacation time, and the richness of academic interaction. Telemedicine can collapse the problems associated with obtaining specialist care in neurologically underserved rural and urban communities. The cost of a telemedicine service to provide "24-7" acute stroke coverage is financially advantageous compared to retaining a full time on-site stroke expert, may support local stroke center designation at the spoke hospital, and prevent re-routing of patients away from the hospital as disease-specific triage algorithms emerge related to stroke. Smaller hospitals can therefore increase operational efficiency, particularly when the need for a specialist is infrequent or when clinical concerns are too urgent to wait for transfer or a visiting consultant.[51,52] Additionally, telemedicine-affiliated community hospitals can offer patients an attractive marriage of convenience and personalized care with access to a comprehensive range of specialists.

Reimbursement, Licensure, and Malpractice Barriers

Nevertheless, multiple challenges persist. Reimbursement on a fee-for-service or contractual basis between institutions may not be feasible for the community hospital. Government reimbursement for telemedicine services may remain limited by interstate commerce restrictions and local practice requirements, and may depend on studies demonstrating that the costs of consultation are counterbalanced by avoiding unnecessary transfers.[53] Additionally, privacy concerns must be properly addressed with secure, encrypted transfer of information and rules governing who may access the patient's medical information from a distance.

Stroke consultants may be deterred from providing telemedicine-based consultation by the requirement of securing licensure in all states in which they provide consultation. However, acute stroke consultation may be exempt from these rules in states that make exceptions for emergency situations, limited duration of clinical care, or consultation to patients in bordering states. Still, other states prohibit ongoing telemedicine relationships, permitting only those consults made on an "irregular basis." Some have argued that patients be "electronically transported" to the state of the consulting physician for legal purposes to alleviate the restrictions of licensure. A national licensure program would be more challenging to implement but would be consistent with the aim of telemedicine consultation to facilitate access by the public to evidence-based care delivered at the highest quality.[54] This mission is reflected in the Telecommunications Reform Act of 1996, which notes that "state regulation designed to protect vital state interests must give way to paramount Federal legislation." Thus, the sovereignty of licensure and malpractice laws in each state may need to yield to the need to provide equality in access to care among patients residing in different states and various geographic or medically isolated communities.

Malpractice laws provide the most difficult challenge to removing the barriers to broad-scale telemedicine consultation. Malpractice claims are governed by the realm of tort law, in which cases are evaluated based on the standard of care available in that local community at that time. States avoid additional expenses when residents are compensated in malpractice suits against providers and, therefore, have an incentive not to compromise standards for malpractice and liability. Nevertheless, malpractice claims require that a relationship between physician and patient have been established when a breach of duty results in damages to a patient. A paradox is thus created in which the state must sanction and facilitate the telemedicine-based physician–patient contract before it can support malpractice claims. It is not clear, however, which standards should be considered when consultation has been expressly requested to obtain an opinion or to achieve standard of care, which is different than that locally available. To make malpractice concerns even more palpable, telemedicine-based consultations are often recorded during the digital encoding.[55] These concerns will likely be muted in national systems of medical care, in which explicit standards of cost and care are centralized. [54]

REFERENCES

1. Tissue plasminogen activator for acute ischemic stroke. The National Institute of Neurological Disorders and Stroke rt-PA Stroke Study Group. *N Engl J Med* 1995; 333:1581–1587.
2. Marler JR, Tilley BC, Lu M, Brott TG, Lyden PC, Grotta JC, Broderick JP, Levine SR, Frankel MP, Horowitz SH, Haley Jr. EC, Lewandowski CA, Kwiatkowski TP. Early stroke treatment associated with better outcome: the NINDS rt-PA stroke study. *Neurology* 2000;55:1649–1655.
3. Alberts MJ, Hademenos G, Latchaw RE, Jagoda A, Marler JR, Mayberg MR, Starke RD, Todd HW, Viste KM, Girgus M, Shephard T, Emr M, Shwayder P, Walker MD. Recommendations for the establishment of primary stroke centers. Brain Attack Coalition. *JAMA* 2000;283:3102–3109.
4. Lacy CR, Suh DC, Bueno M, Kostis JB. Delay in presentation and evaluation for acute stroke: Stroke Time Registry for Outcomes Knowledge and Epidemiology (S.T.R.O.K.E.). *Stroke* 2001;32:63–69.

5. Burgin WS, Staub L, Chan W, Wein TH, Felberg RA, Grotta JC, Demchuk AM, Hickenbottom SL, Morgenstern LB. Acute stroke care in non-urban emergency departments. *Neurology* 2001;57:2006–2012.

6. Grotta JC, Burgin WS, El-Mitwalli A, Long M, Campbell M, Morgenstern LB, Malkoff M, Alexandrov AV. Intravenous tissue-type plasminogen activator therapy for ischemic stroke: Houston experience 1996 to 2000. *Arch Neurol* 2001;58:2009–2013.

7. Katzan IL, Furlan AJ, Lloyd LE, Frank JI, Harper DL, Hinchey JA, Hammel JP, Qu A, Sila CA. Use of tissue-type plasminogen activator for acute ischemic stroke: the Cleveland area experience. *JAMA* 2000;283:1151–1158.

8. Katzan IL, Hammer MD, Furlan AJ, Hixson ED, Nadzam DM. Quality improvement and tissue-type plasminogen activator for acute ischemic stroke: a Cleveland update. *Stroke* 2003;34:799–800.

9. Hanson SK, Brauer DJ, Anderson DC, Koller RL, Davenport JG, Ramirez-Lassepas M, Klassen AC, Altafullah IM, Brown RD. Stroke Treatment in the Community (STIC)—intravenous rt-PA in clinical practice. *Neurology* 1998;50:A155–A156 [abstract].

10. Bravata DM, Kim N, Concato J, Krumholz HM, Brass LM. Thrombolysis for acute stroke in routine clinical practice. *Arch Intern Med* 2002;162:1994–2001.

11. Silliman SL, Quinn B, Huggett V, Merino JG. Use of a field-to-stroke center helicopter transport program to extend thrombolytic therapy to rural residents. *Stroke* 2003;34:729–733.

12. Schwamm LH, Pancioli A, Acker 3rd, JE, Goldstein LB, Zorowitz RD, Shephard TJ, Moyer P, Gorman M, Johnston SC, Duncan PW, Gorelick P, Frank J, Stranne SK, Smith R, Federspiel W, Horton KB, Magnis E, Adams RJ. Recommendations for the establishment of stroke systems of care: recommendations from the American Stroke Association's task force on the development of stroke systems. *Stroke* 2005;36:690–703.

13. Lattimore SU, Chalela J, Davis L, DeGraba T, Ezzeddine M, Haymore J, Nyquist P, Baird AE, Hallenbeck J, Warach S. Impact of establishing a primary stroke center at a community hospital on the use of thrombolytic therapy: the NINDS suburban hospital stroke center experience. *Stroke* 2003;34:e55–e57.

14. Gropen TI, Gagliano PJ, Blake CA, Sacco RL, Kwiatkowski T, Richmond NJ, Leifer D, Libman R, Azhar S, Daley MB. Quality improvement in acute stroke: the New York State Stroke Center Designation Project. *Neurology* 2006;67:88–93.

15. Mavrogeni SI, Tsirintani M, Kleanthous C, Vranakis K, Secheta E, Mihelakis D, Sotiriou D, Gatzonis M, Tsolas C, Kontaratos AN, Cokkinos DV. Supervision of thrombolysis of acute myocardial infarction using telemedicine. *J Telemed Telecare* 2000;6:54–58.

16. Pysher L, Harlow C. Teleradiology using low-cost consumer-oriented computer hardware and software. *AJR Am J Roentgenol* 1999;172:1181–1184.

17. Apple SL, Schmidt JH. Technique for neurosurgically relevant CT image transfers using inexpensive video digital technology. *Surg Neurol* 2000;53:411–416.

18. Levine SR, Gorman M. "Telestroke": the application of telemedicine for stroke. *Stroke* 1999;30:464–469.

19. Craig JJ, McConville JP, Patterson VH, Wootton R. Neurological examination is possible using telemedicine. *J Telemed Telecare* 1999;5:177–181.

20. Shafqat S, Kvedar JC, Guanci MM, Chang Y, Schwamm LH. Role for telemedicine in acute stroke. Feasibility and reliability of remote administration of the NIH stroke scale. *Stroke* 1999;30:2141–2145.

21. Goldstein LB, Bertels C, Davis JN. Interrater reliability of the NIH stroke scale. *Arch Neurol* 1989;46:660–662.
22. Wang S, Lee SB, Pardue C, Ramsingh D, Waller J, Gross H, Nichols 3rd, FT, Hess DC, Adams RJ. Remote evaluation of acute ischemic stroke: Reliability of National Institutes of Health Stroke Scale via telestroke. *Stroke* 2003;34:e188–e191.
23. Handschu R, Littmann R, Reulbach U, Gaul C, Heckmann JG, Neundorfer B, Scibor M. Telemedicine in emergency evaluation of acute stroke: interrater agreement in remote video examination with a novel multimedia system. *Stroke* 2003;34: 2842–2846.
24. American Heart Association. Heart disease and stroke statistics—2003 update. Dallas: American Heart Association; 2002; p. 15–17.
25. Von Kummer R, Allen KL, Holle R, Bozzao L, Bastianello S, Manelfe C, Bluhmki E, Ringleb P, Meier DH, Hacke W. Acute stroke: usefulness of early CT findings before thrombolytic therapy. *Radiology* 1997;205:327–333.
26. Hacke W, Kaste M, Fieschi C, Toni D, Lesaffre E, von Kummer R, Boysen G, Bluhmki E, Hoxter G, Mahagne MH, et al. Intravenous thrombolysis with recombinant tissue plasminogen activator for acute hemispheric stroke. The European Cooperative Acute Stroke Study (ECASS). *JAMA* 1995;274:1017–1025.
27. Buchan AM, Barber PA, Newcommon N, Karbalai HG, Demchuk AM, Hoyte KM, Klein GM, Feasby TE. Effectiveness of t-PA in acute ischemic stroke: outcome relates to appropriateness. *Neurology* 2000;54:679–684.
28. Kalafut MA, Schriger DL, Saver JL, Starkman S. Detection of early CT signs of >1/3 middle cerebral artery infarctions: interrater reliability and sensitivity of CT interpretation by physicians involved in acute stroke care. *Stroke* 2000;31:1667–1671.
29. Johnston KC, Worrall BB. Teleradiology assessment of computerized tomographs online reliability study (tractors) for acute stroke evaluation. *Telemed J E Health* 2003;9: 227–233.
30. Schwamm LH, Rosenthal ES, Hirshberg A, Schaefer PW, Little EA, Kvedar JC, Petkovska I, Koroshetz WJ, Levine SR. Virtual telestroke support for the emergency department evaluation of acute stroke. *Acad Emerg Med* 2004;11:1193–1197.
31. Audebert HJ, Wimmer ML, Hahn R, Schenkel J, Bogdahn U, Horn M, Haberl RL. Can telemedicine contribute to fulfill WHO Helsingborg Declaration of specialized stroke care? *Cerebrovasc Dis* 2005;20:362–369.
32. Audebert HJ, Clarmann von Clarenau S, Schenkel J, Furst A, Ziemus B, Metz C, Haberl RL. Problems of emergency transfers of patients after a stroke. Results of a telemedicine pilot project for integrated stroke accommodation in southeast Bavaria (TEMPiS). *Dtsch Med Wochenschr* 2005;130:2495–2500.
33. Wiborg A, Widder B. Teleneurology to improve stroke care in rural areas: the Telemedicine in Stroke in Swabia (TESS) project. *Stroke* 2003;34:2951–2956.
34. Audebert HJ, Kukla C, Clarmann von Claranau S, Kuhn J, Vatankhah B, Schenkel J, Ickenstein GW, Haberl RL, Horn M. Telemedicine for safe and extended use of thrombolysis in stroke. the Telemedic Pilot Project for Integrative Stroke Care (TEMPiS) in Bavaria. *Stroke* 2005;36:287–291.
35. Wang S, Gross H, Lee SB, Pardue C, Waller J, Nichols 3rd, FT, Adams RJ, Hess DC. Remote evaluation of acute ischemic stroke in rural community hospitals in Georgia. *Stroke* 2004;35:1763–1768.

36. LaMonte MP, Bahouth MN, Hu P, Pathan MY, Yarbrough KL, Gunawardane R, Crarey P, Page W. Telemedicine for acute stroke: triumphs and pitfalls. *Stroke* 2003;34:725–728.
37. Nesbitt TS, Hilty DM, Kuenneth CA, Siefkin A. Development of a telemedicine program: a review of 1,000 videoconferencing consultations. *West J Med* 2000;173: 169–174.
38. Hess DC, Wang S, Hamilton W, Lee S, Pardue C, Waller JL, Gross H, Nichols F, Hall C, Adams RJ. REACH: clinical feasibility of a rural telestroke network. *Stroke* 2005;36:2018–2020.
39. Audebert HJ, Kukla C, Vatankhah B, Gotzler B, Schenkel J, Hofer S, Furst A, Haberl RL. Comparison of tissue plasminogen activator administration management between telestroke network hospitals and academic stroke centers: the Telemedical Pilot Project for Integrative Stroke Care in Bavaria/Germany. *Stroke* 2006;37:1822–1827.
40. Merino JG, Silver B, Wong E, Foell B, Demaerschalk B, Tamayo A, Poncha F, Hachinski V. Extending tissue plasminogen activator use to community and rural stroke patients. *Stroke* 2002;33:141–146.
41. Audebert HJ, Schenkel J, Heuschmann PU, Bogdahn U, Haberl RL. Effects of the implementation of a telemedical stroke network: the Telemedic Pilot Project for Integrative Stroke Care (TEMPiS) in Bavaria/Germany. *Lancet Neurol* 2006;5: 742–748.
42. Choi JY, Porche NA, Albright KC, Khaja AM, Ho VS, Grotta JC. Using telemedicine to facilitate thrombolytic therapy for patients with acute stroke. *J Comm J Qual Patient Saf* 2006;32:199–205.
43. Craig J, Russell C, Patterson V, Wootton R. User satisfaction with realtime teleneurology. *J Telemed Telecare* 1999;5:237–241.
44. Craig J, Chua R, Russell C, Wootton R, Chant D, Patterson V. A cohort study of early neurological consultation by telemedicine on the care of neurological inpatients. *J Neurol Neurosurg Psychiatry* 2004;75:1031–1035.
45. Crome O, Bahr M. Editorial comment—remote evaluation of acute ischemic stroke: a reliable tool to extend tissue plasminogen activator use to community and rural stroke patients? *Stroke* 2003;34:e191–e192.
46. Barber M, Stott DJ. Validity of the telephone interview for cognitive status (TICS) in post-stroke subjects. *Int J Geriatr Psychiatry* 2004;19:75–79.
47. Grant JS, Elliott TR, Weaver M, Bartolucci AA, Giger JN. Telephone intervention with family caregivers of stroke survivors after rehabilitation. *Stroke* 2002;33:2060–2065.
48. Holden MK, Dyar T, Schwamm L, Bizzi E. Home-based telerehabilitation using a virtual environment system. *Proceedings of the 2nd International Workshop on Virtual Rehabilitation*; 2003; p 4–12.
49. Meyer BC, Lyden PD, Al-Khoury L, Cheng Y, Raman R, Fellman R, Beer J, Rao R, Zivin JA. Prospective reliability of the STRokE DOC wireless/site independent telemedicine system. *Neurology* 2005;64:1058–1060.
50. Choi JY, Wojner AW, Cale RT, Gergen P, DeGioanni J, Grotta JC. Telemedicine physician providers: augmented acute stroke care delivery in rural Texas: An initial experience. *Telemed J E Health* 2004;10:S90–S94.
51. McCue MJ, Mazmanian PE, Hampton CL, Marks TK, Fisher EJ, Parpart F, Malloy WN, Fisk KJ. Cost-minimization analysis: A follow-up study of a telemedicine program. *Telemed J* 1998;4:323–327.

52. Adelman SH, McBryde Jr. AM, Can using emergent technology incur liability? *Bull Am Coll Surg* 1998;83:18–23, 41.

53. Medicare program; revisions to payment policies under the physician fee schedule for calendar year 2003 and inclusion of registered nurses in the personnel provision of the critical access hospital emergency services requirement for frontier areas and remote locations. Final rule with comment period. *Fed Regist* 2002;67:79965–80184.

54. Sanders JH, Bashshur RL. Challenges to the implementation of telemedicine. *Telemed J* 1995;1:115–123.

55. Caryl CJ. Malpractice and other legal issues preventing the development of telemedicine. *J Law Health* 1997;12:173–204.

56. Audebert HJ, Kukla C, Clarmann von Claranau S, Kuhn J, Vatankhah B, Schenkel J, Ickenstein GW, Haberl RL, Horn M. Telemedicine for safe and extended use of thrombolysis in stroke: the Telemedic Pilot Project for Integrative Stroke Care (TEMPiS) in Bavaria. *Stroke* 2005;36:287–291.

57. Hess DC, Wang S, Gross H, Nichols FT, Hall CE, Adams RJ. Telestroke: extending stroke expertise into underserved areas. *Lancet Neurol* 2006;5:275–278.

INDEX

Acute Ischemic Stroke: An Evidence-based Approach, Edited by David M. Greer.